Understanding Developmental Disorders

Edited by Jonathan Glazzard

Published in London, United Kingdom

Understanding Developmental Disorders
http://dx.doi.org/10.5772/intechopen.1004681
Edited by Jonathan Glazzard

Contributors
Arezousadat Razavi, Arzu Selamioglu, Claudia D. Tesche, Daphne Golden, Filippos Vlachos, Hagit Friedman, Hojjatollah Siavoshy, Joan Esse Wilson, Laura Berteotti, Maria Chalmpe, Rituparna Sahana, Sambhu Prasad, Simone Zorzi, Soni Kisku, Sweta Gupta, Wenn B. Lawson, Xiang-Jiao Yang

First published in London, United Kingdom, 2026 by IntechOpen
IntechOpen is the global imprint of INTECHOPEN LIMITED, registered in England and Wales, registration number: 11086078, 167-169 Great Portland Street, London, W1W 5PF, United Kingdom

For EU product safety concerns: IN TECH d.o.o., Prolaz Marije Krucifikse Kozulić 3, 51000 Rijeka, Croatia, info@intechopen.com or visit our website at intechopen.com.

British Library Cataloguing-in-Publication Data
A catalogue record for this book is available from the British Library

Understanding Developmental Disorders
Edited by Jonathan Glazzard
p. cm.

This title is part of the Nervous System and Mental Health Book Series, Volume 5
Series Editor: Toshikazu Shinba

Print ISBN 978-1-83634-284-7
Online ISBN 978-1-83634-283-0
eBook (PDF) ISBN 978-1-83634-285-4
ISSN 3050-2985

If disposing of this product, please recycle the paper responsibly.

IntechOpen Book Series

Nervous System and Mental Health

Volume 5

Aims and Scope of the Series

Mental health is frequently linked to the nervous system. Conversely, disturbances in the nervous system often lead to mental health problems. However, this linkage is not as clear as it is commonly accepted. Mental health is usually described using subjective terms, which are based on psychological and psychiatric symptomatology. Diagnosis of a mental illness is made through the presence of the subjective symptoms characterizing the illness.

On the other hand, the nervous system has been deeply investigated using objective measures, including molecular, genetic, imaging, pharmacological and physiological ones. It is essential to combine objective views of the nervous system with subjective perspectives on mental health to develop an integrative approach to understanding human cognitive functions and achieving overall well-being. In this book series, experts in various fields of the nervous system and mental health will present their views on these challenging topics.

Meet the Series Editor

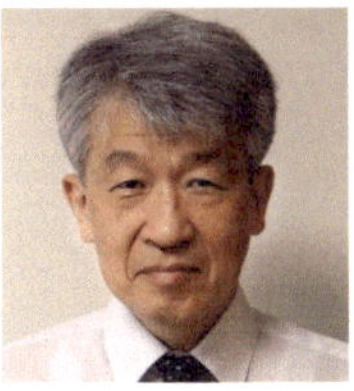

Dr. Toshikazu Shinba is a psychiatrist and neuroscientist who has been working in both clinical and basic research fields. He has been affiliated with the Tokyo Institute of Psychiatry, Department of Neurophysiology and Stress Disorders Project, and now works as a psychiatrist at Shizuoka Saiseikai General Hospital, Department of Psychiatry. The primary focus of his research is the electrophysiological analysis of attention and arousal in both humans and rodents. In clinical research, EEG, heart rate variability and skin conductance have been measured in mental disorders and arousal/consciousness disturbances. In basic research, single neuronal firing and EEG recordings have been assessed in rats. His research interests cover physiological rhythms related to attention, arousal, and consciousness in both the central and peripheral nervous systems, with a focus on understanding mental states.

Meet the Volume Editor

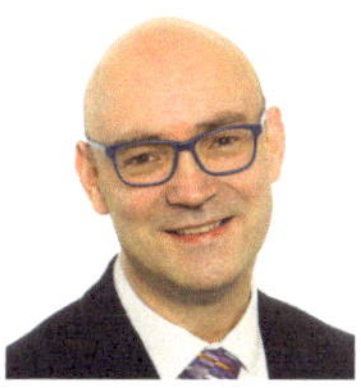

Prof. Glazzard is the Rosalind Hollis Professor of Education for Social Justice at the University of Hull. He is a co-convenor of the British Educational Research Association Special Interest Group, Mental Health and Wellbeing. Prof. Glazzard holds visiting professorships in England at Bishop Grosseteste University (BGU), Birmingham Newman University, and the University of Northampton. His research focuses on the experiences of minoritized individuals and groups. He sits on the editorial boards of several journals, including the International Journal of Educational and Life Transitions and Equity in Education & Society. He is a co-convenor of the British Educational Research Association Special Interest Group, Mental Health and Wellbeing in Education. His current research focuses on the experiences of LGBTQ+, disabled youth. Recent publications have focused on mental health, educational and life transitions, and early reading development in children.

Contents

Preface

This Edited Volume is a collection of peer-reviewed, relevant research chapters that explore key developments in the field of Developmental Disorders. The book includes scholarly contributions from various authors and is edited by an expert in the field. Each contribution comes as a separate chapter complete in itself but directly related to the book's topics and objectives.

The book includes 10 chapters:

1. A Mechanistic Common Denominator of Neurodevelopmental Disorders and a Therapeutic Approach

2. The Metabolic Evaluation of the Patient with a Developmental Disorder

3. Independent Living for Persons with Neurodevelopmental Disorders

4. Lysine Acetyltransferase 6A and Its Paralog: From Biological Functions to Neurodevelopmental Disorders, Cancer and New Therapeutics

5. Neuromuscular Adaptations to Exercise Training in People with Intellectual Disabilities

6. Motor Developmental Delay

7. Heterogeneity in the Neurocognitive Characteristics of Developmental Dyslexia: Theoretical Approaches and Research Findings

8. Autism: Its Foundation and Practical Implications

9. Autism Spectrum Condition: An Update on its Understanding and Clinical Perspective

10. Utilizing Transcranial Electrical Stimulation (TES) to Individualize Social Learning Therapy with Autistic Adults and Adults with High Traits of Autism

IntechOpen

Chapter 1

A Mechanistic Common Denominator of Neurodevelopmental Disorders and a Therapeutic Approach

Hagit Friedman

Abstract

Neural development is a highly intricate process that begins at the molecular level and culminates in the formation of complex neural circuits. This developmental journey involves a cascade of events influenced, synchronized, and controlled by genetic, epigenetic, and ambient factors. The enigma of developmental disorders is a continuously growing scientific and clinical issue. Various fetal injuries and birth trauma increase babies' vulnerability to developmental problems. These pronounce impairments in the proliferation and plasticity of synapses and brain circuits. Developmental impairments manifest in delayed developmental milestones, sensory dysregulation, cognitive difficulties, seizures, abnormal muscle tone, and more. The DSM-5 sorts developmental disorders into clusters, appearing with high comorbidity among themselves: intellectual developmental disability, communication disorder, ASD, ADHD, motor disorders affecting developmental milestones since infancy, and specific learning disorders. Individuals affected with developmental disorders may exhibit a spectrum of impairment severity and experience varying degrees of symptoms and deficits, despite having the same diagnosis. The wide range of associated symptoms and severity result in various levels of mental, emotional, and physical consequences. Despite the diverse expressions, developmental disorders share a common cellular mechanistic denominator—intracellular mitochondrial function, affecting a variety of intra—and intercellular functions. A mechanism-oriented intervention would minimize developmental neurological and functional deficits. Low-power laser therapy is a nonintrusive painless therapeutic tool. Employing laser acupoint stimulation to auricular and body clinically proven locations generates a novel and powerful, neuro-based therapeutic approach, to improve neurodevelopmental track of infants and children. In the chapter, I discuss and analyze these scientific clinical issues.

Keywords: neurodevelopmental disorder, brain development, child development, acupoint laser stimulation, low-power laser therapy, laser acupuncture, auricular laser acupuncture

1. Introduction

1.1 Neurodevelopmental syndromes

Neurodevelopmental syndromes, a continuously growing issue, are impairments in the growth and development of the brain and CNS that are pronounced in a variety of emotional, cognitive, motor, and social skills [1]. Neurodevelopmental disorders are a heterogeneous assemblage of early onset mental and physical impairments negatively impacting the nervous system development [2], causing one's malfunction in various domains of life (i.e., personal, social, academic, and occupational) depending on the deficits caused. Individuals affected with developmental disorders may exhibit a spectrum of impairment severity and experience varying degrees of symptoms and deficits, despite having the same diagnosis. The wide range of associated symptoms and severity result in various levels of mental, emotional, and physical consequences [3].

The DSM-5 sorts neurodevelopmental disorders into six key clusters, appearing with high comorbidity among themselves as follows:

Intellectual developmental disability, also termed general learning disability, influences learning ability, information processing, abstract thinking, and problem-solving. It is expressed in typically limited adaptive behavior through daily living activities. Global developmental delay is categorized under intellectual disability and is diagnosed when various areas of intellectual functioning are involved [4].

Communication disorder influences one's ability to understand or apply language and speech to efficiently participate in a conversation [5]. It also involves deficiencies in verbal and nonverbal communication [6]. Communication delays/disorders can range from sound substitution to the failure to understand or use one's mother tongue [7].

Autism spectrum disorder (ASD) is the joint name for neurodevelopmental injuries characterized by abnormal social interaction, communication problems, restricted variety of repetitive and inflexible patterns of behavior and areas of interest, and typical motor impairments. ASD severity and specific symptoms vary widely, modifying a person's ability to understand and interact with others and to adapt to common circumstances. A result of autism dimensionality is considerable variability in the nature and extent of support required. ASD diagnosis is based on the presence of ASD symptoms, causing significant impairment in multiple functional aspects [8].

Attention deficit hyperactivity disorder (ADHD) is a neurodevelopmental disorder characterized by interrupted executive function, inducing prevalent and persistent symptoms of inattention, hyperactivity, impulsivity and emotional dysregulation [9–11]. ADHD emotional regulation core symptom [12, 13] stems from disturbed executive function [14–20]. Additional difficulties in self-regulation (i.e., management, inhibition, and sustained attention) may cause inadequate professional accomplishment and social difficulties [21, 22], leading to diminished quality of life [23]. ADHD is associated with other neurodevelopmental and mental disorders and nonpsychiatric disorders, which can cause additional impairment [11].

Motor disorders affect developmental milestones since infancy including developmental coordination disorder, stereotypic movement disorder, tic disorders (i.e., Tourette's syndrome), and apraxia of speech.

Specific learning disorders are difficulties in information processing that can display in various learning disabilities. When someone has multiple learning difficulties, it is named comorbidity of learning disabilities or dual diagnosis of learning disabilities.

2. Nervous system development: From molecules and synapses to cells and circuits

Neural development is a highly intricate process that begins at the molecular level and culminates in the formation of complex neural circuits. This developmental journey involves a cascade of events influenced, synchronized and controlled by genetic, epigenetic, and ambient factors.

The molecular foundation of brain neural development lies in gene expression and signaling pathways. Gene regulatory networks orchestrate the differentiation of neural stem cells into neurons and glial cells, for maintaining the balance between proliferation and differentiation in neural progenitors [24–26].

Signaling molecules, including the Wnt, Sonic Hedgehog (Shh), and Bone Morphogenetic Protein (BMP) pathways, play pivotal roles in directing cell fate. These pathways guide neurogenesis, shaping the developing brain's architecture. Neurotrophic factors like Brain-Derived Neurotrophic Factor (BDNF) are essential for neuronal survival and synaptic plasticity, support neuron survival, and drive the growth and differentiation of neuronal circuits [27–29].

Neurogenesis and gliogenesis, the generation of neurons and glia cells, occurs through a tightly regulated process involving neural stem cells that provide the necessary signals for the transition from a proliferative state to differentiation [30]. Glial cells, which include astrocytes, oligodendrocytes, and microglia, develop concurrently with neurons. These cells are critical for normal neuronal function, maintaining homeostasis, and modulating synaptic activity [31–33]. The collaborative interplay between neurons and glia is essential for healthy brain development [34].

Synaptogenesis, the formation of synapses, is a defining phase of neural development, in which neurons establish connections through the sprouting and elongation of axons and dendrites, guided by molecular cues and adhesion proteins. The establishment of developed neuronal connections depends on synchronized action of many distinct molecules, including any of which could potentially be changed by genetic variation and mutation. During this step, excitatory and inhibitory synapses are formed, allowing for the integration of information. The balance between these synapses is crucial for proper circuit development and function, directing behavior and cognition [35–39].

As neurons mature, they connect to form complex circuits. Circuit formation is a complex interplay of guidance cues and synaptic selection, ultimately leading to the functional connectivity that underpins behavior. Axonal guidance mechanisms ensure that connections are made accurately, leading to the establishment of functional networks. This process involves a combination of molecular signals and cellular performance [40–46].

Following initial synapse formation, a refinement process occurs where excess connections are pruned. This "use it or lose it" principle is essential for optimizing network efficiency and functionality. The maturation of neural circuits is marked by myelination (formation and wrapping of myelin sheaths around axons by oligodendrocytes), enhancing the speed and accuracy of electrical transmission. This process is critical for efficient communication between neurons [47–51].

Neural plasticity, particularly during critical periods of development, allows circuits to adapt based on experience, shaping the neural architecture in response to environmental input. Factors such as stress, nutrition, and exposure to toxins can disrupt normal developmental processes, emphasizing the importance of a supportive environment for optimal brain development [52].

Hence, normal neural development is a complex interplay of molecular signals, cellular processes, and environmental influences to establish functional neural circuits. Understanding this dynamic process is essential for unraveling the mechanisms underlying brain development and function and the potential consequences of neurodevelopmental disorders. As we continue to explore this intricate normal route, the integration of molecular, cellular, and circuit-level insights paves the way for advancements in understanding developmental pathology and efficient intervention.

Major anomalies from the proper developmental route in early brain development may cause damage to neural proliferation and synapse formation [53].

There may be various internal and external causes for neurodevelopmental disorders, influencing the development of brain circuits during various developmental time windows—before or after birth. These include genetic abnormalities, metabolic diseases, immune syndromes, infection, placental function, birth trauma, damaged microbiome, nutritional aspects, physical trauma, toxic environmental factors, and more [54–63].

During the many years of research, conducted using many scientific approaches and numerous scientific tools, multiple factors involved in neurodevelopmental disorders were identified (i.e., missing or abnormal synaptic proteins and enzymes, deformed neural circuits, and more) [64–71]. This yielded an insight that neurodevelopmental disorders are multifactorial. Yet recently, it has become evident that there is one basic, active, long-lasting common denominator that links between the injured factors in the developmental path.

3. Mitochondria: Neural common denominator of neurodevelopmental impairments

Mitochondria are important factors in neuronal development and function. Often referred to as the powerhouses of the cell, mitochondria are essential for producing the energy required for neural development and for various cellular functions. Beyond energy metabolism, mitochondria are involved in processes such as iron metabolism and calcium homeostasis. Moreover, mitochondria are associated with normal and defective cell proliferation and participate in cellular apoptosis. Each eukaryotic cell may have hundreds to tens of thousands of mitochondria, depending on cellular function and energy consumption. Brain cells, being experts in cellular communication, require a lot of energy for their development, circuit wiring and message transfer. Therefore, brain cells contain many mitochondria. Recent studies have highlighted the mitochondrial critical role in the wiring of human brain circuits, indicating that proper mitochondrial function is fundamental for normal neuronal development and function [52].

Mitochondrial diseases are common faults, with approximately 0.02% prevalence in population and up to 0.5% of infants with mtDNA mutations [72, 73]. Main mitochondrial syndromes have been traditionally defined as rising from mitochondrial DNA mutations (mtDNA) or nuclear DNA (nDNA). In fundamental mitochondrial syndromes, high energy demand tissues are affected, causing neurologic, vision, hearing, neuromuscular, neurodevelopmental, and behavioral abnormalities.

Mitochondrial function can be influenced by environmental stimuli producing reactive oxygen species (ROS) that, with stress, trigger a lack of energy causing a primary mitochondrial disorder [74]. Mitochondrial disfunction can affect DNA, protein, and lipids.

Mitochondrial disorders include a decrease or increase in mitochondrial function, depending on the cause and the developmental time window, and may lead to neuronal damage. It was found that neurodevelopmental impairment (or susceptibility to mental-emotional injury) may be the result of mitochondrial disorder and abnormal mitochondrial physiology [52, 75–78].

Recent studies have highlighted the role of mitochondrial disorder/dysfunction in neurodevelopmental disorders, such as ASD, ADHD, intellectual disability, and speech delay. Moreover, specific mitochondrial disorders and dysfunctions have been identified in connection with certain neurodevelopmental disorders [72–74, 79–81].

Specifically, of the above DSM mentioned NDD's sections, creatine formation involves the mitochondria, and creatine is necessary in the use of ATP. Hence, in cases of mitochondrial disturbance of the creatine pathway, individuals exhibit intellectual and language disorders [82]. Additionally, ADHD and ASD were found to have several biological factors, including increased oxidative stress, increased toxic metal burden, decreased methylation, mitochondrial dysfunction, and cerebral hypoperfusion. These mutual features imply mitochondrial dysfunction plays a key role in the development of both conditions [83], probably with distinction depending on the lesion developmental time window and specific brain circuits involved.

Hence, the etiology of neurodevelopmental disorders involves damage to the neural mitochondria and inflammation, which causes neural circuits' injury—impaired proliferation of contact points (= synapses) between neural cells and impaired neural circuits construction plasticity. In other words, damage to mitochondrial function, causing reduced cellular energy production, may lead to neural deterioration. As cells of the nervous system contain a lot of mitochondria, this is especially significant for neurons and glial cells [84–86].

Mitochondrial function is greatly affected by environmental factors, and impaired mitochondrial function is linked to environmental triggers [87–93]. Therefore, it is important to focus intervention and therapy on improving patient's mitochondrial function, using a safe and noninvasive tool that has been scientifically proven to overcome the environmental impact.

4. Novel therapeutic approach

4.1 Acupoint stimulation

Despite recent technological and scientific advances, there is currently no definite cure for neurodevelopmental impairments. Recent studies have shown that acupoint stimulation has promising results improving clinical symptoms of various cognitive injuries (memory impairment, language impairment, executive dysfunction, and decreased functional capacity) and enhancing brain function, significantly outperforming other interventions (including western pharmacology) [94–105].

At the intracellular level, one of the neuroprotective mechanisms by acupoint stimulation in the treatment of cognitive injury is anti-apoptosis (= anti-programed cell death), as apoptosis of hippocampal or cortical neurons is an important factor in cognitive injury [106, 107]. Programmed cell death consists of mitochondrial receptor tracks—intracellular and the cell membrane tracks. Injury signs by inflammation, poisonous proteins, and oxidative stress, may cause apoptotic cascade tracks, triggering neural apoptosis and cognitive injury. Acupoint stimulation accelerates neural survival mainly by adjusting genes and factors that participate in the mitochondria-dependent intracellular tracks of programed cell death, such as NF-κB, Bax, Fas, p53, and Noxa [108–117].

Another intracellular neuroprotective mechanism by acupoint stimulation in the treatment of cognitive injury is anti-oxidation, as the imbalance between oxidative and antioxidant systems leads to damage in hippocampal neurons. Acupoint stimulation regulates the production of pro-oxidative stress factors (NO and iNOS) [118–120], and hippocampal superoxide anions, thereby reducing oxidative stress [121, 122].

Moreover, acupoint stimulation was shown to have anti neuroinflammation properties. A key component of neuroinflammation in the central nervous system is microglial activation, causing the release of large quantities of inflammatory mediators and the induction of neuronal apoptosis [123, 124]. Acupoint stimulation regulates microglial polarization [125], decreases microglial activation in the hippocampal CA1 region [113, 126], and reduces the production of pro-inflammatory cytokines such as (TNF-α), IL-6, and IL-1β [126–128].

In the neural inter-cellular and circuit level, acupoint stimulation was shown to modulate neural regeneration and neuroplasticity, by enhancing growth factors BDNF, bFGF, and EGF. Moreover, acupoint stimulation has influenced synaptic functional plasticity and structure by monitoring the cAMP/PKA/CREB, BDNF/TrkB-PI3K/AKT/GSK-3β, signaling tracks, and excitatory transmitter innervation (glutamatergic, dopaminergic, noradrenergic, and cholinergic), promoting neural regeneration [129–136], sprouting of neural extensions, and modulating synaptic plasticity [137–164].

These effects of acupoint stimulation contribute to the recovery of hippocampal and cortical cells and restore their activity and connectivity. These pathways, as shown by molecular, cellular, and neuroimaging findings, facilitate the amelioration of cognitive injury by acupoint stimulation [165–178].

Our low power laser protocol is based on:

Physics characteristics of laser beam (including wavelength and frequency)—These are selected in accordance with patient's signs and symptoms.

Suitable acupoints for laser stimulation—These acupoints are selected in accordance with western auricular findings, traditional Chinese/Korean/Japanese medicine, and neuroanatomy and neurophysiology, relating to the patient's clinical picture.

4.2 Low power laser approach: Physics characteristics of the LASER tool

Employing low power laser, we use an innovative and well-known scientific and therapeutic approach to solve neural developmental injury.

Laser acupoint stimulation is a nonintrusive approach that has been successfully adopted and developed in recent years, with scientific documentation in high-level journals and books. Laser acupoint stimulation is widely used in clinical practice, being employed to decrease inflammation, edema, and chronic injuries; to advance healing of lesions, deep tissues, and neural extensions; and to reduce nerve damage and pain.

Low-power laser heals neural injuries, including neurodevelopmental disorders, through targeting the main elements of the pathological mechanism—reducing tissue oxidative stress and reducing the concentration of inflammatory proteins, tuning mitochondria energy production, and accelerating the creation of ATP and nerve growth factors.

LASER apparatuses produce electromagnetic radiation with constant wavelength, phase, and polarization, affecting living tissues and biological systems by nonthermal means [179]. Hence, applying this noninvasive procedure is safe even for the care of high-risk patients [180–182].

Acupoint stimulation using a low-power laser device begins exact changes in brain action, which are sensed by the patient as a recovery (i.e., no pain, no neural inflammation, etc.). These changes are measured and quantified by brain imaging [183, 184]. Hence, when the right therapeutic features are activated (laser capacity, beam wavelength, rate, interval, and acupoint settings), the laser beam decreases tissue oxidative stress and rises cellular ATP production, upgrading cell metabolism, and decreasing inflammation [185, 186].

As the aim of low-power laser are basic units of body cells, it successfully fights many injuries and ailments, including healing of soft tissues, reducing inflammation, and relieving chronic and acute physical and mental pain [187–192] (additional low-power laser clinical applications are detailed in Ref. [52]).

Our laser system creates beams with wavelengths in the range of red and blue light.

In addition to raising the construction of cellular energetic coin = ATP, as mentioned above, low-power laser Infrared beam can encourage the release of NO (nitric oxide) and CCO (cytochrome c oxidase) and regulate ROS, intracellular organelles' membrane activity (mainly the mitochondria), transmembrane calcium flux, and more [193–197].

Moreover, in eukaryote cells, low-power laser creates a shift toward higher oxidation in the total redox potential of the mitochondria; as a result, ATP levels and blood flow increase, and the availability of oxygen in damaged brain circuits is improved [198].

Red to near-infrared wavelength laser beam has a healing effect on local and systemic injuries and affects the functioning of the brain and additional internal organs. Moreover, red/NIR wavelengths are within the living tissue "optical window," allowing optimal tissue penetration depth, into shallow to deeper tissue layers.

Blue wavelength (405 nm) laser beam improves therapy energetic results, being absorbed by NADH (1st unit of the cellular respiratory chain), showing five times higher absorption compared to red laser wavelength [199].

Hence, bichromate laser radiation (red and blue wavelength range) yields a bigger change in the mitochondria redox potential, increasing the proton-motive force and thereby ATP cycle is enhanced [200] (for additional physics details see in Ref. [52]). This change at the cellular-molecular level is manifested clinically and functionally.

4.3 Clinical considerations: Specific locations for acupoint stimulation

Acupuncture, an old therapeutic approach, has been long used by clinicians around the world to overcome and cure chronic/acute medical situations, using intrusive metal needles. World Health Organization recommended acupuncture for the treatment of at least 20 pathologies, including pain, in patients at risk [201–203]. In addition, acupuncture has been shown to have potential benefits for a variety of mental disorders [204–208].

Therapy of cognitive impairment using acupoint stimulation shows promising results. The acupoints chosen in scientific publications were mostly found on upper and lower limbs and the head and neck (GV20, ST36, GV24, GV14, HT7), with GV20 being most popular. Stimulation of acupoints centered on GV20 showed the best therapeutic effect in clinical studies [209, 210], with high degree of similarity. For coping with cognitive impairment and neuroinflammation, stimulation of acupoints GV20 and ST36 was most efficient.

However, these most efficient acupoints for cognitive impairment [208, 211] are located near skull vertex, on fontanels and along cranial suture lines, and were punctured to depth of 20–25 mm obliquely [212, 213]. With young age patients, needle acupuncture/direct laser stimulation over skull acupoints and open suture fontanels should be avoided. Hence, instead of over-fontanelle skull direct acupoint needling, we use laser acupoint stimulation over distal and auricular acupoints [52, 214, 215].

5. Conclusion and recommendation

Low-power laser is an appropriate therapeutic tool for all patient populations. Laser acupoint stimulation is noninvasive, flexible, and diverse yet always based on the physical characteristics of the laser beam and its therapeutic effects on human body cells through specific somatotopic skin locations. Hence, even patients at risk, including old and sick or fragile babies with neurodevelopmental injury, may be suitable candidates for laser therapy, using evidence-based protocols tailored for their needs.

As we know, the molecular and cellular mechanisms of laser acupoint stimulation and as it has been proven clinically efficient with no damage or pain, we conclude that it is the kindest therapy we may offer patients with neurodevelopmental injuries.

Author details

Hagit Friedman[1,2]

1 Simaney Derech, Zichron-Yaakov, Israel

2 Haifa University, Haifa, Israel

*Address all correspondence to: drhagitfriedman@gmail.com

References

[1] Friedman H, Soloveichick M, Barak S, et al. Neuroplasticity in young age: Computer-based early neurodevelopment classifier. In: Neuroplasticity—Insights of Neural Organization. London, UK: IntechOpen; 2018

[2] American Psychiatric Association, DSM-5 Task Force. Diagnostic and Statistical Manual of Mental Disorders: DSM-5. 5th ed. Washington, DC: American Psychiatric Association; 2013. pp. 31-33

[3] Morris-Rosendahl DJ, Crocq MA. Neurodevelopmental disorders-the history and future of a diagnostic concept. Dialogues in Clinical Neuroscience. 2020;**22**(1):65-72

[4] American Psychiatric Association, DSM-5 Task Force. Diagnostic and Statistical Manual of Mental Disorders: DSM-5. 5th ed. Washington, DC: American Psychiatric Association; 2013. pp. 58-65

[5] Collins JW. The Greenwood Dictionary of Education. Santa Barbara, USA: Bloomsbury Publishing Plc.; 2011. p. 86

[6] Ad Hoc Committee on Service Delivery in the Schools. Definitions of Communication Disorders and Variations. Rockville, Maryland, USA: American Speech-Language-Hearing Association; 1993

[7] Gleason JB. The Development of Language. Boston: Allyn and Bacon; 2001

[8] Friedman H. Autism spectrum disorder (ASD): From mechanism to novel therapeutic approach. In: Learning Disabilities. IntechOpen; 2021

[9] American Psychiatric Association. Diagnostic and Statistical Manual of Mental Disorders (Fifth, Text Revision (DSM-5-TR) ed.). Washington, DC: American Psychiatric Association; 2022

[10] Foreman DM. Attention deficit hyperactivity disorder: Legal and ethical aspects. Archives of Disease in Childhood. 2006;**91**(2):192-194

[11] Faraone SV, Banaschewski T, Coghill D, et al. The world federation of ADHD international consensus statement: 208 evidence-based conclusions about the disorder. Neuroscience and Biobehavioral Reviews. 2021:128, 789-818

[12] Faraone SV, Rostain AL, Blader J, et al. Practitioner review: Emotional dysregulation in attention-deficit/hyperactivity disorder—Implications for clinical recognition and intervention. Journal of Child Psychology and Psychiatry, and Allied Disciplines. 2019;**60**(2):133-150

[13] Shaw P, Stringaris A, Nigg J, et al. Emotion dysregulation in attention deficit hyperactivity disorder. The American Journal of Psychiatry. 2014;**171**(3):276-293

[14] Pievsky MA, McGrath RE. The neurocognitive profile of attention-deficit/hyperactivity disorder: A review of meta-analyses. Archives of Clinical Neuropsychology. 2018;**33**(2):143-157

[15] Hart H, Radua J, Nakao T, et al. Meta-analysis of functional magnetic resonance imaging studies of inhibition and attention in attention-deficit/hyperactivity disorder: Exploring task-specific, stimulant medication, and age effects. JAMA Psychiatry. 2013;**70**(2):185-198

[16] Hoogman M, Muetzel R, Guimaraes JP, et al. Brain imaging of the

cortex in ADHD: A coordinated analysis of large-scale clinical and population-based samples. The American Journal of Psychiatry. 2019;**176**(7):531-542

[17] Brown TE. ADD/ADHD and impaired executive function in clinical practice. Current Psychiatry Reports. 2008;**10**(5):407-411

[18] Malenka RC, Nestler EJ, Hyman SE. In: Sydor A, Brown RY, editors. Molecular Neuropharmacology: A Foundation for Clinical Neuroscience. 2nd ed. New York: McGraw-Hill Medical; 2009. pp. 266, 315, 318-323

[19] Diamond A. Executive functions. Annual Review of Psychology. 2013;**64**:135-168

[20] Antshel KM, Hier BO, Barkley RA. Executive functioning theory and ADHD. In: Goldstein S, Naglieri JA, editors. Handbook of Executive Functioning. New York, NY: Springer; 2014. pp. 107-120

[21] Barkley RA, Murphy KR. The nature of executive function (EF) deficits in daily life activities in adults with ADHD and their relationship to performance on EF tests. Journal of Psychopathology and Behavioral Assessment. 2011;**33**(2):137-158

[22] Fleming M, Fitton CA, Steiner MF, et al. Educational and health outcomes of children treated for attention-deficit/ hyperactivity disorder. JAMA Pediatrics. 2017;**171**(7):e170691

[23] Lee YC, Yang HJ, Chen VC, et al. Meta-analysis of quality of life in children and adolescents with ADHD: By both parent proxy-report and child self-report using PedsQL™. Research in Developmental Disabilities. 2016;**51-52**:160-172

[24] Gage FH, Temple S. Neural stem cells: Generating and regenerating the brain. Neuron. 2013;**80**(3):588-601

[25] Temple S. The development of neural stem cells. Nature. 2001;**414**(6859):112-117

[26] Temple S. Stem cell plasticity—Building the brain of our dreams. Nature Reviews. Neuroscience. 2001;**2**:513-520

[27] Skaper SD. Neurotrophic factors: An overview. Methods in Molecular Biology. 2018;**1727**:1-17

[28] Skaper SD. The neurotrophin family of neurotrophic factors: An overview. Methods in Molecular Biology. 2012;**846**:1-12

[29] Huang EJ, Reichardt LF. Neurotrophins: Roles in neuronal development and function. Annual Review of Neuroscience. 2001;**24**:677-736

[30] Lamkin ER, Heiman MG. Coordinated morphogenesis of neurons and glia. Current Opinion in Neurobiology. 2017;**47**:58-64

[31] Vieira R, Mariani JN, Huynh NPT, et al. Young glial progenitor cells competitively replace aged and diseased human glia in the adult chimeric mouse brain. Nature Biotechnology. 2024;**42**:719-730

[32] Zhong S, Kiyoshi CM, Du Y, et al. Genesis of a functional astrocyte syncytium in the developing mouse hippocampus. Glia. 2023;**71**(4):1081-1098

[33] Miller FD et al. Timing is everything: Making neurons versus glia in the developing cortex. Neuron. 2007;**54**(3):357-369

[34] Lago-Baldaia I, Fernandes VM, Ackerman SD. More than mortar:

Glia as architects of nervous system development and disease. Frontiers in Cell and Development Biology. 2020;**8**:611269

[35] Hastings MH, Gilbert J, Huo Y, Man HY. Synaptogenesis. In: Eisenstat DD, Goldowitz D, Oberlander TF, Yager JY, editors. Neurodevelopmental Pediatrics. Cham: Springer; 2023

[36] Qi C, Luo LD, Feng I, Ma S. Molecular mechanisms of synaptogenesis. Frontiers in Synaptic Neuroscience. 2022;**14**:939793

[37] Friedman H et al. Assembly of new individual excitatory synapses: Time course and temporal order of synaptic molecule recruitment. Neuron. 2000;**27**:57-69

[38] Zhai RG, Friedman H, et al. Assembling the presynaptic active zone, the characterization of an active zone precursor vesicle. Neuron. 2001;**29**:131-143

[39] Sanes JR, Zipursky SL. Synaptic specificity, recognition molecules, and assembly of neural circuits. Cell. 2020;**181**(3):536-556

[40] Dorskind JM, Kolodkin AL. Revisiting and refining roles of neural guidance cues in circuit assembly. Current Opinion in Neurobiology. 2021;**66**:10-21

[41] Blockus H, Rolotti SV, Szoboszlay M, et al. Synaptogenic activity of the axon guidance molecule Robo2 is critical for hippocampal circuit function. bioRxiv. 2019. 840710

[42] Velten J, Agarwal R, Dosch K, et al. The molecular logic of synaptic wiring at the single cell level. bioRxiv. 2020.11.30.402057

[43] Zhu JJ. Architectural organization of ~1,500-neuron modular minicolumnar disinhibitory circuits in healthy and Alzheimer's cortices. Cell Reports. 2023;**42**(8):112904

[44] Chou Y, Nawabi H, Li J. Research hotspots and trends for axon regeneration (2000-2021): A bibliometric study and systematic review. Inflammation and Regeneration. 2022;**42**(1):60

[45] Pasterkamp RJ, Burk K. Axon guidance receptors: Endocytosis, trafficking and downstream signaling from endosomes. Progress in Neurobiology. 2021;**198**:101916

[46] Yam PT, Charron F. Signaling mechanisms of non-conventional axon guidance cues: The Shh, BMP and Wnt morphogens. Current Opinion in Neurobiology. 2013;**23**(6):965-973

[47] Kelley KW, Pașca SP. Human brain organogenesis: Toward a cellular understanding of development and disease. Cell. 2022;**185**(1):42-61

[48] Lu B, Wang KH, Nose A. Molecular mechanisms underlying neural circuit formation. Current Opinion in Neurobiology. 2009;**19**(2):162-167

[49] Nakadate K, Kawakami K. Molecules affecting brain development and nervous system. International Journal of Molecular Sciences. 2023;**24**(10):8691

[50] Zhang C, Ko J. Editorial: Synaptic assembly and neural circuit development. Frontiers in Synaptic Neuroscience. 2018;**10**:30

[51] Ko J, Kim E. Special issue on synapse assembly, neural circuit development, and brain disorders. Experimental & Molecular Medicine. 2018;**50**:1-2

[52] Friedman H. Early trauma, brain development, and a novel therapeutic approach. In: Friedman H, editor. Neuropediatrics—Recent Advances and Novel Therapeutic Approaches. London, UK: IntechOpen; 2024

[53] Pletikos M, Sousa AM, Sedmak G, et al. Temporal specification and bilaterality of human neocortical topographic gene expression. Neuron. 2014;**81**(2):321-332

[54] Brown AS. Prenatal infection as a risk factor for schizophrenia. Schizophrenia Bulletin. 2006;**32**(2):200-202

[55] Richardson AJ, Ross MA. Fatty acid metabolism in neurodevelopmental disorder: A new perspective on associations between attention-deficit/hyperactivity disorder, dyslexia, dyspraxia and the autistic spectrum. Prostaglandins, Leukotrienes, and Essential Fatty Acids. 2000;**63**(1-2):1-9

[56] Skeaff SA. Iodine deficiency in pregnancy: The effect on neurodevelopment in the child. Nutrients. 2011;**3**(2):265-273

[57] Collins KA, Popek E. Birth injury: Birth asphyxia and birth trauma. Academic Forensic Pathology. 2018;**8**(4):788-864

[58] Kratimenos P, Penn AA. Placental programming of neuropsychiatric disease. Pediatric Research. 2019;**86**(2):157-164

[59] Borrego-Ruiz A, Borrego JJ. Neurodevelopmental disorders associated with gut microbiome dysbiosis in children. Children. 2024;**11**(7):796

[60] Iliodromiti Z, Triantafyllou AR, Tsaousi M, et al. Gut microbiome and neurodevelopmental disorders: A link yet to be disclosed. Microorganisms. 2023;**11**(2):487

[61] Forsberg H. Microbiome programming of brain development: Implications forneurodevelopmental disorders. Developmental Medicine and Child Neurology. 2019;**61**:744-749

[62] Lacorte E, Gervasi G, Bacigalupo I, et al. A systematic review of the microbiome in children with neurodevelopmental disorders. Frontiers in Neurology. 2019;**10**:727

[63] Laue HE, Coker MO, Madan JC. The developing microbiome from birth to 3 years: The gut-brain axis and neurodevelopmental outcomes. Frontiers in Pediatrics. 2022;**10**:815885

[64] Boivin MJ, Kakooza AM, Warf BC, et al. Reducing neurodevelopmental disorders and disability through research and interventions. Nature. 2015;**527**(7578):S155-S160

[65] Monteiro P, Feng G. SHANK proteins: Roles at the synapse and in autism spectrum disorder. Nature Reviews. Neuroscience. 2017;**18**(3):147-157

[66] Vyas Y, Cheyne JE, Lee K, et al. Shankopathies in the developing brain in autism spectrum disorders. Frontiers in Neuroscience. 2021;**15**:775431

[67] Huang M, Qi Q, Xu T. Targeting Shank3 deficiency and paresthesia in autism spectrum disorder: A brief review. Frontiers in Molecular Neuroscience. 2023;**16**:1128974

[68] Kaizuka T, Takumi T. Postsynaptic density proteins and their involvement in neurodevelopmental disorders. The Journal of Biochemistry. 2018;**163**(6):447-455

[69] Williams JHG. Self–other relations in social development and autism: Multiple roles for mirror neurons and other brain bases. Autism Research. 2008;**1**:73-90

[70] Hamilton AF. Reflecting on the mirror neuron system in autism: A systematic review of current theories. Developmental Cognitive Neuroscience. 2013;**3**:91-105

[71] Lust JM, van Schie HT, Wilson PH, et al. Activation of mirror neuron regions is altered in developmental coordination disorder (DCD)-neurophysiological evidence using an action observation paradigm. Frontiers in Human Neuroscience. 2019;**13**:232

[72] Rahman S. Mitochondrial disease in children. Journal of Internal Medicine. 2020;**287**:609-633

[73] Parikh S, Goldstein A, Koenig MK, et al. Diagnosis and management of mitochondrial disease: A consensus statement from the mitochondrial medicine society. Genetics in Medicine. 2015;**17**:689-701

[74] Suomalainen A, Battersby BJ. Mitochondrial diseases: The contribution of organelle stress responses to pathology. Nature Reviews. Molecular Cell Biology. 2018;**19**(2):77-92

[75] Friedman H. Autism spectrum disorder (ASD): From molecular mechanism to novel therapeutic approach. In: Learning Disabilities—Neurobiology, Assessment, Clinical Features and Treatments. London, UK: IntechOpen; 2022

[76] Singh K et al. Developmental regression and mitochondrial function in children with autism. Annals of Clinical Translational Neurology. 2020;**7**:683-694

[77] Hassan H et al. Alterations in mitochondrial respiratory capacity and membrane potential: A link between mitochondrial dysregulation and autism. MitoFit Preprint Arch. Current Issues in Molecular Biology. 2021;**43**(3):2238-2252

[78] Nguyen A et al. Mechanisms of mitochondrial oxidative stress in brain injury: From pathophysiology to therapeutics. Oxygen. 2023;**3**(2): 163-178

[79] Haas RH. Autism and mitochondrial disease. Developmental Disabilities Research Reviews. 2010;**16**:144-153

[80] Falk MJ. Neurodevelopmental manifestations of mitochondrial disease. Journal of Developmental and Behavioral Pediatrics. 2010;**31**:610-621

[81] Rossignol DA, Frye RE. Mitochondrial dysfunction in autism spectrum disorders: A systematic review and meta-analysis. Molecular Psychiatry. 2012;**17**:290-314

[82] Joncquel-Chevalier CM, Voicu PM, Fontaine M, et al. Creatine biosynthesis and transport in health and disease. Biochimie. 2015;**119**:146-165

[83] Bradstreet JJ, Smith S, Baral M, Rossignol DA. Biomarker-guided interventions of clinically relevant conditions associated with autism spectrum disorders and attention deficit hyperactivity disorders. Alternative Medicine Review. 2010;**15**:15-32

[84] Shen X et al. Mitochondrial quality control in the brain: The physiological and pathological roles. Frontiers in Neuroscience. 2022;**16**:1075141

[85] Anitha A, Thanseem I, Iype M, Thomas SV. Mitochondrial dysfunction in cognitive neurodevelopmental disorders: Cause or effect? Mitochondrion. 2023;**69**:18-32

[86] Pinto Payares DV, Spooner L, Vosters J, et al. A systematic review on the role of mitochondrial dysfunction/disorders in neurodevelopmental disorders and psychiatric/behavioral

disorders. Frontiers in Psychiatry. 2024;**15**:1389093

[87] Frye RE et al. Mitochondria may mediate prenatal environmental influences in autism spectrum disorder. Journal of Personalized Medicine. 2021;**11**:218

[88] Byun HM, Baccarelli AA. Environmental exposure and mitochondrial epigenetics: Study design and analytical challenges. Human Genetics. 2014;**133**(3):247-257

[89] Meyer JN et al. Mitochondria as a target of environmental toxicants. Toxicological Sciences. 2013;**134**(1):1-17

[90] Reddam A et al. Environmental chemical exposures and mitochondrial dysfunction: A review of recent literature. Current Environmental Health Reports. 2022;**9**:631-649

[91] Duarte-Hospital C et al. Mitochondrial dysfunction as a Hallmark of environmental injury. Cell. 2022;**11**(1):110

[92] Jayasundara N. Ecological significance of mitochondrial toxicants. Toxicology. 2017;**391**(1):64-74

[93] Helley MP et al. Mitochondria: A common target for genetic mutations and environmental toxicants in Parkinson's disease. Frontiers in Genetics. 2017;**8**:177

[94] Lu L, Zhang Y, Tang X, et al. Evidence on acupuncture therapies is underused in clinical practice and health policy. BMJ. 2022;**376**:e0674

[95] Huang Q, Luo D, Chen L, et al. Effectiveness of acupuncture for Alzheimer's disease: An updated systematic review and metanalysis. Current Medical Science. 2019;**39**(3):500-511

[96] Li W, Wang Q, Du S, et al. Acupuncture for mild cognitive impairment in elderly people: Systematic review and meta-analyses. Medicine (Baltimore). 2020;**99**(39):e22365

[97] Tang Y, Wang T, Yang L, et al. Acupuncture for postoperative cognitive dysfunction: A systematic review and meta-analysis of randomized controlled trials. Acupuncture in Medicine. 2021;**39**:423-431

[98] Tong T, Pei C, Chen J, et al. Efficacy of acupuncture therapy for chemotherapy-related cognitive impairment in breast cancer patients. Medical Science Monitor. 2018;**24**:2919-2927

[99] Yang X, Gong W, Ma X, et al. Factor analysis of electroacupuncture and selective serotonin reuptake inhibitors for major depressive disorder: An 8-week controlled clinical trial. Acupuncture in Medicine. 2020;**8**:45-52

[100] Sun ZL, Liu J, Guo W, et al. Serum brain-derived neurotrophic factor levels associate with cognitive improvement in patients with schizophrenia treated with electroacupuncture. Psychiatry Research. 2016;**244**:370-375

[101] Zhou J, Peng W, Xu M, et al. The effectiveness and safety of acupuncture for patients with Alzheimer disease: A systematic review and meta-analysis of randomized controlled trials. Medicine (Baltimore). 2015;**94**(22):e933

[102] Zhou S, Dong L, He Y, Xiao H. Acupuncture plus herbal medicine for Alzheimer's disease: A systematic review and meta-analysis. The American Journal of Chinese Medicine. 2017;**45**(7):1327-1344

[103] Yang JW, Shi GX, Zhang S, et al. Effectiveness of acupuncture for vascular cognitive impairment no dementia: A

randomized controlled trial. Clinical Rehabilitation. 2019;**33**(4):642-652

[104] Zhang H, Zhao L, Yang S, et al. Clinical observation on effect of scalp electroacupuncture for mild cognitive impairment. Journal of Traditional Chinese Medicine. 2013;**33**(1):46-50

[105] Wang S, Yang H, Zhang J, et al. Efficacy and safety assessment of acupuncture and nimodipine to treat mild cognitive impairment after cerebral infarction: A randomized controlled trial. BMC Complementary and Alternative Medicine. 2016;**16**(1):361

[106] Obulesu M, Lakshmi MJ. Apoptosis in Alzheimer's disease: An understanding of the physiology, pathology and therapeutic avenues. Neurochemical Research. 2014;**39**(12):2301-2312

[107] Sairanen T, Karjalainen-Lindsberg ML, Paetau A, et al. Apoptosis dominant in the periinfarct area of human ischaemic stroke–a possible target of antiapoptotic treatments. Brain. 2006;**129**(Pt1):189-199

[108] Zhang J, Tang C, Liao W, et al. The anti-apoptotic and antioxidative stress effects of Zhisanzhen in the Alzheimer's disease model rat. Neuroreport. 2019;**30**:628-636

[109] Guo HD, Tian JX, Zhu J, Li L, et al. Electroacupuncture suppressed neuronal apoptosis and improved cognitive impairment in the AD model rats possibly via downregulation of notch signaling pathway. Evidence-Based Complementary and Alternative Medicine. 2015;**2015**:3935

[110] Liu F, Jiang YJ, Zhao HJ, et al. Electroacupuncture ameliorates cognitive impairment and regulates the expression of apoptosis related genes Bcl-2 and Bax in rats with cerebral ischaemia-reperfusion injury. Acupuncture in Medicine. 2015;**33**:478-484

[111] Yun YC, Jang D, Yoon SB, et al. Laser acupuncture exerts neuroprotective effects via regulation of CREB, BDNF, Bcl-2, and Bax gene expressions in the hippocampus. Evidence-Based Complementary and Alternative Medicine. 2017;**2017**:7181637

[112] Zhang Q, Li Y, Yin C, et al. Electro-acupuncture pretreatment ameliorates anesthesia and surgery-induced cognitive dysfunction via inhibiting mitochondrial injury and neuro-apoptosis in aged rats. Neurochemical Research. 2022;**47**:1751-1764

[113] Feng S, Wang Q, Wang H, et al. Electroacupuncture pretreatment ameliorates hypergravity-induced impairment of learning and memory and apoptosis of hippocampal neurons in rats. Neuroscience Letters. 2010;**478**:150-155

[114] Du Y, Liu R, Sun G, Meng P, Song J. Pre-moxibustion and moxibustion prevent Alzheimer's disease. Neural Regeneration Research. 2013;**8**:2811-2819

[115] Feng X, Yang S, Liu J, et al. Electroacupuncture ameliorates cognitive impairment through inhibition of NF-κB-mediated neuronal cell apoptosis in cerebral ischemia-reperfusion injured rats. Molecular Medicine Reports. 2013;**7**:1516-1522

[116] Wawryk-Gawda E, Chylińska-Wrzos P, Lis-Sochocka M, et al. P53 protein in proliferation, repair and apoptosis of cells. Protoplasma. 2014;**251**:525-533

[117] Zhu Y, Zeng Y. Electroacupuncture protected pyramidal cells in hippocampal CA1 region of vascular dementia

rats by inhibiting the expression of p53 and Noxa. CNS Neuroscience & Therapeutics. 2011;**17**:599-604

[118] Su X, Wu Z, Mai F, et al. 'Governor vessel-unblocking and mind-regulating' acupuncture therapy ameliorates cognitive dysfunction in a rat model of middle cerebral artery occlusion. International Journal of Molecular Medicine. 2019;**43**:221-232

[119] Chen Y, Zhou J, Li J, Yang SB, et al. Electroacupuncture pretreatment prevents cognitive impairment induced by limb ischemia-reperfusion via inhibition of microglial activation and attenuation of oxidative stress in rats. Brain Research. 2012;**1432**:36

[120] Wu G, Li L, Li HM, et al. Electroacupuncture ameliorates spatial learning and memory impairment via attenuating NOX2-related oxidative stress in a rat model of Alzheimer's disease induced by Aβ1-42. Cellular and Molecular Biology. 2017;**63**:38-45

[121] Li H, Wang Y, Feng D, Liu Y, et al. Alterations in the time course of expression of the Nox family in the brain in a rat experimental cerebral ischemia and reperfusion model: Effects of melatonin. Journal of Pineal Research. 2014;**57**:110-119

[122] Wang J, Liu Y, Shen H, et al. Nox2 and Nox4 participate in ROS-induced neuronal apoptosis and brain injury during ischemia reperfusion in rats. Acta Neurochirurgica. Supplement. 2020;**127**:47-54

[123] Yirmiya R, Goshen I. Immune modulation of learning, memory, neural plasticity and neurogenesis. Brain, Behavior, and Immunity. 2011;**25**(2):181-213

[124] Jazwa A, Cuadrado A. Targeting heme oxygenase-1 for neuroprotection and neuroinflammation in neurodegenerative diseases. Current Drug Targets. 2010;**11**:1517-1531

[125] Li L, Li L, Zhang J, et al. Disease stage-associated alterations in learning and memory through the electroacupuncture modulation of the cortical microglial M1/M2 polarization in mice with Alzheimer's disease. Neural Plasticity. 2020;**2020**:8836173

[126] Cai M, Lee JH, Yang EJ. Bee venom ameliorates cognitive dysfunction caused by neuroinflammation in an animal model of vascular dementia. Molecular Neurobiology. 2017;**54**:5952-5960

[127] Fang Y, Sui R. Electroacupuncture at the Wangu acupoint suppresses expression of inflammatory cytokines in the hippocampus of rats with vascular dementia. African Journal of Traditional, Complementary, and Alternative Medicines. 2016;**13**:17-24

[128] Wang Y, Wang Q, Ren B, et al. "Olfactory three-needle" enhances spatial learning and memory ability in SAMP8 mice. Behavioural Neurology. 2020;**2020**:2893289

[129] Li F, Yan CQ, Lin LT, et al. Acupuncture attenuates cognitive deficits and increases pyramidal neuron number in hippocampal CA1 area of vascular dementia rats. BMC Complementary and Alternative Medicine. 2015;**15**:133

[130] Li G, Zhang X, Cheng H, et al. Acupuncture improves cognitive deficits and increases neuron density of the hippocampus in middle-aged SAMP8 mice. Acupuncture in Medicine. 2012;**30**:339-345

[131] Zhao L, Zhou C, Li L, Liu J, et al. Acupuncture improves cerebral microenvironment in mice with Alzheimer's disease treated with

hippocampal neural stem cells. Molecular Neurobiology. 2017;**54**:5120-5130

[132] Fan XW, Liu HH, Wang HB, et al. Electroacupuncture improves cognitive function and hippocampal neurogenesis after brain irradiation. Radiation Research. 2017;**187**:672-681

[133] Li X, Guo F, Zhang Q, et al. Electroacupuncture decreases cognitive impairment and promotes neurogenesis in the APP/PS1 transgenic mice. BMC Complementary and Alternative Medicine. 2014;**14**:37

[134] Zhang S, Xie R, Zhao T, et al. Neural stem cells preferentially migrate to glioma stem cells and reduce their stemness phenotypes. International Journal of Oncology. 2014;**45**:1989-1996

[135] Li L, Li J, Dai Y, et al. Electro-acupuncture improves the early pattern separation in Alzheimer's disease mice via basal forebrain-hippocampus cholinergic neural circuit. Frontiers in Aging Neuroscience. 2021;**13**:770948

[136] Ahn SM, Kim YR, Kim HN, et al. Electroacupuncture ameliorates memory impairments by enhancing oligodendrocyte regeneration in a mouse model of prolonged cerebral hypoperfusion. Scientific Reports. 2016;**6**:28646

[137] Gutiérrez-Vargas JA, Múnera A, Cardona-Gómez GP. CDK5 knockdown prevents hippocampal degeneration and cognitive dysfunction produced by cerebral ischemia. Journal of Cerebral Blood Flow and Metabolism. 2015;**35**:1937-1949

[138] Xu B, Sun A, He Y, et al. Loss of thin spines and small synapses contributes to defective hippocampal function in aged mice. Neurobiology of Aging. 2018;**71**:91-104

[139] Zhao L, Liu JW, Kan BH, et al. Acupuncture accelerates neural regeneration and synaptophysin production after neural stem cells transplantation in mice. World Journal of Stem Cells. 2020;**12**:1576-1590

[140] Cai M, Lee JH, Yang EJ. Electroacupuncture attenuates cognition impairment via anti-neuroinflammation in an Alzheimer's disease animal model. Journal of Neuroinflammation. 2019;**16**:264

[141] Dong W, Yang W, Li F, Guo W, et al. Electroacupuncture improves synaptic function in SAMP8 mice probably via inhibition of the AMPK/eEF2K/eEF2 signaling pathway. Evidence-Based Complementary and Alternative Medicine. 2019;**2019**:8260815

[142] Ma C, Zhou Y, Yi W, et al. Electroacupuncture of the Baihui and Shenting acupoints for vascular dementia in rats through the miR-81/IL-16/PSD-95 pathway. Annals of Translational Medicine. 2022;**10**:540

[143] Lin R, Li X, Liu W, et al. Electro-acupuncture ameliorates cognitive impairment via improvement of brain-derived neurotropic factor-mediated hippocampal synaptic plasticity in cerebral ischemia-reperfusion injured rats. Experimental and Therapeutic Medicine. 2017;**14**:2373-2379

[144] Pei W, Meng F, Deng Q, et al. Electroacupuncture promotes the survival and synaptic plasticity of hippocampal neurons and improvement of sleep deprivation-induced spatial memory impairment. CNS Neuroscience & Therapeutics. 2021;**27**:1472-1482

[145] Maqbool M, Mobashir M, Hoda N. Pivotal role of glycogen synthase kinase-3: A therapeutic target for Alzheimer's disease. European Journal

of Medicinal Chemistry. 2016;**107**: 63-81

[146] Yu CC, Wang Y, Shen F, et al. High-frequency (50 Hz) electroacupuncture ameliorates cognitive impairment in rats with amyloid beta 1-42-induced Alzheimer's disease. Neural Regeneration Research. 2018;**13**:1833-1841

[147] Wang Y, Zheng A, Yang H, et al. "Olfactory three needle" acupuncture enhances synaptic function in Aβ(1-42)-induced Alzheimer's disease via activating PI3K/AKT/GSK-3β signaling pathway. Journal of Integrative Neuroscience. 2021;**20**:55-65

[148] Lin R, Wu Y, Tao J, Chen B, et al. Electroacupuncture improves cognitive function through Rho GTPases and enhances dendritic spine plasticity in rats with cerebral ischemia-reperfusion. Molecular Medicine Reports. 2016;**13**:2655-2660

[149] Herring BE, Nicoll RA. Long-term potentiation: From CaMKII to AMPA receptor trafficking. Annual Review of Physiology. 2016;**78**:351-365

[150] Zheng Y, Qin Z, Tsoi B, et al. Electroacupuncture on trigeminal nerve-innervated acupoints ameliorates poststroke cognitive impairment in rats with middle cerebral artery occlusion: Involvement of neuroprotection and synaptic plasticity. Neural Plasticity. 2020;**2020**:8818328

[151] Dai Y, Zhang Y, Yang M, et al. Electroacupuncture increases the hippocampal synaptic transmission efficiency and long-term plasticity to improve vascular cognitive impairment. Mediators of Inflammation. 2022;**2022**:5985143

[152] Li QQ, Shi GX, Yang JW, et al. Hippocampal cAMP/PKA/CREB is required for neuroprotective effect of acupuncture. Physiology & Behavior. 2015;**139**:482-490

[153] Zheng CX, Lu M, Guo YB, et al. Electroacupuncture ameliorates learning and memory and improves synaptic plasticity via activation of the PKA/CREB signaling pathway in cerebral hypoperfusion. Evidence-Based Complementary and Alternative Medicine. 2016;**2016**:7893710

[154] Treu SP, Plante DT. Cerebrospinal fluid orexin in Alzheimer's disease: A systematic review and meta-analysis. Sleep Medicine. 2021;**85**:230-238

[155] Hou Z, Yang X, Li Y, Chen J, Shang H. Electroacupuncture enhances neuroplasticity by regulating the orexin A-mediated cAMP/PKA/CREB signaling pathway in senescence-accelerated mouse prone 8 (SAMP8) mice. Oxidative Medicine and Cellular Longevity. 2022;**2022**:8694462

[156] Ye Y, Li H, Yang JW, Wang XR, et al. Acupuncture attenuated vascular dementia-induced hippocampal long-term potentiation impairments via activation of D1/D5 receptors. Stroke. 2017;**48**:1044-1161

[157] Xiao LY, Wang XR, Yang JW, et al. Acupuncture prevents the impairment of hippocampal LTP through β1-AR in vascular dementia rats. Molecular Neurobiology. 2018;**55**:7677-7690

[158] Xiao LY, Yang JW, Wang XR, et al. Acupuncture rescues cognitive impairment and upregulates dopamine-βhydroxylase expression in chronic cerebral hypoperfusion rats. BioMed Research International. 2018;**2018**:5423961

[159] Nguyen PV, Gelinas JN. Noradrenergic gating of

long-lasting synaptic potentiation in the hippocampus: From neurobiology to translational biomedicine. Journal of Neurogenetics. 2018;**32**:171-182

[160] Zhang Y, Mao X, Lin R, et al. Electroacupuncture ameliorates cognitive impairment through inhibition of Ca(2+)-mediated neurotoxicity in a rat model of cerebral ischemia-reperfusion injury. Acupuncture in Medicine. 2018;**36**:401-407

[161] Lee B, Sur BJ, Kwon S, Jung E, et al. Acupuncture stimulation alleviates corticosterone-induced impairments of spatial memory and cholinergic neurons in rats. Evidence-Based Complementary and Alternative Medicine. 2012;**2012**:670536

[162] Lee B, Sur B, Shim J, et al. Acupuncture stimulation improves scopolamine-induced cognitive impairment via activation of cholinergic system and regulation of BDNF and CREB expressions in rats. BMC Complementary and Alternative Medicine. 2014;**14**:338

[163] Liu PR, Zhou Y, Zhang Y, Diao S. Electroacupuncture alleviates surgeryinduced cognitive dysfunction by increasing α7-nAChR expression and inhibiting inflammatory pathway in aged rats. Neuroscience Letters. 2017;**659**:1-6

[164] Picciotto MR, Higley MJ, Mineur YS. Acetylcholine as a neuromodulator: Cholinergic signaling shapes nervous system function and behavior. Neuron. 2012;**76**:116-129

[165] Escobar I, Xu J, Jackson CW, Perez-Pinzon MA. Altered neural networks in the papez circuit: Implications for cognitive dysfunction after cerebral ischemia. Journal of Alzheimer's Disease. 2019;**67**:425-446

[166] Vann SD, Nelson AJ. The mammillary bodies and memory: More than a hippocampal relay. Progress in Brain Research. 2015;**219**:163-185

[167] Zarei M, Patenaude B, Damoiseaux J, Morgese C, Smith S, Matthews PM, et al. Combining shape and connectivity analysis: An MRI study of thalamic degeneration in Alzheimer's disease. NeuroImage. 2010;**49**:1-8

[168] Jang SH, Kwon HG. Neural injury of the Papez circuit following hypoxic-ischemic brain injury: A case report. Medicine (Abingdon). 2016;**95**:e5173

[169] Lin B, Zhang L, Yin X, et al. Modulation of entorhinal cortex-hippocampus connectivity and recognition memory following electroacupuncture on 3×Tg-AD model: Evidence from multimodal MRI and electrophysiological recordings. Frontiers in Neuroscience. 2022;**16**:968767

[170] Lu Y, Huang Y, Tang C, et al. Brain areas involved in the acupuncture treatment of AD model rats: A PET study. BMC Complementary and Alternative Medicine. 2014;**14**:178

[171] Zhang Q, Li J, Huang S, Yang M, et al. Functional connectivity of the retrosplenial cortex in rats with ischemic stroke is improved by electroacupuncture. Acupuncture in Medicine. 2021;**39**:200-207

[172] Zheng W, Su Z, Liu X, Zhang H, et al. Modulation of functional activity and connectivity by acupuncture in patients with Alzheimer disease as measured by resting-state fMRI. PLoS ONE. 2018;**13**:e0196933

[173] Wang Z, Liang P, Zhao Z, et al. Acupuncture modulates resting state hippocampal functional connectivity

in Alzheimer disease. PLoS ONE. 2014;**9**:e91160

[174] Liang P, Wang Z, Qian T, Li K. Acupuncture stimulation of Taichong (Liv3) and Hegu (LI4) modulates the default mode network activity in Alzheimer's disease. American Journal of Alzheimer's Disease and Other Dementias. 2014;**29**:739-748

[175] Lai X, Ren J, Lu Y, et al. Efects of acupuncture at HT7 on glucose metabolism in a rat model of Alzheimer's disease: An 18F-FDG-PET study. Acupuncture in Medicine. 2016;**34**:215-222

[176] Chen S, Xu M, Li H, et al. Acupuncture at the Taixi (KI3) acupoint activates cerebral neurons in elderly patients with mild cognitive impairment. Neural Regeneration Research. 2014;**9**:1163-1168

[177] Wang Z, Nie B, Li D, et al. Effect of acupuncture in mild cognitive impairment and Alzheimer disease: A functional MRI study. PLoS ONE. 2012;**7**:e42730

[178] Tan TT, Wang D, Huang JK, et al. Modulatory effects of acupuncture on brain networks in mild cognitive impairment patients. Neural Regeneration Research. 2017;**12**: 250-258

[179] Zein R et al. Review of light parameters and photobiomodulation efficacy: Dive into complexity. Journal of Biomedical Optics. 2018;**23**(12):12090

[180] Kurath-Koller S et al. Changes of locoregional skin temperature in neonates undergoing laser needle acupuncture at the acupuncture point large intestine. Evidence-based Complementary and Alternative Medicine. eCAM. 2015;**2015**:571857

[181] Raith W et al. Thermographic measuring of skin temperature using laser needle acupuncture in preterm neonates. Evidence-based Complementary and Alternative Medicine. eCAM. 2012;**2012**:614210

[182] Raith W et al. Near-infrared spectroscopy for objectifying cerebral effects of laser acupuncture in term and preterm neonates. Evidence-based Complementary and Alternative Medicine. eCAM. 2013;**2013**:346852

[183] Siedentopf CM et al. fMRI detects activation of the visual association cortex during laser acupuncture of the foot in humans. Neuroscience Letters. 2002;**327**:53-56

[184] Litcher G et al. Acupuncture using laser needles modulates brain function: First evidence from functional transcranial Doppler sonography and fMRI. Lasers in Medical Science. 2004;**19**:6-11

[185] de Freitas LF et al. Proposed mechanisms of photobiomodulation or low-level light therapy. IEEE Journal of Selected Topics in Quantum Electronics. 2016;**22**(3):7000417

[186] Mussttaf RA et al. Assessing the impact of low-level laser therapy (LLLT) on biological systems: A review. International Journal of Radiation Biology. 2019;**95**(2):120-143

[187] Fulop AM et al. A meta-analysis of the efficacy of laser phototherapy on pain relief. The Clinical Journal of Pain. 2019;**26**:729-736

[188] Chow RT et al. 830 nm laser irradiation induces varicosity formation, reduces mitochondrial membrane potential, and blocks fast axonal flow in small and medium diameter rat dorsal root ganglion neurons: Implications

for the analgesic effects of 830 nm laser. Journal of the Peripheral Nervous System. 2007;**12**:28-39

[189] Xu S, Wan B. Recent advances in lowlevel laser therapy on depression. Stress and Brain. 2022;**2**(4):123-138

[190] Chow R, Armati P, Laakso EL, Bjorda JM, Baxter GD. Inhibitory effects of laser irradiation on peripheral mammalian nerves and relevance to analgesic effects: A systematic review. Photomedicine and Laser Surgery. 2011;**29**(6):365-381

[191] Yan W, Chow R, Armati PJ. Inhibitory effects of visible 650-nm and infrared 808 nm laser irradiation on somatosensory and compound muscle action potentials in rat sciatic nerve: Implications for laser-induced analgesia. Journal of the Peripheral Nervous System. 2011;**16**(2):130-135

[192] Masoumipoor M, Jameie S, Janzadeh A, et al. Effects of 660-and 980-nm low-level laser therapy on neuropathic pain relief following chronic constriction injury in rat sciatic nerve. Lasers in Medical Science. 2014;**29**(5):1593-1598

[193] Farivar S et al. Biological effects of low-level laser therapy. Journal of Lasers in Medical Sciences. 2014;**5**(2):58-62

[194] Ferraresi C et al. Time response of increases in ATP and muscle resistance to fatigue after low-level laser (light) therapy (LLLT) in mice. Lasers in Medical Science. 2015;**30**(4):1259-1267

[195] Huang YY et al. Transcranial lowlevel laser (light) therapy for traumatic brain injury. Journal of Biophotonics. 2012;**5**:827-837

[196] Khuman J et al. Low-level laser light therapy improves cognitive deficits and inhibits microglial activation after controlled cortical impact in mice. Journal of Neurotrauma. 2012;**29**:408-417

[197] Osipov AN et al. Effects of laser radiation on mitochondria and mitochondrial proteins subjected to nitric oxide. Frontiers in Medicine. 2018;**5**:112

[198] Thunshelle C, Hamblin MR. Transcranial low-level laser (light) therapy for brain injury. Photomedicine and Laser Surgery. 2016;**34**:587-598

[199] Sies H, Jones DP. Reactive oxygen species (ROS) as pleiotropic physiological signaling agents. Nature Reviews. Molecular Cell Biology. 2020;**21**:363-383

[200] Berry BJ et al. Use the protonmotive force: Mitochondrial uncoupling and reactive oxygen species. Journal of Molecular Biology. 2018;**430**(21):3873-3891

[201] Stahler van Amerongen K et al. Ear acupuncture points in neonates. The Journal of Alternative and Complementary Medicine. 2008;**14**(1):47-52

[202] Ecevit A et al. Acupuncture in preterm babies during minor painful procedures. Journal of Traditional Chinese Medicine. 2011;**31**(4): 308-310

[203] Landgren K, Kvorning N, Hallström I. Acupuncture reduces crying in infants with infantile colic: A randomized, controlled, blind clinical study. Acupuncture in Medicine. 2010;**28**(4):174-179

[204] Errington-Evans N. Acupuncture for anxiety. CNS Neuroscience and Therapeutics. 2012;**18**(4):277-284

[205] Lee S, Kim S. The effects of acupuncture on sleep disorders and its underlying mechanism: A literature review of rodent studies. Frontiers in Neuroscience, Section Translational Neuroscience. 2023;**8**(17):1243029

[206] Grant S, Colaiaco B, Motala A, Shanman R, et al. Acupuncture for the treatment of adults with posttraumatic stress disorder: A systematic review and meta-analysis. Journal of Trauma & Dissociation. 2018;**19**(1):39-58

[207] Ding N, Li L, Song K, Huang A, Zhang H. Efficacy and safety of acupuncture in treating posttraumatic stress disorder: A protocol for systematic review and meta-analysis. Medicine. 2020;**99**(26):e20700

[208] Tang X, Lin S, Fang D, Lin B, et al. Efficacy and underlying mechanisms of acupuncture therapy for PTSD: Evidence from animal and clinical studies. Frontiers in Behavioral Neuroscience. 2023;**17**:1163718

[209] Feng S, Ren Y, Fan S, Wang M, et al. Discovery of acupoints and combinations with potential to treat vascular dementia: A data mining analysis. Evidence-Based Complementary and Alternative Medicine. 2015;**2015**:310591

[210] Yu C, Wang L, Kong L, Shen F, et al. Acupoint combinations used for treatment of Alzheimer's disease: A data mining analysis. Journal of Traditional Chinese Medicine. 2018;**38**:943-952

[211] Kwon CY, Leem J, Kim DW, et al. Effects of acupuncture on earthquake survivors with major psychiatric disorders and related symptoms: A scoping review of clinical studies. PLoS ONE. 2023;**18**(6):e0286671

[212] Li H. A Study of Acupuncturing "Chou's Tiaoshen" Acupoints on Patients in Subacute Insomnia. ISRCTN Registry. UK: The UK's Clinical Study Registry; 2018

[213] Jialing Z, Zongshi Q, Tsz HS, et al. Electroacupuncture plus auricular acupressure for chemotherapy associated insomnia in breast cancer patients: A pilot randomized controlled trial. Integrative Cancer Therapies. 2021;**20**:1-11

[214] Mercane B, Ginatempo F, Manca A, et al. Anatomo-physiologic basis for auricular stimulation. Acupunture in Medicine. 2018;**30**:141-150

[215] Alimi D, Chelly JE. New universal nomenclature in auriculotherapy. Journal of Alternative and Complementary Medicine. 2018;**24**:7-14

Chapter 2

The Metabolic Evaluation of the Patient with a Developmental Disorder

Arzu Selamioglu

Abstract

Metabolic evaluation plays a critical role in the diagnosis and management of patients with developmental disorders. This process involves a thorough assessment of the patient's medical history, physical examination, and a series of specialized laboratory tests. Key tests typically include blood and urine analyses to measure amino acids, organic acids, and other metabolic markers, alongside genetic testing to identify mutations linked to metabolic disorders. This chapter provides an in-depth examination of the metabolic evaluation process, detailing the tools used and the interpretation of the resulting metabolic profiles. Additionally, it explores the metabolic diseases most commonly associated with developmental disorders and emphasizes the importance of early detection. Identifying metabolic abnormalities early can lead to targeted interventions, such as dietary modifications, enzyme replacement therapies, and other medical treatments, which significantly improve clinical outcomes. In patients with developmental disorders, timely and accurate metabolic evaluation not only aids in diagnosis but also facilitates personalized treatment plans, ultimately improving quality of life and long-term prognosis.

Keywords: inborn metabolic disorder, developmental delay, intellectual disability, autism spectrum disorder, diagnostic evaluation, metabolic screening, remove metabolic screening

1. Introduction

Developmental disorders, as categorized in the Diagnostic and Statistical Manual of Mental Disorders, 5th Edition (DSM-5), encompass a wide range of neurodevelopmental conditions. These include intellectual disability (ID), global developmental delay (GDD), communication disorders (such as language disorder, speech sound disorder, childhood-onset fluency disorder, and social/pragmatic communication disorder), autism spectrum disorder (ASD), attention deficit/hyperactivity disorder (ADHD), specific learning disorders (including difficulties in reading, written expression, and mathematics), and motor disorders (such as developmental coordination disorder, stereotypic movement disorder, and tic disorders) [1].

Inborn metabolic disorders (IMDs) are caused by genetic defects in enzymes or carrier proteins involved in the synthesis or breakdown of proteins, carbohydrates, or fatty acids. While each inherited metabolic disorder is rare individually, their collective incidence ranges from 1:800 to 1:2500, showing significant phenotypical and genetic heterogeneity [2]. The latest classifications list nearly 1500 IMDs across 124 categories, with new conditions regularly being discovered [3].

Developmental delay is a key symptom of various IEMs that manifest at an early age. Routine metabolic testing in children with GDD has shown a diagnosis rate of 0.8–2.5% for IEMs. However, a detailed metabolic reassessment has identified the causative IEM in up to 14% of patients previously classified as having GDD of unknown origin [4]. Understanding the general characteristics of developmental delays due to IEMs is crucial for accurate identification and appropriate follow-up through metabolic evaluations.

Firstly, developmental delays caused by IEMs are often global, meaning they affect all areas of development to some extent. Behavioral issues such as severe irritability, impulsivity, aggression, and hyperactivity are common, with typical examples seen in disorders like Krabbe disease (globoid cell leukodystrophy), Sanfilippo disease (mucopolysaccharidosis (MPS) type III), and Hunter disease (MPS type II). Motor automatisms and stereotypic behaviors are also frequently observed. Self-harm, such as compulsive thumb or finger chewing, which can lead to severe injuries, is a hallmark symptom of Lesch-Nyhan syndrome in boys. Secondly, developmental delays in children with IEMs are generally progressive. These children may initially experience a normal developmental period, followed by a gradual regression of milestones. While this progression may be subtle at first, it eventually becomes more noticeable as the gap between children with GDD and their healthy peers widens over time. Thirdly, delayed development is often accompanied by other neurological dysfunctions such as abnormal muscle tone, sensory deficits, seizures, pyramidal tract signs, and extrapyramidal or cranial nerve impairments [4].

IMDs have been identified in patients previously misdiagnosed with intellectual developmental disorders (IDD), ASD, or ADHD of unknown etiology. Early diagnosis of IMDs is crucial, as many of these disorders are progressive, deteriorating, and often treatable. Timely identification in newborns allows for prompt interventions, which can significantly reduce morbidity, mortality, and disability [5]. Metabolic diseases can be the underlying cause of developmental disorders, and evaluating these disorders from a metabolic perspective creates opportunities for treatment that could vastly improve patient outcomes. Developmental disorders often have complex neurodevelopmental, biochemical, and genetic components. Thorough metabolic evaluations not only help ensure accurate diagnosis but also expand treatment options and improve the quality of life for affected individuals.

2. Key considerations in patient history for metabolic disease

In view of the non-specific presentation of many IMDs, it is necessary to search for metabolic clues to initiate specific IMD investigations. As with all disorders, the basis of diagnosis relies on a good history and careful examination with subsequent investigations [6]. A comprehensive medical history, including a three-generation family tree and examination, is necessary prior to considering any investigations. Hereditary factors can potentially be inferred from the family history, especially if there are patterns of recurrent miscarriages, stillbirths, or deaths during infancy or childhood.

Additionally, if other children in the family show signs of developmental delays or learning disabilities, particularly among first- and second-degree relatives, this may further suggest a genetic component. In males with GDD or learning difficulties, special attention should be given to maternal male relatives with similar challenges, as this could indicate an X-linked genetic cause. Ethnic background is also important, as certain rare recessive disorders tend to occur more frequently in endogamous populations, such as the Irish Traveler or Roma communities. For example, the Irish Traveler population exhibits a higher prevalence of conditions like galactosemia, MPS type I, I-cell disease, glutaric aciduria type I, and Cohen syndrome, all of which are associated with developmental delays or learning difficulties, sometimes with only subtle clinical signs [7].

It is important to diagnose IMDs because there are many effective treatments, and early diagnosis greatly enhances the chance of a better outcome. These molecules are key to cell-cell signaling and embryogenesis, and therefore, they are present in the neonatal period with dysmorphic features. Such conditions include the peroxisomal disorders—for example, Zellweger syndrome and the congenital disorders of glycosylation (CDG). The failure to break down complex molecules results in their accumulation, which presents with dysmorphic features. These are not obvious at birth, with a few exceptions such as I-cell disease, although rarely, storage disorders can present as hydrops fetalis.

Further clues may be gained from the obstetric history. Previous multiple spontaneous abortions may indicate previously affected fetuses that were non-viable. Hyperemesis is associated with fat oxidation disorders, as are frank hepatic symptoms such as acute fatty liver of pregnancy and the more severe HELLP syndrome (hemolysis, elevated liver enzymes, and low platelets).

Children may also unknowingly avoid certain foods as they feel unwell and therefore self-treat to some degree. Classic examples include low-protein intake in children with urea cycle defects and the avoidance of sweets, resulting in perfect dentition in hereditary fructose intolerance. IMDs have an associated impact on development. This impact may be minor, so direct inquiry into all areas of development is important. It is also crucial to remember that IMDs can present at any age and are not restricted to neonates and young infants [6].

Seizures in IMDs, often myoclonic or partial complex, are frequently resistant to anticonvulsant therapy. Movement disorders such as dystonia and chorea may be associated with inherited metabolic diseases. Diseases affecting the white matter may present as changes in muscle tone, either hypotonia or hypertonia, and may manifest as delays or loss of motor functions. Examples of such diseases include leukodystrophies such as Canavan disease and Alexander disease, as well as certain lysosomal disorders. Some inherited metabolic diseases can cause neuronal migration defects. Peroxisomal disorders and CDG are part of this group. Stroke is an unusual condition in children and should raise suspicion of homocystinuria and MELAS (mitochondrial encephalopathy, lactic acidosis, and stroke-like episodes). Fabry disease and some CDG are also associated with stroke [8].

A detailed patient history can also reveal cases where neonatal metabolic screening was insufficient. This is particularly relevant for individuals born before newborn screening programs were established or for immigrants from countries with inadequate screening protocols. Disorders like phenylketonuria, homocystinuria, galactosemia, congenital hypothyroidism, and mild forms of maple syrup urine disease can cause GDD or ID, sometimes without obvious symptoms. These conditions should be considered in patients fitting the aforementioned scenarios, especially since treatments are available. Early detection of these conditions can significantly improve patient outcomes, making thorough assessment critical. Additionally, it is important to note that around 20% of homocystinuria cases may go undetected by standard newborn screenings conducted on days 3–4 due to insufficient protein exposure [7].

3. Key considerations in physical examination

A comprehensive examination of all systems, along with a current developmental, functional, or cognitive skills assessment, should be performed. This includes noting any abnormal growth measurements, dysmorphic features, or congenital abnormalities that might suggest a syndromic etiology. Neurocutaneous markers may indicate phakomatoses such as neurofibromatosis type 1, tuberous sclerosis, or Sturge–Weber syndrome. Subtle signs of spinal dysraphism are often associated with developmental abnormalities. Additionally, hepatosplenomegaly or cardiomyopathy may suggest an IMD [7].

The physical examination should assess for possible dysmorphology, hepatosplenomegaly, and cutaneous markers of neurocutaneous syndromes, as well as the presence of dermal sinuses, hair tufts, or other subtle signs of spinal dysraphism in the sacral region. Furthermore, height, weight, and head circumference should be measured. In patients with developmental disorders, measuring head circumference is crucial for assessing possible underlying conditions such as microcephaly. A notable genetic factor associated with microcephaly is the loss of function in the SMPD4 gene, which has been linked to a specific developmental disorder. This disorder is characterized by microcephaly, arthrogryposis, and other congenital abnormalities, often accompanied by a simplified gyral pattern in the brain, cerebellar hypoplasia, and hypomyelination. SMPD4 regulates critical cellular pathways involving sphingolipids, which impact cell proliferation and differentiation. Loss of function in this gene disrupts these processes, leading to severe developmental outcomes [9].

Additional signs and symptoms can help identify the causes of GDD. Most IMDs do not have specific features easily identifiable through examination and present with generalized symptoms secondary to metabolic decompensation. Classical dysmorphic syndromes resulting from defects in embryogenesis include peroxisomal disorders such as Zellweger syndrome (large fontanelle, bulbous forehead, profound hypotonia, ptosis, and jaundice), CDG (e.g., inverted nipples, fat pads, cerebellar dysgenesis, pericardial and pleural effusions, and ascites), and sterol synthesis defects (Smith-Lemli-Opitz syndrome—upturned nose, prominent forehead, syndactyly of the second and third toes, hypotonia, and genital anomalies). Storage disorders that develop coarse features and hepatosplenomegaly include the MPSs, such as Hurler and Hunter syndromes.

Ophthalmic examination is critical because many disorders exhibit ocular signs. Oil-drop cataracts are present at birth in most infants with galactosemia, which can be easily missed as only the edge of the cataract is visible due to their transparency. If untreated, these cataracts will mature, but early treatment usually results in complete resolution. In sphingolipidoses, a cherry red spot develops due to abnormal lipid deposition around the fovea. The contrast between the pale lipid deposits and the red fovea creates this characteristic appearance. Pigmentary retinopathy is seen in many IMDs, including mitochondrial cytopathies, fatty acid oxidation defects, and peroxisomal disorders. Eye movements may also be abnormal, including external ophthalmoplegia in mitochondrial cytopathies, leading to reduced eye movement in all planes of gaze. Limitation of downward gaze is a feature of Gaucher disease, particularly noticeable when descending stairs, leading to unsteadiness and compensatory head-thrusting. In the late-infantile/juvenile forms of Niemann-Pick type C, vertical supranuclear gaze palsy may also be an early sign. Ptosis is found in many conditions, including peroxisomal and mitochondrial disorders [6].

Cardiac manifestations in IMDs include cardiomyopathy and arrhythmias. Arrhythmias may be episodic, as seen in fatty acid oxidation defects, or persistent, such as heart block in Kearns-Sayre syndrome, a mitochondrial disorder. Cardiomyopathy may present with signs of heart failure, including excessive sweating and shortness of breath while feeding. Patients typically present with chest symptoms, and an x-ray revealing cardiomegaly indicates cardiomyopathy. Both dilated and hypertrophic cardiomyopathies are seen in IMDs, and it is essential to recognize that dilated cardiomyopathy may have originated as hypertrophic. Thus, it is prudent to investigate both causes of hypertrophic and dilated cardiomyopathies. Myopathy is commonly associated with IMDs, such as infantile Pompe disease (glycogen storage disease type II (GSDII)), characterized by marked hypertrophic cardiomyopathy, hypotonia, myopathic facies, and a prominent tongue. However, sick children with cardiomyopathy tend to be hypotonic, making the distinction less obvious. The presence or absence of organomegaly may provide clues when considering an IMD. It is important to remember that glycogen is stored in the liver, muscles, and kidneys. A child presenting with marked hepatomegaly in the absence of splenomegaly should raise suspicion of a GSD. Splenomegaly can occur in GSDs, particularly type IV, secondary to liver disease. Massive hepatomegaly and splenomegaly are suggestive of a storage disorder, such as the MPSs. Splenomegaly greater than hepatomegaly is seen in storage disorders, particularly Gaucher disease. Neurological features of IMDs are extremely varied, but it should be remembered that a sick neonate usually presents with hypotonia, so normal or increased tone may indicate an IMD. Odors are also often reported as helpful in diagnosing an IMD [6].

4. Diagnostic evaluation of patients with developmental disorders for inborn metabolic diseases

4.1 Biochemical and metabolic analyses

For the first tier non-targeted screening, a range of blood and urine tests are recommended. Blood tests include ammonia, lactate, plasma amino acids, total homocysteine, acylcarnitine profile, copper, folate, and ceruloplasmin. Urine tests should assess organic acids, purines and pyrimidines, creatine metabolites, oligosaccharides, and glycosaminoglycans (GAGs). These tests provide a comprehensive screening approach to identify potential metabolic abnormalities. After conducting a clinical assessment, the use of appropriate diagnostic laboratory tests, brain imaging, and other evidence-based evaluations is essential for establishing a diagnosis and creating a care plan. Furthermore, there is an increased focus on identifying "treatable" causes of GDD, recommending metabolic screening for IEM in children with GDD of unknown origin. For the second tier targeted testing, the following biochemical and molecular analyses should be considered: whole blood manganese levels, plasma cholesterol, the plasma 7-dehydroxy-cholesterol to cholesterol ratio, plasma pipecolic acid and urine amino adipic semialdehyde, plasma very long-chain fatty acids, plasma vitamin B12 and folate, and the serum and cerebrospinal fluid (CSF) lactate to pyruvate ratio. Enzyme activities in leukocytes, including arylsulfatase A, biotidinase, glucocerebrosidase, and fatty aldehyde dehydrogenase, should also be evaluated. Additional tests include urine deoxypyridinoline, CSF amino acids, CSF neurotransmitters, and the CSF to plasma glucose ratio. Coenzyme Q measurement in fibroblasts is recommended, along with molecular analyses for specific genes such as CA5A, NPC1, NPC2, SC4MOL, SLC18A2, SLC19A3, SLC30A10, SLC52A2, SLC52A3, PDHA1, DLAT, PDHX, SPR, and TH. These tests provide more targeted insights into potential metabolic and genetic disorders. Certain tests, such as plasma homocysteine, ammonia, and acylcarnitine profiling, were not included in first-line investigations. These tests should only be performed in specific clinical scenarios, such as elevated plasma methionine or in cases with suspected fatty acid oxidation disorders (FAODs). Plasma ammonia analysis is not recommended as a first-line test due to the risk of false positives. Plasma acylcarnitine profiling should be considered for cases with hypoglycemia, hypotonia, or cardiomyopathy, as it helps identify disorders related to energy metabolism [7].

Folate plays a crucial role in several metabolic processes, including nucleotide synthesis, amino acid metabolism, and methylation reactions, which are essential for normal brain development. Disruptions in folate transport or metabolism, such as genetic abnormalities or the presence of autoantibodies to folate receptor alpha (FRα), can impair these processes, leading to developmental disorders. Folate deficiency during pregnancy has been associated with an increased risk of neural tube defects and other neurodevelopmental disorders, including autism. Furthermore, conditions like cerebral folate deficiency syndrome, characterized by low levels of 5-methyltetrahydrofolate (5-MTHF) in cerebrospinal fluid, have been linked to severe neurological symptoms in children. Supplementation with folinic acid has been shown to reverse or alleviate symptoms in many cases, particularly in individuals with autoantibodies to FRα [10].

Key metabolic tests include qualitative urinary organic acids (UOA), which are diagnostic for organic acidurias and certain other disorders. Plasma amino acids (AA), collected pre-prandial, are critical for diagnosing aminoacidopathies and helpful in identifying mitochondrial and urea cycle defects. Plasma lactate, which must be collected under specific conditions for accuracy, can indicate mitochondrial disorders, organic acidemias, and FAODs. Venous blood gas with an anion gap calculation may reveal metabolic acidosis or lactic acidosis, while plasma creatine phosphokinase levels may be elevated in muscular dystrophies, mitochondrial diseases, and FAODs. Plasma glucose levels are also informative, as low levels can indicate FAODs or organic acidemias, and post-prandial elevations may suggest glycogen synthase deficiency. A full blood count and blood film can reveal abnormalities like macrocytic or normocytic anemia, neutropenia, or thrombocytopenia, often linked to metabolic conditions. Plasma liver function tests can help diagnose disorders like tyrosinemia, UCDs, or mitochondrial diseases, while plasma urea and electrolytes provide insights into renal tubular dysfunction. Plasma bone profiles assess phosphate resorption, which may be reduced in mitochondrial or renal tubular disorders. Thyroid function tests can detect hypothyroidism, which can contribute to GDD or LD. Paired plasma and urine urate/creatinine ratios can indicate defects in purine metabolism or kidney function, while total urine GAGs screen for MPS [11].

To facilitate the diagnosis of treatable conditions, several specialized tests should be performed depending on the suspected disorder. For CDG, serum transferrin or N-glycan profiling is indicated. Disorders of amino acid metabolism require plasma amino acids, plasma ammonia, and plasma acylcarnitine testing. Plasma total homocysteine levels are essential for diagnosing methionine synthase deficiency (homocystinuria with megaloblastic anemia). For glycine encephalopathy due to aminomethyltransferase or glycine decarboxylase deficiency (nonketotic hyperglycinemia), CSF and plasma amino acids should be evaluated. GLUT1 deficiency can be detected using the CSF to blood glucose ratio. Urine oligosaccharides and GAGs testing help diagnose disorders of complex molecule degradation, while plasma (oxy-)sterols screening is important for Niemann-Pick disease types C1 and C2. For pyruvate dehydrogenase complex deficiencies, both CSF and blood lactate ratios are critical. Plasma very long chain fatty acids should be measured for X-linked adrenoleukodystrophy and plasma cholestanol for diagnosing cerebrotendinous xanthomatosis. Urine purines and pyrimidines testing is required for disorders of nucleobase, nucleotide, and nucleic acid metabolism, and copper and ceruloplasmin levels are vital for identifying hereditary ceruloplasmin deficiency, Menkes disease, and Wilson disease. Disorders of trace elements and metals necessitate testing of serum zinc, sialotransferrins, manganese, and CSF lactate, while CSF neurotransmitter analysis is essential for neurotransmitter disorders and disorders of vitamin and cofactor metabolism [11].

4.2 Genetic analyses

The comprehensive care for individuals with neurodevelopmental disorders primarily involves the pursuit of an underlying etiological diagnosis, typically through genetic evaluation, alongside appropriate diagnostic explanations and referrals to evidence-based treatments and supports for families. Identifying a genetic etiology can provide insight into prognosis, clarify recurrence risk, guide clinical management, and connect patients and families to condition-specific resources and support. Given the diagnostic yield and potential clinical and personal benefits of genetic testing, there is a consensus that all individuals with GDD, ID, and/or autism spectrum disorder should undergo genetic testing. Despite this recommendation, data suggest that only a small proportion of children with ASD and ID receive genetic testing. Genetic testing has become the standard practice for diagnosing various neurodevelopmental disorders, and it is highly likely that the criteria for testing will expand in the near future. Clinically, a genetic etiology might be suspected and verified through gene-specific testing or, more frequently, through chromosomal microarray (CMA) analysis, exome sequencing (ES), or FMR1 CGG repeat analysis for Fragile X syndrome. These tests are typically conducted as a routine part of the assessment for patients with ID, GDD, or ASD, particularly in cases where no clinically recognizable syndrome is present. Genome-wide chromosomal microarray (CMA) is recommended as a first-line test for patients with ASD, ID, GDD, and/or multiple congenital anomalies. CMA detects copy number variants (CNVs), which are gains or losses of chromosomal material. In certain cases, these gains or losses can affect gene function, potentially impacting health and development. Additionally, CMA can identify regions of homozygosity, which may aid in the detection of genetic conditions caused by uniparental disomy, such as Silver–Russell syndrome or Angelman syndrome. While CMA can detect CNVs, it has limited capability in identifying balanced chromosomal rearrangements (e.g., translocations, inversions), mitochondrial genome imbalances, epigenetic abnormalities, or low-level mosaicism. CMA detects copy number variants (CNVs) with a diagnostic yield ranging between 15 and 20%. Exome sequencing (ES), on the other hand, examines the protein-coding regions of the genome to identify genetic variants, with a diagnostic yield of 31–36%. ES is particularly effective in diagnosing patients with ID, GDD, and ASD. In contrast, gene panel testing is more targeted and can detect genetic variants such as mosaicism with greater depth, but it lacks the broad scope of ES. Additionally, ES offers the advantage of reanalysis over time, allowing for an increase in diagnostic yield as new genetic information emerges. Fragile X syndrome, caused by the loss of function of the FMR1 gene, is considered one of the most common inherited genetic causes associated with ID and ASD. Approximately 99% of Fragile X syndrome cases result from the expansion of the unstable CGG repeat sequence in the 5′ untranslated region (UTR) of the FMR1 gene. In the general population, individuals typically have 44 or fewer CGG repeats, while more than 200 repeats lead to methylation and transcriptional silencing of the gene. Since the FMR1 gene is located on the X chromosome, mutations can result in variable phenotypes in males and females. FMR1 CGG repeat analysis is commonly performed using PCR and Southern Blot techniques and yields four main categories of results: normal (≤44 repeats), intermediate (45–54 repeats), pre-mutation (55–200 repeats), and full mutation (>200 repeats) [1].

The diagnostic yield of Fragile X testing varies depending on study design and the characteristics of the population being tested. In individuals with ID, the diagnostic yield ranges between 0.5 and 6%, whereas in ASD populations, this rate is generally lower, ranging between 0.23 and 1.2%.

These include chromosome microarray, Fragile X (FMR1 gene) testing, Rett syndrome testing, brain MRI/spectroscopy, electroencephalography and other neurophysiological tests, and thyroid function assessments. Additionally, comprehensive audiological and ophthalmological screening should be conducted to rule out any treatable primary sensory deficits in all patients presenting with IDD [1].

For many years, biochemical screening has been recommended as a first-line etiological investigation for individuals with GDD or ID. However, in cases of isolated ID, the diagnostic yield of initial biochemical screening is very low, around 1%, rising to 5% when specific neurological features are present. ES has now emerged as one of the most cost-effective and powerful diagnostic tools for ID, with an average diagnostic yield of 36%. It has significantly enhanced the identification of unspecific or atypical phenotypes and led to the discovery of hundreds of previously unknown genes [12].

It is important for clinicians providing care to children and adolescents with neurodevelopmental disorders to understand these common tests and their role in delivering the best medical care and to facilitate the genetic etiologic evaluation of these patients by ordering tests or collaborating with genetic specialists.

5. Multisystem evaluation in developmental disorders

The age of onset and clinical progression provide key insights into the metabolic nature of the disease, with multisystem involvement being common. Organs such as the liver, spleen, muscles, bones, skin, and connective tissues are frequently affected. A comprehensive initial evaluation for children with undifferentiated developmental delay should include a thorough developmental assessment, neurological examination, brain imaging, electrophysiological studies (such as auditory brainstem responses, visual and somatosensory evoked potentials, nerve conduction studies, and electromyogram), and radiographs of the hands, chest, and spine to check for dysostosis multiplex. Additionally, a range of metabolic tests including plasma and urinary amino acid analysis, urinary organic acid analysis (even in the absence of metabolic acidosis), plasma ammonia levels (preferably 2 hours after a protein meal), plasma lactate, urinary MPS screening, and urinary oligosaccharide screening should be conducted. This evaluation helps in detecting early-stage, treatable IEMs and establishes a baseline for monitoring the disease's natural progression [4].

In patients with developmental disorders, metabolic diseases should be strongly suspected when findings such as ID, epilepsy, coma episodes, specific lesions on MRI, hearing defects, fundoscopic abnormalities, or signs of cerebral ischemia are present. Additionally, if the patient presents with symptoms such as splenomegaly, skeletal anomalies, muscle involvement, elevated transaminases, hepatomegaly, liver diseases like cirrhosis, dilated/hypertrophic cardiomyopathy, heart failure, arrhythmias, or hematological disorders (such as cytopenias, vacuoles on peripheral smear, hemolysis, bone marrow abnormalities, or thrombosis), they should be further evaluated for potential metabolic diseases [8].

6. Inborn metabolic diseases associated with developmental disorders

Disorders of amino acid metabolism, such as phenylketonuria, homocystinurias, and maple syrup urine disease, typically present after birth with white matter changes in the brain. These conditions may resemble behavioral disorders like ADHD or ASD, and neuropsychiatric symptoms such as anxiety and depression are also common. While dietary restrictions help stabilize many patients, the long-term outcomes, particularly in older individuals, are not well documented.

Organic acidurias, such as propionic acidemia and methylmalonic acidemia, are often associated with abnormalities in the basal ganglia and white matter lesions. These disorders may resemble cerebral palsy or other motor disorders. Despite strict management, patients may continue to experience ADHD, learning disabilities, and optic atrophy, and exacerbations can lead to motor delays during adolescence.

Neurodegenerative diseases such as glutaric aciduria types 1, 2 and Canavan disease are marked by severe postnatal brain abnormalities, including cerebellar atrophy and cortical damage. These disorders often cause early developmental regression, spasticity, seizures, and premature death.

Metal accumulation disorders, such as Wilson disease (copper) and neurodegeneration with brain iron accumulation (NBIA), lead to progressive neurodegeneration. Wilson disease can cause motor dysfunction, tremors, and psychiatric symptoms if untreated. NBIA disorders are similarly severe, progressing to motor dysfunction and cognitive decline despite treatment efforts.

Inborn errors of amino acid transport, such as those affecting the large neutral amino acid transporter or glutamine synthetase, result in significant neurological outcomes. These conditions may involve hypomyelination, cerebral atrophy, and congenital microcephaly. They frequently present with ID or ASD-like features, and while treatment can provide stability, the long-term outlook remains uncertain.

Neurotransmitter metabolism defects, such as those affecting monoamine synthesis, typically manifest early in life with dystonia, seizures, and developmental delays. These conditions can mimic Parkinsonism or cerebral palsy. Treatments, such as L-Dopa, may stabilize the disease, though severe forms may not be compatible with life.

Metabolic epilepsy syndromes, such as SSADH deficiency, present with seizures, ataxia, and ASD-like features. While treatments can help manage seizures, the progression of neurological impairment continues, and mortality rates remain high in severe cases.

Disorders of glycine and lipoate metabolism, including nonketotic hyperglycinemia, result in profound neurological symptoms such as neonatal encephalopathy, epilepsy, and severe ID. While milder forms of these diseases may lead to moderate ID, severe forms often result in early death.

Disorders that affect GABA, glutamate, and glycine receptor function, such as mutations in SLC25A12 or NMDA receptor defects, cause a range of neurological and psychiatric symptoms, including epilepsy, ID, and behavioral issues like ADHD. While treatments such as clonazepam can alleviate some symptoms, severe mutations can result in fatal outcomes.

Copper and manganese deficiency disorders lead to severe early encephalopathies. For instance, Menkes disease, resulting from copper deficiency, leads to seizures and developmental delays, often resulting in early death without treatment. In contrast, manganese deficiency causes cerebellar atrophy and profound ID, though treatment may stabilize the condition [13].

Fatty acid metabolism disorders, such as DHA transporter defects, present with microcephaly, developmental delays, and spasticity. These conditions are often fatal without intervention. Similarly, vitamin and cofactor deficiencies, such as biotinidase or B12 deficiencies, can result in seizures and developmental delays, though these conditions are often treatable with appropriate supplementation [14].

Defects in phospholipid metabolism, such as those caused by mutations in PLA2G6, result in neurodegeneration, dystonia-parkinsonism, cognitive decline, and psychiatric symptoms. While treatments may stabilize some symptoms, neurodegeneration often progresses, and long-term outcomes are poor.

CDG significantly interfere with brain development, particularly in fetal life. These disorders often present with cerebellar involvement and structural abnormalities. CDG should be considered in any case of unexplained multi-organ involvement and neurological symptoms, as early intervention can be life-saving in some forms of the disease [13].

Mitochondrial disorders, such as those caused by SLC25A19 mutations, result in severe neurodevelopmental abnormalities, including microcephaly and basal ganglia necrosis. While some forms can be treated with thiamine supplementation, severe cases are often fatal [15].

GAG and oligosaccharide catabolism disorders, such as Sanfilippo disease (MPS type III), which lead to progressive cortical and subcortical atrophy with symptoms like behavioral problems and cognitive decline. Sialidosis and mucolipidosis cause myoclonic epilepsy, developmental delays, and progressive blindness. These disorders typically show no antenatal abnormalities but progress after birth, with neurodegeneration leading to death.

Complex molecule synthesis defects related to phospholipid metabolism, such as choline kinase deficiency, SERAC1, and ABHD12, result in a range of neurodevelopmental issues, including ID, ASD-like symptoms, spasticity, and dystonia. Most of these disorders mimic neurodevelopmental conditions early on but later progress into neurodegenerative diseases, with few effective treatments available.

Disorders involving phospholipid inositides (PI3K/AKT) regulate cell growth and brain development. Mutations in genes like PLA2G6 result in neurodegeneration due to iron accumulation in the brain, leading to symptoms like dystonia-parkinsonism, cognitive decline, and psychiatric disorders. Another example is PNPLA6, which causes cerebellar atrophy and is associated with several neurodegenerative disorders, including hereditary spastic paraplegia and Gordon-Holmes syndrome. These disorders lead to progressive neurological decline, with varying severity and outcomes based on the specific mutation.

Sphingolipid metabolism defects, such as CERS1 and FAHN, primarily result in late-onset neurodevelopmental disorders and neurodegeneration. These disorders typically present in childhood with symptoms like progressive myoclonic epilepsy, cognitive decline, and spastic paraplegia. GM3 synthase deficiency presents with early symptoms resembling Rett syndrome, such as profound developmental regression and stagnation, and typically evolves into a neurodegenerative disorder.

AKT3, PIK3R2, and PIK3CA mutations, which cause congenital macrocephaly and overgrowth disorders. These conditions result in abnormally enlarged brain size and ID, but their progression tends to be more stable, behaving similarly to neurodevelopmental (NDEV) disorders rather than progressive neurodegeneration.

SNAP29 (CEDNIK syndrome), a neurocutaneous syndrome characterized by cerebral dysgenesis, early severe ID, microcephaly, ichthyosis, and keratoderma. Patients show cortical dysplasia and polymicrogyria. Although the long-term outcomes are uncertain, the condition is generally considered stable. Disorders involving SNARE proteins such as NAPB, STXBP1, and others, present with microcephaly, hypomyelination, and cerebellar atrophy. These disorders frequently result in early-onset epileptic encephalopathy, ID, neuropsychiatric signs, and movement disorders. They are classified as neurodevelopmental disorders, but long-term data on their progression are limited.

SV protein dysfunctions also impact endocytosis and trafficking, as shown by disorders like Rabenosyn-5 deficiency, which leads to complex phenotypes, including early infantile spasms, epilepsy, ID, and vitamin B12 deficiency with methylmalonic acidemia accumulation. These conditions can lead to stability with appropriate management. VPS15 deficiency causes severe cortical and optic nerve atrophy, spasticity, pseudobulbar palsy, hearing deficits, and late-onset epilepsy, but stability may be achieved with treatment.

Autophagy disorders, such as AP-5 (SPG48) and EPG5 (Vici syndrome), prominently affect the central nervous system. SPG48 causes hereditary spastic paraplegia with ID and white matter lesions, initially presenting as a neurodevelopmental disorder but later evolving into a neurodegenerative disease. Vici syndrome is a multisystem disorder with progressive postnatal microcephaly, profound developmental delay, motor impairment, nystagmus, and sensorineural deafness, often leading to neurodegeneration.

WDR45 (BPAN: SENDA syndrome) can present with neurodegeneration with brain iron accumulation (NBIA) features, including ID, seizures, spastic paraplegia, and Rett-like symptoms. In adolescence, these patients may experience a progression to parkinsonism, dystonia, and optic atrophy, evolving from neurodevelopmental disorders to neurodegeneration.

SNX14 is another disorder listed, associated with cerebellar atrophy, GDD, ASD, hypotonia, absent speech, and progressive cerebellar atrophy. Patients often present with progressive neurological symptoms, including ataxia, seizures, and a storage disease phenotype.

The section on tRNA synthetases describes how mutations in mitochondrial tRNA (mt-tRNA) synthetases lead to severe neurological diseases that typically evolve toward neurodegeneration. These disorders involve white matter, cerebellar, and brain stem abnormalities. For example, RARS2 (mt arginyl-tRNA synthetase) presents with perinatal encephalopathy, lethargy, hypotonia, epilepsy, and microcephaly. Similarly, DARS2 (mt aspartyl-tRNA synthetase) causes childhood to adulthood-onset leukencephalopathy, cerebellar ataxia, and spinal cord dysfunction, often with elevated lactate levels. TARS2 (mt threonyl-tRNA synthetase) leads to early psychomotor delay and hypotonia, while VARS2 (mt valyl-tRNA synthetase) causes developmental delay, seizures, facial dysmorphism, and lactic acidosis in childhood.

Sytoplasmic tRNA synthetase disorders result in severe neurological phenotypes, including hypomyelination, microcephaly, seizures, sensorineural hearing loss, and developmental delay. These disorders, in addition to neurological symptoms, can also involve liver dysfunction and lung disease. Mutations in five ARS genes have been implicated in dominant Charcot-Marie-Tooth (CMT) disease and related neuropathies. Specific tRNA synthetases mentioned include glycyl (GARS), tyrosyl (YARS), alanyl (AARS), histidyl (HARS), and tryptophanyl (WARS), with disease mechanisms often involving defects in peripheral nerve axons [13].

In patients with ADHD, certain IMDs should be considered, including X-linked adrenoleukodystrophy, phenylketonuria, metachromatic leukodystrophy, Niemann–Pick disease type C, 4-hydroxybutyric aciduria, Sanfilippo A and B syndromes, beta-mannosidosis, and atypical nonketotic hyperglycinemia. For patients presenting with mania or bipolar disorder, metabolic conditions like ornithine transcarbamylase deficiency, acute intermittent porphyria, and Wilson disease should be considered. Additionally, in patients exhibiting psychosis, possible metabolic conditions to consider include metachromatic leukodystrophy, Niemann-Pick type C, Wilson disease, occipital horn syndrome, Hartnup disease, and methylenetetrahydrofolate reductase deficiency [8].

7. Treatment options

After a diagnosis of an inborn metabolic disease, the patient should be evaluated for specific treatment options. Early and accurate diagnosis through metabolic and genetic testing is critical to effective intervention. The treatment landscape for IEM spans various approaches, including dietary management, cofactor supplementation, enzyme replacement, stem cell transplantation, and emerging gene therapies. By 2011, 81 treatable IEMs were identified as causes of ID, with more recent discoveries such as dihydrofolate reductase deficiency and hypermanganesemia now treatable with interventions like folinic acid and chelation therapy [8]. Currently, 89 treatable IEMs are recognized, covering a broad spectrum of metabolic categories, including amino acid and organic acid metabolism, mitochondrial disorders, lysosomal storage diseases, urea cycle disorders, and vitamin/cofactor-related conditions [11].

Mitochondrial and metabolic disorders are increasingly understood to contribute to neurodevelopmental disorders like ASD, ADHD, GDD, and ID. As the "powerhouses" of cells, mitochondria play a crucial role in brain development and function. When mitochondrial dysfunction occurs, it can lead to reduced energy production, increased oxidative stress, and neuroinflammation, negatively affecting cognitive and motor abilities.

Research also indicates that abnormalities in fatty acid metabolism may play a role in conditions like ADHD, dyslexia, dyspraxia, and ASD. Essential fatty acids, such as omega-3 and omega-6, are vital for brain development, and disruptions in their metabolism can lead to cognitive and behavioral challenges. Studies show that individuals with these conditions often have lower levels of highly unsaturated fatty acids and elevated enzyme activity, such as phospholipase A2. Early detection of fatty acid imbalances, coupled with targeted supplementation, may help mitigate these symptoms. For example, NAXD deficiency leads to severe neurodevelopmental issues such as neurological regression, cardiomyopathy, seizures, and skin lesions, which

DOI: http://dx.doi.org/10.5772/intechopen.1008936

worsen during periods of illness. While treatments like vitamin B3 supplementation show promise, further research is needed to confirm their efficacy.

Defects in fatty acid oxidation and amino acid metabolism disrupt cellular energy balance, resulting in developmental regression, motor impairments, and cognitive deficits. Early detection enables timely intervention, slowing disease progression, and improving long-term neurological outcomes. Patients with neurodevelopmental disorders, particularly those with suspected metabolic origins, should undergo thorough metabolic assessments. Tailored mitochondrial therapies could greatly enhance the quality of life for affected individuals.

8. Conclusion

The metabolic evaluation of patients with developmental disorders is an essential process for identifying underlying inborn errors of metabolism (IEM) that could contribute to neurodevelopmental delays and dysfunctions. Early and precise diagnosis of these metabolic conditions allows for the implementation of tailored interventions, including dietary modifications, enzyme replacement, and emerging therapies such as gene therapy. These treatments can significantly enhance patient outcomes, reducing the morbidity and mortality associated with many IEMs.

The body of research and clinical data supporting the integration of metabolic and genetic testing into the diagnostic process for developmental disorders provides a strong case for the inclusion of these evaluations in standard medical practice. By embracing a comprehensive, multidisciplinary approach to diagnosis and treatment, clinicians can offer more effective care, ultimately improving the quality of life and prognosis for individuals affected by metabolic diseases and related neurodevelopmental conditions.

Conflict of interest

The authors declare no conflict of interest.

Nomenclature

5-MTHF	methyltetrahydrofolate
AA	amino acids
ADHD	attention deficit/hyperactivity disorder
ASD	autism spectrum disorder
CDG	congenital disorders of glycosylation
CMA	chromosomal microarray
CNVs	copy number variants
CSF	cerebrospinal fluid
DSM-5	diagnostic and statistical manual of mental disorders, 5th edition
ES	exome sequencing
FAODs	fatty acid oxidation disorders
FRα	folate receptor alpha
GAGs	glycosaminoglycans
GDD	global developmental delay

HELLP	haemolysis, elevated liver enzymes, low platelets
ID	intellectual disability
IDD	intellectual developmental disorders
IEM	inborn errors of metabolism
IMD	inborn metabolic disease
MELAS	mitochondrial encephalopathy, lactic acidosis, and stroke-like episodes
MPS	Mucopolysaccharidoses
NBIA	brain iron accumulation
TARS2	mt threonyl-tRNA synthetase
VARS2	mt valyl-tRNA synthetase

Author details

Arzu Selamioglu
Bağcılar Training and Research Hospital, Istanbul, Turkey

*Address all correspondence to: arzuceyln@hotmail.com

References

[1] Savatt JM, Myers SM. Genetic testing in neurodevelopmental disorders. Frontiers in Pediatrics. 2021;**9**:526779

[2] Senarathne UD, Indika NLR, Jezela-Stanek A, Ciara E, Frye RE, Chen C, et al. Biochemical, genetic and clinical diagnostic approaches to autism-associated inherited metabolic disorders. Genes. 2023;**14**(4):803

[3] Ferreira CR, Rahman S, Keller M, Zschocke J, ICIMD Advisory Group, Abdenur J, et al. An international classification of inherited metabolic disorders (ICIMD). Journal of Inherited Metabolic Disease. 2021;**44**(1):164-177

[4] Eun SH, Hahn SH. Metabolic evaluation of children with global developmental delay. Korean Journal of Pediatrics. 2015;**58**(4):117

[5] Márquez-Caraveo ME, Ibarra-González I, Rodríguez-Valentín R, Ramírez-García MÁ, Pérez-Barrón V, Lazcano-Ponce E, et al. Brief report: Delayed diagnosis of treatable inborn errors of metabolism in children with autism and other neurodevelopmental disorders. Journal of Autism and Developmental Disorders. 2021;**51**:2124-2131

[6] Champion MP. An approach to the diagnosis of inherited metabolic disease. Archives of Disease in Childhood. Education and Practice Edition. 2010;**95**(2):40-46

[7] O'Byrne JJ, Lynch SA, Treacy EP, King MD, Betts DR, Mayne PD, et al. Unexplained developmental delay/learning disability: Guidelines for best practice protocol for first line assessment and genetic/metabolic/radiological investigations. Irish Journal of Medical Science. 2016;**185**:241-248

[8] Van Karnebeek CD, Shevell M, Zschocke J, Moeschler JB, Stockler S. The metabolic evaluation of the child with an intellectual developmental disorder: Diagnostic algorithm for identification of treatable causes and new digital resource. Molecular Genetics and Metabolism. 2014;**111**(4):428-438

[9] Magini P, Smits DJ, Vandervore L, Schot R, Columbaro M, Kasteleijn E, et al. Loss of SMPD4 causes a developmental disorder characterized by microcephaly and congenital arthrogryposis. American Journal of Human Genetics. 2019;**105**(4):689-705

[10] Desai A, Sequeira JM, Quadros EV. The metabolic basis for developmental disorders due to defective folate transport. Biochimie. 2016;**126**:31-42

[11] Hoytema van Konijnenburg EM, Wortmann SB, Koelewijn MJ, Tseng LA, Houben R, Stöckler-Ipsiroglu S, et al. Treatable inherited metabolic disorders causing intellectual disability: 2021 review and digital app. Orphanet Journal of Rare Diseases. 2021;**16**:1-35

[12] Delanne J, Bruel AL, Huet F, Moutton S, Nambot S, Grisval M, et al. The diagnostic rate of inherited metabolic disorders by exome sequencing in a cohort of 547 individuals with developmental disorders. Molecular Genetics and Metabolism Reports. 2021;**29**:100812

[13] Saudubray JM, Garcia-Cazorla A. An overview of inborn errors of metabolism affecting the brain: From neurodevelopment to neurodegenerative disorders. Dialogues in Clinical Neuroscience. 2018;**20**(4):301-325

[14] Richardson AJ, Ross MA. Fatty acid metabolism in neurodevelopmental

disorder: A new perspective on associations between attention-deficit/hyperactivity disorder, dyslexia, dyspraxia and the autistic spectrum. Prostaglandins, Leukotrienes, and Essential Fatty Acids. 2000;**63**(1-2):1-9

[15] Frye RE, Rossignol DA. Mitochondrial and metabolic abnormalities in neurodevelopmental disorders. Journal of Pediatric Biochemistry. 2012;**2**(4):177-180

Chapter 3

Independent Living for Persons with Neurodevelopmental Disorders

Simone Zorzi and Laura Berteotti

Abstract

Independent living is essential for individuals with neurodevelopmental disorders, as it directly enhances their dignity and well-being. This chapter introduces a groundbreaking redefinition of independence, moving beyond mere physical autonomy to focus on the critical aspects of decision-making, daily life management, and active community participation. It offers a novel view of independence as a continuum, where individuals with neurodevelopmental disabilities require varying degrees of support. Autonomy is achieved through a dynamic, personalized process involving self-determination, tailored assistance, and environmental adaptations, empowering individuals to live according to their unique preferences and fully engage in society. What sets this approach apart is its emphasis on independence not as a fixed end goal but as a flexible, evolving process that adapts to the strengths and needs of each individual. The chapter highlights the critical role of adaptable support systems—such as life skills education, community services, and vocational programs—as essential components for fostering greater independence. The innovative focus on person-centered planning ensures that support is customized to the individual, moving away from outdated, one-size-fits-all models. Moreover, this chapter addresses societal barriers and attitudes, particularly in employment and housing, that restrict opportunities for these individuals. It also explores the transformative potential of assistive technologies, such as communication devices and smart home systems, as powerful tools that can significantly enhance independence and overall quality of life for individuals with neurodevelopmental disorders.

Keywords: neurodevelopmental disorders, independence, assistive technology, person-centered planning, inclusion

1. Introduction

This chapter introduces a novel dimension of independence taking into consideration that independent living is a fundamental aspect of human dignity and well-being, particularly for individuals with neurodevelopmental disorders (NDDs). The concept of independent living encompasses more than just the ability to live alone; it involves the capacity to make personal choices, manage one's own life, and participate fully in the community. For NDDs—such as autism spectrum disorder (ASD), attention-deficit hyperactivity disorder (ADHD), intellectual disabilities (ID), and specific learning disorders achieving a level of independence is both a significant personal milestone and a broader societal challenge. NDDs encompass a range of conditions marked by abnormal development of the central nervous system (CNS), resulting in brain dysfunctions that emerge later in life. These disorders may be linked to neuropsychiatric issues or difficulties with motor skills, learning, language, or non-verbal communication [1]. The impact of these disorders varies widely among individuals, with some experiencing mild difficulties that require minimal support, while others face profound challenges that necessitate extensive assistance throughout their lives [2]. Despite these challenges, the desire for independence is a common goal among NDDs. Independence in this context does not necessarily mean complete autonomy, but rather the ability to live a life that is self-directed and fulfilling. This includes managing daily tasks such as cooking, cleaning, and personal hygiene, making decisions about one's own life, engaging in social relationships, and participating in the workforce. Independence is understood as a continuum where individuals achieve autonomy through a dynamic process of self-determination, personalized assistance, and environmental adjustments, which allow them to live according to their preferences and fully engage in society. This flexible and person-centered approach reflects the importance of tailoring interventions to individual strengths and goals. The need for adaptable support systems is critical, including life skills education, vocational programs, and community-based services, which help individuals achieve greater autonomy. Achieving such independence can significantly enhance the quality of life and contribute to a sense of self-worth and purpose [3]. However, the path to independent living for NDDs is often obstructed by a variety of barriers [4]. As noted by Jeste [5], cognitive ability plays a crucial role in determining the potential of individuals with ID to live independently. This is closely tied to self-determination, competence, self-esteem, and self-advocacy [6]. Cognitive impairments can make decision-making and problem-solving difficult, while social communication challenges can hinder interactions with others. Health significantly impacts the ability of individuals with ID to manage their lives with minimal support from others. However, from birth, ID face challenges, as they may encounter physical and mental health issues, including cognitive decline [7]. Behavioral issues, such as impulsivity, anxiety, or difficulty in managing stress, can further complicate daily living. Additionally, sensory processing difficulties can make routine activities, such as shopping or using public transportation, overwhelming and stressful [8]. These challenges underscore the need for comprehensive support systems designed to help NDDs achieve as much independence as possible. Over the past several decades, there has been a growing recognition of the importance of such support, leading to the development of a wide range of services and interventions. These include specialized education programs that focus on life skills training, community-based support services that provide assistance with daily living, and the use of assistive technologies that help individuals communicate, learn, and manage tasks more effectively [9]. Agarwal [10] highlighted that education plays a key role in improving the ability of individuals with ID to achieve greater freedom and employment opportunities, as it is fundamental to leading a meaningful life. This involves experiences centered on social inclusion, skill development, integrated work opportunities, and career training, all of which contribute to independent living. Academic support and training have shown significant improvements in various aspects of independence, such as enhancing self-advocacy, functional communication, self-determination, daily living skills, building confidence, and better community engagement [11]. One of the key strategies in promoting independent living is person-centered planning. This approach involves tailoring support to the individual's unique strengths, preferences, and goals. Rather than focusing solely on the limitations imposed by the disorder, person-centered planning emphasizes the individual's capabilities and potential. This approach not only empowers individuals to take control of their lives but also ensures that the support they receive is aligned with their personal aspirations and needs [12]. In addition to individualized support, the broader social context plays a crucial role in enabling independent living. Societal attitudes toward disability have evolved considerably, with an increasing emphasis on inclusion and accessibility. This shift has been reflected in policies and legislation designed to protect the rights of individuals with disabilities and to ensure their access to the same opportunities as everyone else. For example, the Americans with Disabilities Act (ADA) [13] in the United States and similar legislation in other countries have been instrumental in removing barriers and promoting equal opportunities for individuals with disabilities [14]. Policies and regulations have been recognized as key elements that can significantly influence the decision for independent living among individuals with ID [15]. Having a safe and comfortable home equipped with good facilities, such as convenient access to transportation and services, is essential for achieving successful independent living for ID [16]. Nevertheless, significant challenges remain in ensuring that these rights are fully realized in practice. Many NDDs still face discrimination and exclusion, particularly in areas such as employment and housing. Furthermore, the transition from childhood to adulthood can be particularly difficult, as many of the supports that are available during school years are no longer accessible once an individual reaches adulthood. This gap in services can make it challenging for individuals to continue progressing toward independence [17]. As we look to the future, it is clear that ongoing efforts are needed to support independent living for NDDs. This includes not only improving existing services and supports but also continuing to advocate for policies that promote inclusion and accessibility. Research and innovation will also play a crucial role, particularly in the development of new technologies and interventions that can enhance independence. Recently, assistive technology has gained popularity for its ability to enhance the functioning and independence of individuals with ID, thereby supporting their well-being and empowerment [18] and increasing the potential to greatly improve the quality of life for NDDs [19]. Mobile technology and gadgets have proven to be effective tools for self-prompting, enabling instructions for daily living skills to be provided in natural settings [20]. Furthermore, technology ensures equitable access and opportunities for ID to engage in society. According to Bennett et al. [21], transportation remains one of the most critical and challenging aspects for ID when it comes to traveling. This chapter will explore the multifaceted nature of independent living for persons with neurodevelopmental disorders. It will examine the specific challenges faced by these individuals, the support systems that have been developed to address these challenges, and the strategies that can be employed to enhance their independence. Through a comprehensive analysis of both individual and societal dimensions, the chapter aims to provide a deeper understanding of what it means to live independently with a neurodevelopmental disorder and how various stakeholders can contribute to making this goal a reality for more individuals.

2. Overview of neurodevelopmental disorders

NDDs represent a broad category of conditions that arise due to atypical development and functioning of the brain and central nervous system. NDDs comprise ID; communication disorders; ASD; attention-deficit/hyperactivity disorder (ADHD); neurodevelopmental motor disorders, including tic disorders; and specific learning disorders [22]. Research has suggested that common molecular pathways may explain the range of clinical symptoms seen in NDDs. As a result, comorbidity of two or more of these conditions is often observed. For example, a combination of ID, ASD, and epilepsy is frequently reported in individual patients [23]. These disorders generally manifest early in childhood, typically before school age, and have a significant impact on a range of developmental domains including cognitive, motor, language, and social functioning.

A key feature of neurodevelopmental disorders is that they usually begin in childhood, before puberty. Unlike many neuropsychiatric conditions, these disorders, including ADHD, ASD, intellectual disability, and learning and communication disorders, tend to follow a stable course rather than the fluctuating pattern of remission and relapse often seen in mood disorders and schizophrenia that emerge after puberty. These conditions are marked by early-onset neurocognitive impairments and are more prevalent in males [24]. The clinical variability seen in NDDs is mirrored by significant genetic diversity, making it difficult to identify a clear genetic cause in most cases. Unlike Mendelian disorders, which are driven by one or two harmful variants in a single gene, NDDs are complex conditions influenced by numerous genetic factors, with environmental elements playing a major role. Only a small portion of NDDs are linked to straightforward genetic causes. This presents the ongoing challenge of developing more effective methods to connect specific phenotypes with their underlying genetic components in NDDs [22]. Moreover, there is significant overlap between these disorders and their associated symptoms, further justifying the need to consider them as a related group [25].

The Diagnostic and Statistical Manual of Mental Disorders, Fifth Edition (DSM-5), provides a comprehensive framework for understanding and classifying neurodevelopmental disorders. The DSM-5, published by the American Psychiatric Association in 2013 [8], categorizes neurodevelopmental disorders into several distinct subtypes, each with specific diagnostic criteria that guide clinicians in diagnosing and managing these conditions [8]. ID are defined by significant limitations in both intellectual functioning, which includes reasoning, learning, and problem-solving, and adaptive behavior, which encompasses a range of everyday social and practical skills. Intellectual functioning is typically measured using standardized tests of intelligence, with disability defined as a score more than two standard deviations below the population mean. Adaptive behavior is assessed across conceptual, social, and practical domains, including skills such as communication, social participation, and independent living. ID originate during the developmental period, and the degree of impairment can range from mild to profound, affecting the level of support an individual may need throughout their life [26]. Other neurodevelopmental disorders categorized under the DSM-5 include specific learning disorders, which involve difficulties in specific areas of academic performance, such as reading (dyslexia), writing, or mathematics (dyscalculia), in the presence of an intelligence quotient (IQ) that falls within the normal range and which are not better accounted for by an uncorrected auditory or visual acuity. Communication disorders encompass a range of deficits affecting language, speech, and communication abilities. Language disorders are characterized by persistent difficulties in acquiring and using language, impacting both verbal and nonverbal forms of communication, and are more commonly expressed as issues with articulation rather than comprehension. Speech sound disorder (SSD) involves challenges in producing speech sounds that are not appropriate for a child's developmental level, while social (pragmatic) communication disorder (SCD) presents difficulties in the social use of language and nonverbal communication, which can lead to challenges in social interactions and relationships; childhood-onset fluency disorder (COFD), commonly known as stuttering, is among the most frequently recognized speech disorders. It is characterized by challenges in maintaining smooth speech and proper timing patterns. Research indicates that communication disorders, along with specific learning disorders and developmental coordination disorders, are among the most common neurodevelopmental conditions. Global prevalence rates for these conditions are estimated to range from 5 to 10% for communication disorders, 5% for specific learning disorders, and 5 to 8% for developmental coordination disorders [27]. Motor disorders, including developmental coordination disorder and tic disorders, affect motor skills development and coordination. Developmental coordination disorder (DCD) is characterized by challenges in gross and fine motor skills; in contrast, tic disorders involve involuntary, repetitive movements or vocalizations known as tics. Both conditions can significantly impact an individual's ability to function effectively in daily life. ADHD is the most common neurodevelopmental disorder in children. It is characterized by symptoms of inattention, hyperactivity, impulsivity, or a mix of these, which must lead to functional difficulties in various areas of life, including home and school environments [5]. ASD is one of the most widely recognized neurodevelopmental disorders. ASD is characterized by persistent deficits in social communication and social interaction across multiple contexts, along with restricted, repetitive patterns of behavior, interests, or activities. These symptoms typically emerge in early childhood, often before the age of three, and vary widely in severity. Some individuals with ASD may have significant intellectual impairments, while others may possess average or even above-average intelligence. The spectrum nature of the disorder means that individuals can experience a wide range of challenges, from difficulties in everyday social interactions to profound impairments in verbal communication and behavior [8]. Due to this variability, the support needs of individuals with ASD can differ dramatically, requiring highly individualized intervention strategies [28].

Each of these disorders, while distinct, shares a common origin in the disruption of typical brain development and function, leading to impairments that can have a profound impact on the individual's ability to navigate daily life [8]. The prevalence of neurodevelopmental disorders has been steadily increasing over the past several decades, a trend that has significant implications for public health, education systems, and social services worldwide. The rise in diagnosis rates can be attributed to a combination of factors, including greater awareness, improved diagnostic criteria, and potential environmental and genetic influences that are not yet fully understood [29]. ASD, for example, has seen a dramatic increase in prevalence rates. According to the Centres for Disease Control and Prevention (CDC), the prevalence of ASD in the United States has risen to approximately 1 in 54 children as of 2020, compared to 1 in 150 children in 2000 [30]. This increase reflects not only improved diagnostic practices but also a broader recognition of the spectrum nature of autism, which includes individuals with a wide range of abilities and challenges. The growing number of individuals diagnosed with ASD highlights the need for expanded services and supports to accommodate this population, from early intervention programs to adult services that promote independent living. ADHD is similarly prevalent, with estimates suggesting that approximately 5% of children worldwide are diagnosed with the disorder [31]. ID affects an estimated 1–3% of the global population, with variations in prevalence rates depending on the criteria and methods used for diagnosis [32] with greater prevalence in developing countries, likely due to a higher number of births and limited availability of adequate healthcare services [27]. The impact of these disorders on individuals and their families is profound, as these conditions often require lifelong support and intervention. Individuals with NDDs are at a higher risk for a range of health problems, including mental health disorders, and may face significant barriers to accessing education, employment, and social inclusion.

These disorders often present with a range of cognitive, behavioral, social, and sensory challenges that interfere with an individual's ability to function independently in everyday life:

- Cognitive challenges: Neurodevelopmental disorders, such as specific learning disabilities, autism spectrum disorder, and attention-deficit/hyperactivity disorder (ADHD), often share a key characteristic: They are commonly linked to impairments in domain-general cognitive functions like attention, memory, and executive functioning [33]. These cognitive deficits are believed to contribute to the various functional challenges experienced by children with these disorders, including academic struggles, behavioral issues, and social isolation. These challenges may include difficulties with attention, executive functioning, memory, and intellectual abilities. For example, children with ADHD often struggle with sustaining attention, organizing tasks, and following through on instructions, which can hinder academic performance and daily task completion [34]. Similarly, individuals with intellectual disability may have limited intellectual functioning, affecting their capacity to understand complex concepts, make decisions, and engage in abstract thinking [26]. These cognitive impairments can lead to significant difficulties in achieving educational goals, maintaining employment, and managing daily responsibilities.

- Behavioural challenges: Behavioural disorders, also known as behavioural challenges, are another critical aspect of neurodevelopmental disorders, often manifesting as hyperactivity, impulsivity, repetitive behaviours, and self-injurious actions, as well as auto- and hetero-aggressive behaviours. In individuals with ASD, repetitive behaviours and insistence on sameness can disrupt daily routines and create challenges in adapting to new environments or changes in routine [8]. Additionally, aggression, tantrums, and noncompliance are common behavioural issues in children with neurodevelopmental disorders, which can strain family dynamics and hinder social interacions [35]. Behavioural interventions are often necessary to manage these behaviours and improve the individual's ability to function in various settings.

- Social interaction difficulties: Social interaction difficulties are a hallmark of many neurodevelopmental disorders, particularly ASD. Individuals with these disorders often struggle with understanding social cues, engaging in reciprocal communication, and forming relationships. For example, individuals with ASD may have difficulty interpreting facial expressions, body language, and tone of voice, leading to challenges in building and maintaining social connections [36]. These social deficits can result in social isolation, difficulties in forming friendships, and challenges in participating in group activities. Moreover, social interaction difficulties can contribute to anxiety, depression, and other mental health issues, further complicating daily living and overall well-being [37].

- Sensory processing issues: Sensory processing issues are prevalent in NDDs, affecting how they perceive and respond to sensory stimuli. Sensory processing difficulties can manifest as hypersensitivity or hyposensitivity to sensory input, such as noise, light, touch, and movement. For instance, individuals with ASD may exhibit extreme sensitivity to sounds, textures, or lights, leading to discomfort, distress, or avoidance behaviors [38]. These sensory challenges can interfere with daily activities, such as dressing, eating, and participating in social events, as well as impact the individual's ability to function in environments like school or the workplace. Sensory processing issues often require specialized interventions, such as occupational therapy, to help individuals manage their sensory responses and improve their participation in daily life [39].

Even though NDDs may experience changes as individuals mature, leading to potential improvements over time, the overall progression of these disorders generally remains stable. As a result, it is common for these conditions to persist into adulthood, and individuals may also develop new, concurrent issues [27]. The early onset and the persistent nature of these disorders throughout an individual's lifespan make them particularly challenging, not only for the individuals affected but also for their families, caregivers, and the broader community. NDDs represent a significant public health concern, affecting more than 3% of children globally [40]. The societal costs associated with these conditions are substantial, encompassing direct costs such as healthcare and special education services, as well as indirect costs related to lost productivity and the need for long-term care [32, 40]. The societal impact of neurodevelopmental disorders extends beyond the individuals and families directly affected. These conditions place a considerable burden on public health systems, educational institutions, and social services [41]. The need for specialized educational programs, early intervention services, and long-term care creates significant economic demands. For example, the lifetime cost of supporting an individual with ASD in the United States is estimated to be between $1.4 million and $2.4 million, depending on the level of intellectual disability [15]. This economic burden is shared by families, who often face significant out-of-pocket expenses, as well as by society, which bears the costs of providing necessary services and support. Furthermore, neurodevelopmental disorders have implications for social policy and advocacy. As the prevalence of these disorders continues to rise, there is an increasing need for policies that promote inclusion, accessibility, and the rights of individuals with disabilities [41]. This includes ensuring that NDDs have access to appropriate educational opportunities, healthcare services, and employment options, as well as supporting their transition to independent living [14]. The growing recognition of the importance of these issues has led to significant advances in legislation and policy, such as the Americans with Disabilities Act (ADA) [13] in the United States that seeks to protect the rights of individuals with disabilities and promote their full participation in society [16]. In summary, the rising prevalence of neurodevelopmental disorders and their significant societal impact underscore the importance of continued research, advocacy, and the development of effective interventions. As our understanding of these disorders grows, so too must our commitment to supporting NDDs in achieving their full potential and leading fulfilling, independent lives.

3. The independent living concept in the neurodevelopmental disorder field

Independence is a central concept in the philosophy of independent living, particularly for individuals with disabilities. It refers to the capacity to make choices and decisions about one's own life, to control one's environment, and to participate fully in society without unnecessary reliance on others [42]. Independence, in this context, is not an absolute state but rather exists on a continuum that ranges from total dependence to complete independence [43, 44]. This continuum acknowledges that while complete independence may be an ideal, in reality, every individual, regardless of their abilities, experiences varying degrees of dependence and interdependence throughout their lives [21]. The concept of independence is deeply tied to the broader goals of self-determination and autonomy. It encompasses a wide range of behaviors and skills that enable individuals to manage their daily lives, make informed decisions, and engage in meaningful activities. These skills include everything from basic self-care and household management to more complex tasks such as financial management, employment, and social participation. The degree of independence that an individual can achieve is influenced by various factors, including personal capabilities, available support, and environmental barriers [43, 44]. In the realm of disability studies and advocacy, independence is not merely about physical or functional autonomy but also about the ability to exert control over one's life and to live according to one's values and preferences [42]. This perspective challenges the traditional medical model of disability, which often focuses on deficits and the need for care, and instead promotes a social model that emphasizes removing societal barriers and providing the necessary support to enable independence [45].

3.1 Historical perspective on independent living for persons with disabilities

The independent living movement has its roots in the broader civil rights movements of the 1960s and 1970s. During this time, there was a significant shift away from the institutionalization of people with disabilities, which had been the dominant approach for much of the twentieth century. Institutionalization often involved isolating individuals with disabilities in large, segregated facilities where they had little control over their lives and few opportunities for personal growth or social participation [45]. In response to these conditions, disability activists, many of whom were individuals with disabilities themselves, began to advocate for the right to live independently in the community. This advocacy led to the development of the independent living philosophy, which asserts that people with disabilities should have the same opportunities as others to live in their communities, make their own decisions, and participate fully in all aspects of life [46, 47]. One of the key milestones in the history of the independent living movement was the establishment of the first Centre for Independent Living (CIL) in Berkeley, California, in 1972. Founded by Ed Roberts, a disability rights advocate who had experienced firsthand the challenges of navigating life with a disability, the Berkeley CIL provided a model for other centers across the United States and around the world. These centers offered a range of services, including peer support, advocacy, and assistance with accessing community resources, all aimed at empowering individuals with disabilities to live independently [48]. The movement gained further momentum with the passage of the Americans with Disabilities Act (ADA) [13] in 1990, which provided legal protections against discrimination and ensured greater access to public spaces, services, and employment opportunities for people with disabilities. The ADA marked a significant victory for the independent living movement, enshrining the principles of independence and inclusion into law. Internationally, the United Nations Convention on the Rights of Persons with Disabilities (CRPD) [49], adopted in 2006, further solidified the right to independent living as a fundamental human right. The CRPD called for the inclusion of people with disabilities in all aspects of society and emphasized the importance of providing the necessary support to enable them to live independently in their communities. The right to independent living (IL) for individuals with ID is explicitly affirmed in Article 19 of the Convention on the Rights of Persons with Disabilities (CRPD) [49], which guarantees the right to choose where and with whom to live. This implies that individuals must be able to exercise their autonomy, with society providing the necessary support to make this possible. At its core, IL emphasizes the right of everyone to have equal opportunities for choice, decision-making, and freedom [50]. The principles of IL uphold the right of every individual to control their own life, live with dignity, and fully participate in society as any other citizen. People should be empowered to take charge of their own journey toward independent living. This global recognition has influenced policies and practices in many countries, leading to a continued shift away from institutional care toward community-based living and independent living programs [51].

3.2 The role of supports in achieving independence

While independence is a central goal of the independent living movement, it is important to recognize that achieving and maintaining independence often requires support. Support can take many forms, including personal assistance services, adaptive technologies, and modifications to the physical environment. These supports are essential for enabling individuals with disabilities to perform daily tasks, manage their lives, and participate in their communities. Personal assistance services, for example, can help individuals with disabilities with tasks such as bathing, dressing, and eating, allowing them to live in their own homes rather than in institutions. Adaptive technologies, such as mobility aids, communication devices, and environmental controls, can empower individuals to interact with their environment more effectively and independently. Environmental modifications, such as ramps, accessible bathrooms, and universal design principles, can remove physical barriers that might otherwise limit a person's ability to live independently [52]. Moreover, the concept of interdependence is crucial in understanding the dynamics of independence. Interdependence acknowledges that all individuals, regardless of ability, rely on others in various ways throughout their lives. This reliance is not a sign of weakness or failure to achieve independence but rather a natural part of the human experience. Recognizing interdependence helps to reframe independence not as an all-or-nothing state but as a process of maximizing personal autonomy while also acknowledging the role of support and relationships in achieving one's goals [21].

3.3 The importance of independence and social inclusion in enhancing quality of life

The emphasis on independence in the independent living philosophy is closely tied to the broader goal of enhancing the quality of life for individuals with disabilities. Several research studies have revealed that gaining independence and having the ability to manage their own lives and disabilities greatly enhances the quality of life for people with disabilities [53]. Independence allows individuals to have greater control over their lives, make decisions that reflect their values and preferences, and engage in activities that are meaningful to them. This autonomy is critical for psychological well-being, as it contributes to a sense of self-efficacy, personal dignity, and fulfillment [47]. Social inclusion is another key component of the independent living philosophy. Inclusion refers to the full participation of individuals with disabilities in all aspects of community life, including education, employment, recreation, and social activities [54]. Social inclusion is essential for breaking down the barriers of isolation and discrimination that have historically marginalized people with disabilities. It promotes a sense of belonging and ensures that individuals with disabilities have the same opportunities to contribute to and benefit from their communities as others [55]. The relationship between independence and social inclusion is reciprocal. While independence empowers individuals to participate in their communities, social inclusion provides the context in which independence can be fully realized. For example, accessible public transportation allows individuals to travel independently, while inclusive workplaces provide opportunities for meaningful employment. Together, independence and inclusion create a foundation for a higher quality of life, enabling individuals with disabilities to lead fulfilling and self-directed lives [51]. Despite the progress made in promoting independent living, there remain significant challenges in achieving full independence and inclusion for all individuals with disabilities, particularly those with ID and autism. Research on the independence of these populations is still limited, with most studies focusing on specific skills and involving small sample sizes. The outcome measures used in these studies are often narrow, limiting the generalizability of the findings [56, 57]. Moreover, while there are tools available to assess adaptive functioning and functional abilities, there is a notable lack of validated instruments specifically designed to evaluate independent living skills on a broad scale. Such tools are crucial for developing personalized programs that support independence by providing detailed information on an individual's abilities, potential barriers, and support needs [58]. Without accurate and comprehensive assessments, it is difficult to design interventions that effectively promote independence and ensure that individuals can achieve the highest possible level of autonomy. To address these challenges, future research should focus on developing and validating tools that can assess independent living skills across a wide range of contexts and populations. Additionally, there is a need for longitudinal studies that examine the long-term outcomes of independent living programs, particularly in terms of quality of life, social inclusion, and psychological well-being. By expanding the research base, it will be possible to create more effective and individualized supports that can help people with disabilities achieve their full potential for independence and inclusion [59]. In conclusion, the concept of independence is at the heart of the independent living philosophy, which seeks to empower individuals with disabilities to lead self-directed lives and participate fully in society. Independence is not an absolute state but exists on a continuum, with varying degrees of dependence and interdependence being a natural part of the human experience. The independent living movement has made significant strides in promoting the rights of people with disabilities to live independently and be included in their communities, but there is still work to be done. Achieving true independence requires not only the removal of societal barriers but also the provision of appropriate supports that enable individuals to exercise autonomy and control over their lives. As research continues to advance, there is a need for more comprehensive tools and studies to better understand the factors that contribute to independence and to develop interventions that can enhance the quality of life for people with disabilities. Ultimately, by embracing the principles of independence and social inclusion, society can create an environment where all individuals, regardless of ability, can thrive and contribute to the richness of the human experience.

4. Challenges to independent living for persons with intellectual disabilities

Independent living for individuals with ID represents an important goal in fostering autonomy and improving quality of life. Achieving this level of independence, however, is fraught with a range of challenges that span cognitive, social, behavioral, and sensory domains. This chapter explores these challenges in depth, highlighting the barriers that individuals with ID face and the implications for their ability to live independently.

4.1 Cognitive and learning challenges

Cognitive challenges are a defining feature of ID and significantly impact an individual's capacity for independent living. One of the primary cognitive challenges is in decision-making and problem-solving. Individuals with ID often exhibit difficulties in evaluating situations, considering the potential consequences of their actions, and making informed decisions [60]. This can manifest in everyday tasks, such as budgeting, where individuals may struggle to prioritize expenses or save for future needs. Similarly, meal planning can become a complex task due to difficulties in selecting appropriate ingredients, balancing nutrition, and managing cooking times. Navigating public transportation is another example, where understanding routes, schedules, and payment methods can be overwhelming, leading to anxiety and avoidance of these essential activities. Memory and information processing are also significantly impaired in individuals with ID. Short-term memory deficits can lead to challenges in retaining important information, such as daily schedules, medication routines, or instructions for using household appliances [61]. These memory issues can result in missed appointments, improper use of medications, or an inability to complete daily tasks effectively. Furthermore, individuals with ID often process information more slowly, which can affect their ability to learn new skills, adapt to changes, or respond to emergency situations [47]. The need for repeated instructions and extended time for task completion can contribute to frustration and a sense of dependency, further complicating the goal of independent living. These cognitive and learning challenges necessitate tailored support strategies, such as the use of visual aids, step-by-step instructions, and frequent repetition to reinforce learning. Cognitive behavioral therapy (CBT) and other structured interventions can also help individuals develop better decision-making and problem-solving skills, enhancing their ability to manage daily life independently [62].

4.2 Social and communication barriers

Social interaction is a critical component of independent living, yet individuals with ID often face significant barriers in this area. Social anxiety and isolation are common among individuals with ID, largely due to difficulties in understanding and interpreting social cues [63]. These individuals may struggle with recognizing facial expressions, interpreting body language, or understanding the tone of voice, which are all crucial for effective communication. As a result, they may misinterpret social situations, leading to misunderstandings and conflicts. For example, a person with ID might perceive neutral feedback as criticism or fail to recognize when someone is being sarcastic, leading to confusion and hurt feelings. The difficulties in social communication often result in social withdrawal, as individuals with ID may choose to avoid interactions altogether rather than risk negative experiences. This isolation can exacerbate feelings of loneliness, depression, and low self-esteem, which are already prevalent in this population [64]. Social isolation can also limit opportunities for learning and practicing social skills, creating a vicious cycle where a lack of social interaction further impedes the development of these essential skills. In addition to social anxiety, individuals with ID often struggle with making and maintaining friendships. The challenges in understanding social norms and expectations can make it difficult to engage in reciprocal relationships. For instance, they may have trouble initiating conversations, maintaining eye contact, or participating in group activities. These social difficulties can lead to exclusion from social groups, further reinforcing feelings of isolation. Communication barriers extend beyond social interactions to include difficulties with both expressive and receptive language. Individuals with ID may have limited vocabulary or struggle with forming coherent sentences, which can make it challenging to express their needs and desires [65]. This can lead to frustration and behavioral issues, as individuals may resort to inappropriate behaviors to communicate when they feel misunderstood. On the other hand, receptive language difficulties can make it hard for individuals to follow instructions, understand rules, or process complex information. This can affect their ability to navigate social situations, follow directions from caregivers, or understand public announcements, such as safety instructions on public transportation. To address these barriers, interventions such as social skills training, speech therapy, and the use of assistive communication devices can be highly effective. These tools can help individuals with ID develop better communication skills, enhance their social interactions, and reduce feelings of isolation, thereby supporting their efforts to live independently.

4.3 Behavioral and emotional regulation

Behavioral and emotional regulation is crucial for the successful management of daily life, but many individuals with ID experience significant challenges in these areas. Managing stress and anxiety is particularly difficult for this population, as they may lack the coping mechanisms necessary to deal with everyday stressors [35]. Individuals with ID often experience heightened levels of anxiety in response to changes in routine, unfamiliar environments, or social interactions. This anxiety can manifest in various ways, such as agitation, withdrawal, or even aggression. For example, an unexpected change in their daily schedule might trigger a severe anxiety response, leading to a meltdown or refusal to participate in activities. Impulsivity and hyperactivity are also common behavioral issues in individuals with ID, particularly those with comorbid conditions such as attention-deficit/hyperactivity disorder (ADHD) [66]. These behaviors can interfere with an individual's ability to focus on tasks, follow through with plans, or adhere to social norms. Impulsivity might lead to rash decisions, such as spending money on unnecessary items or engaging in risky behaviors without considering the consequences. Hyperactivity, on the other hand, can make it difficult for individuals to sit still, concentrate on tasks, or engage in activities that require sustained attention, such as reading or attending appointments. Emotional dysregulation can further complicate efforts to live independently. Many individuals with ID struggle with identifying and expressing their emotions appropriately, leading to difficulties in managing anger, frustration, or sadness [63]. This emotional instability can result in outbursts, self-harm, or withdrawal, which can strain relationships with caregivers, peers, and community members. Moreover, the inability to regulate emotions effectively can make it challenging to maintain employment, adhere to daily routines, or engage in social activities, all of which are essential components of independent living. Addressing these behavioral and emotional challenges often requires a multifaceted approach. Behavioral interventions, such as applied behavior analysis (ABA), can help individuals develop better self-regulation skills by reinforcing positive behaviors and reducing maladaptive ones. Additionally, therapeutic approaches, such as cognitive-behavioral therapy (CBT) and mindfulness training, can teach individuals coping strategies for managing anxiety and stress, improving their overall emotional well-being. Medication may also be prescribed in some cases to manage symptoms of hyperactivity, impulsivity, or anxiety, though this should be part of a broader, individualized treatment plan.

4.4 Sensory processing issues

Sensory processing issues are another significant barrier to independent living for individuals with ID. Sensory processing refers to the way the nervous system receives and interprets sensory information from the environment, such as sights, sounds, smells, tastes, and touch [67]. Many individuals with ID experience either hypersensitivity (over-responsiveness) or hyposensitivity (under-responsiveness) to sensory stimuli, which can interfere with their ability to perform daily tasks and participate in social activities. Hypersensitivity can make certain environments or activities overwhelming for individuals with ID. For example, loud noises, bright lights, or crowded spaces might be intolerable, leading to anxiety, distress, or avoidance behaviors. This hypersensitivity can make it difficult for individuals to engage in everyday activities such as grocery shopping, attending social events, or even using public transportation. In some cases, hypersensitivity to touch might make tasks like dressing or grooming uncomfortable, leading to challenges in maintaining personal hygiene. Conversely, hyposensitivity can result in a lack of awareness or response to sensory stimuli that others might find uncomfortable or even painful. Individuals with hyposensitivity might not notice when they are too cold or too hot, leading to inappropriate clothing choices. They might also have a high tolerance for pain, which can be dangerous if it leads to injuries going unnoticed and untreated. Additionally, hyposensitivity can affect proprioception (the sense of body position), making it difficult for individuals to navigate spaces, perform coordinated movements, or engage in fine motor tasks such as cooking or writing. Sensory processing issues can also impact sleep, which is essential for overall health and well-being. Individuals with ID might experience difficulties falling asleep or staying asleep due to sensory sensitivities, such as being disturbed by minor noises or changes in temperature. Poor sleep can exacerbate other challenges, such as cognitive impairments, emotional dysregulation, and behavioral issues, further complicating efforts to achieve independent living.

To address sensory processing challenges, occupational therapy (OT) can be highly beneficial. OT interventions often include sensory integration therapy, which helps individuals develop a more balanced response to sensory stimuli. Environmental modifications, such as creating sensory-friendly living spaces with dim lighting, soundproofing, or weighted blankets, can also help individuals manage sensory sensitivities. Additionally, sensory diets—planned activities that provide the sensory input individuals need—can help regulate their sensory systems, improving their ability to function independently.

5. Support systems for independent living

The ability of NDDs to live independently is greatly influenced by the availability and effectiveness of various support systems. These systems, which include family and caregiver involvement, educational support, community-based services, and assistive technology, are crucial for promoting autonomy and improving quality of life. This chapter provides an in-depth exploration of these support mechanisms, highlighting their roles in fostering independent living for individuals with ID.

5.1 Educational support: Importance of individualized education programs (IEPs)

Education is a critical component of preparing individuals with ID for independent living, and individualized education programs (IEPs) are central to this process. IEPs are customized educational plans that address the specific academic and functional needs of students with disabilities [68]. These plans are developed collaboratively by educators, parents, and specialists, ensuring that the student receives the support necessary to succeed academically and develop essential life skills [68]. IEPs play a pivotal role in ensuring that students with ID are equipped with the tools they need for independent living. Beyond academic goals, IEPs often include objectives related to daily living skills, such as personal care, money management, and social interaction. These skills are crucial for helping students transition from the structured environment of school to the more independent setting of adult life [69]. Moreover, the legal framework provided by the Individuals with Disabilities Education Act (IDEA) ensures that schools are obligated to provide these tailored services, thus reinforcing the importance of education in promoting independence [70]. Life skills training is an integral component of educational support for individuals with ID. This training provides students with practical skills that are directly applicable to everyday life, including cooking, budgeting, personal hygiene, and communication. Educational programs that incorporate life skills training into their curriculum play a crucial role in preparing students for the challenges of independent living [71]. The three key areas of daily living skills (DLS), as outlined by Sparrow et al. [72], include personal skills (like brushing teeth, showering, taking medication, and managing one's health), domestic skills (such as cleaning, cooking, and doing laundry), and community skills (like managing time, budgeting, and securing and maintaining a job). Developing DLS usually involves receiving instruction, practicing, and getting feedback from others before achieving independence. Mastery of DLS is crucial for reaching adult milestones, such as managing college courses, holding a job, and living independently. For instance, skills like washing work uniforms, showering, keeping track of a work schedule, and arranging transportation are necessary for holding part-time or full-time employment [73]. Life skills training is typically delivered through a combination of classroom instruction, hands-on practice, and real-world experiences. For example, students may learn cooking techniques in a classroom setting and then apply these skills in a kitchen environment, with the support of instructors. This approach not only reinforces learning but also builds confidence as students successfully complete tasks on their own [73, 74].

Additionally, life skills training often includes community-based experiences, such as shopping or using public transportation, which are essential for achieving independence in adult life [75]. The transition from school to adult life is a particularly critical period, and life skills training during this time is essential for ensuring that individuals with ID are prepared for the responsibilities of independent living. Programs that focus on transition planning, including job training, independent living skills, and community integration, are vital for helping students make a successful transition to adulthood [75].

6. Community-based support services

Community-based support services are fundamental to enabling independent living for individuals with ID. Supported living arrangements are a key component of these services, offering individuals the opportunity to live independently while receiving the support they need [73]. These arrangements can vary widely, from shared housing with other individuals with disabilities to independent apartments with visiting support staff, or living in a family home with assistance from caregivers [46]. Supported living is designed to promote autonomy by allowing individuals to make decisions about their daily lives while having access to support when necessary. This model encourages the development of self-care skills and decision-making abilities, as individuals are responsible for managing their household, finances, and personal care, with support provided based on their level of need [76]. Research has shown that individuals in supported living arrangements experience higher levels of satisfaction with their living situation and demonstrate improved social and life skills compared to those in more restrictive settings [52]. The success of supported living arrangements often depends on the quality of the support provided [77]. Effective support includes not only assistance with daily tasks but also opportunities for socialization, community participation, and personal growth. Programs that emphasize the development of social networks and community ties are particularly successful in promoting long-term independence and quality of life [46].

6.1 Community integration programs

Community integration programs are another crucial aspect of community-based support services. These programs are designed to facilitate the full participation of individuals with ID in their communities by providing opportunities for socialization, recreation, and employment. Integration into the community is essential for reducing social isolation and fostering a sense of belonging, which are important for independent living [78]. Community integration programs may include a variety of activities, such as social clubs, sports teams, volunteer opportunities, and cultural events. These activities provide individuals with ID the chance to interact with others, develop social skills, and build relationships. Furthermore, these programs often include support for accessing public services, such as transportation, healthcare, and education, which are essential for independent living [79]. Effective community integration also involves addressing barriers to participation, such as physical accessibility, transportation, and social stigma. Programs that proactively work to remove these barriers and provide inclusive opportunities are crucial for enabling individuals with ID to live independently and fully participate in society [80].

6.2 Vocational training and employment support

Vocational training and employment support are key components of community-based services that promote independent living. Employment provides individuals with ID not only with financial independence but also with a sense of purpose, self-esteem, and social connection. Vocational training programs are designed to equip individuals with the skills necessary to obtain and maintain employment, whether in supported or competitive work environments [75]. These programs often include job coaching, on-the-job training, and ongoing support to ensure that individuals with ID can succeed in the workplace. Additionally, employment support services assist with job placement, helping individuals find positions that match their skills, interests, and abilities. The availability of vocational training and employment support is critical for enhancing the independence and quality of life of individuals with ID [81]. The employment rates and labor force participation of individuals with intellectual and developmental disabilities (IDD) present significant challenges across various national contexts. Research indicates a lack of common definitions and metrics in studies, complicating comparisons of outcomes [82]. The criteria for identifying this population often vary widely, with many studies suffering from inadequate characterization of participants regarding comorbidities and ability levels. Disability status is frequently self-reported rather than clinically confirmed, which affects the accuracy of employment data [83]. Common terminology, including "intellectual disability," "developmental disability," and "autism," often lacks clarity, blurring distinctions between clinical diagnoses and functional profiles. Additionally, employment outcomes are conceptualized differently across countries, particularly where segregated work environments, such as sheltered workshops, exist, leading to inflated statistics on employment rates. Francescutti et al. [84] highlight that individuals with IDD face lower employment rates compared to other disability groups. Their work underscores the impact of co-occurring intellectual and psychiatric disorders on employment outcomes, emphasizing the need for contextual factors to be considered in understanding labor market participation. For example, their analysis points out that only 24.1% of Canadians with developmental disabilities were employed, with even lower rates for those with autism [85]. In the United States, only 27.8% of adults with developmental disabilities were employed at any time, and their earnings were typically much lower than those of their non-disabled peers. Furthermore, the presence of co-occurring conditions, such as mental health disorders, complicates employment prospects. Research has shown that individuals with both ID and psychiatric conditions encounter additional barriers, resulting in even lower rates of labor force participation [84]. This evidence emphasizes the necessity for tailored employment support programs that consider the unique needs of individuals with IDD, aiming to foster greater inclusivity and improve overall employment outcomes.

6.3 Role of family and caregivers

Individuals with ID and their families can contribute to promoting independent living (IL). The transition from a welfare model to a community-based one requires a change in the role of families, who need to support the path to autonomy for people with ID [50]. Family support is often the bedrock upon which the lives of individuals with ID are built. Families provide not only practical assistance but also emotional and psychological support, which is essential for the development of independence. Family members frequently act as advocates, ensuring that individuals with ID have access to necessary services and opportunities that promote autonomy [86]. The involvement of families is particularly crucial during transitional periods, such as moving from school to adult life, where the focus shifts toward independent living. However, families often find this process complex and stressful, and they are concerned that the available options are not adequate [50]. Research has consistently demonstrated that individuals with strong family support systems exhibit better outcomes in terms of social integration, life skills development, and overall well-being [70]. The transition to adulthood is a critical time when the role of the family often expands to include helping the individual navigate complex systems, such as healthcare, housing, and employment. Families that actively engage in planning and preparation during this phase are instrumental in ensuring a smoother transition to independent living [87]. However, the demands on families can be intense, leading to stress and potential burnout. Therefore, access to respite care and external support services is crucial to sustaining family involvement over the long term [88]. Additionally, training programs designed to enhance the skills of family members in supporting independence can be highly beneficial. These programs equip families with strategies to encourage self-reliance while providing the necessary support [89]. Caregivers, whether they are family members or professionals, are essential in fostering independence among individuals with ID. They provide direct support in daily activities, such as personal care, meal preparation, and medication management, while also encouraging the development of life skills that are critical for independent living [90]. The approach that caregivers take can significantly impact the individual's ability to live independently. A person-centered approach, which focuses on the strengths and preferences of the individual, is particularly effective in promoting autonomy [89]. Professional caregivers are often trained to use specific techniques that help individuals with ID develop and maintain independence. These techniques might include using visual schedules, breaking tasks into manageable steps, and providing consistent routines that foster a sense of control and confidence in the individual [90]. The relationship between the caregiver and the individual is also crucial; a relationship based on trust and mutual respect can greatly enhance the individual's confidence and willingness to take on new challenges [90]. Furthermore, the concept of "dignity of risk" is increasingly recognized in caregiving practices. This concept involves allowing individuals with ID to take reasonable risks as part of their growth toward independence rather than overprotecting them. While safety is always a concern, allowing individuals to make decisions, even if they might fail, is essential for building self-confidence and problem-solving skills [91]. However, the low expectations of families and professionals regarding the success of these paths often lead them to make decisions on behalf of individuals with ID, limiting their ability to express their own desires. The lack of communicative support and adequate information are further obstacles that prevent people with ID from taking control of their own lives [50]. Experts note that professionals are concerned about the risks associated with individuals with ID living independently, despite some authors, like Hawkins et al. [92], arguing that risk is a necessary aspect of services. Additionally, professionals tend to have low expectations about the ability of people with ID to create and follow through on plans for independent living. This combination of low expectations and risk aversion can lead to a preference for institutional settings and for professionals and organizations to take over decision-making.

6.4 Use of technology to aid communication, daily living, and learning

Assistive technology plays a pivotal role in supporting individuals with ID in their pursuit of independent living. These technologies range from simple tools that aid in daily living tasks to sophisticated devices and software that enhance communication, learning, and mobility [93]. The use of assistive technology can significantly improve the quality of life for individuals with ID by enabling them to perform tasks independently, communicate more effectively, and participate more fully in educational and community settings [94]. For individuals with communication difficulties, assistive technology can provide vital support. Augmentative and alternative communication (AAC) devices, for example, allow individuals to express themselves and interact with others more easily. These devices range from simple picture boards to complex speech-generating devices that can be customized to the user's specific needs [95]. The use of AAC devices has been shown to improve communication outcomes and social participation for individuals with ID [96]. In educational settings, assistive technology can facilitate learning by providing students with tools that accommodate their specific needs. For example, software programs that offer text-to-speech, voice recognition, or visual aids can help students with ID engage with academic content more effectively. These technologies can also be used to teach life skills, such as money management or cooking, through interactive and accessible formats [97]. Assistive technology also supports independent living by aiding in daily tasks. Devices such as medication reminders, automated home systems, and adaptive cooking tools enable individuals with ID to manage their daily routines with greater independence [98]. These tools not only enhance independence but also provide a sense of control and confidence in one's ability to manage life's challenges. The range of assistive devices and software available for individuals with ID is vast and continues to grow as technology advances. Some commonly used devices include the following:

- Communication devices: Speech-generating devices, such as Dynavox or iPads with communication apps, enable individuals with speech impairments to express themselves and interact with others.

- Daily living aids: Tools such as adaptive utensils, dressing aids, and medication dispensers help individuals perform daily tasks independently.

- Learning tools: Educational software, such as Clicker 7 or Boardmaker, offers visual and interactive learning opportunities that cater to the needs of students with ID.

- Mobility aids: Devices such as adapted bicycles, walkers, and wheelchair-accessible technology allow individuals with physical disabilities to move around more freely and safely.

- Environmental control systems: Smart home technologies, including voice-activated lights, thermostats, and security systems, provide individuals with ID greater control over their living environment.

The effectiveness of these technologies depends on their proper use and the support provided to individuals in learning how to use them. Training and ongoing support are essential to ensure that individuals can maximize the benefits of these devices and incorporate them into their daily lives [98]. In conclusion, assistive technology is a powerful tool that can significantly enhance the independence and quality of life for individuals with ID. By providing support in communication, daily living, and learning, these technologies enable individuals to participate more fully in society and achieve their goals of independent living.

7. Strategies for promoting independent living

Promoting independent living for individuals with ID involves a multi-dimensional approach that includes person-centered planning, life skills training, behavioral interventions, social skills development, employment and vocational training, and appropriate housing options. This section delves into these strategies in detail, providing a comprehensive overview of how they contribute to enhancing the autonomy and quality of life for individuals with ID.

7.1 Person-centered planning

Person-centered planning (PCP) is a core strategy for supporting individuals with ID in achieving independent living. PCP focuses on aligning support services with the individual's personal goals, preferences, and values rather than applying a uniform set of interventions. This approach ensures that the individual's voice is central to the planning process, leading to support strategies that are both meaningful and effective [99]. By fostering active participation in decision-making, PCP enhances engagement and satisfaction, contributing to better overall outcomes for individuals with ID [80]. Before setting goals, it is essential to conduct a thorough assessment to identify the individual's needs, preferences, and quality of life. Assessments should focus on various dimensions, including functional abilities, social participation, and personal aspirations. The Quality of Life and Support Needs Model provides a comprehensive framework for evaluating these aspects, emphasizing the importance of both subjective and objective measures [9]. One valuable assessment tool in this context is the Adult Independent Living Measurement Scales (AILMS), which evaluates individuals' abilities across multiple domains critical for independent living, such as self-care, household management, and community involvement [100]. The AILMS provides a structured approach to measuring progress and identifying areas where additional support may be needed. By integrating these assessments into the PCP process, support plans can be more accurately tailored to the individual's current capabilities and goals. Effective goal setting is integral to PCP. Goals should be specific, measurable, attainable, relevant, and time-bound (SMART) to facilitate clear planning and progress tracking [101]. Goal setting involves not only identifying desired outcomes but also outlining the steps necessary to achieve them. This process requires regular monitoring and evaluation to ensure that the plan remains relevant and responsive to the individual's evolving needs and circumstances [16]. Regular progress reviews are essential for assessing whether goals are being met and for making adjustments as needed. These reviews help in recognizing achievements, addressing barriers, and refining the support plan to better align with the individual's changing aspirations and needs.

7.2 Life skills training

Life skills training is a critical component in fostering independence. By teaching essential skills such as cooking, cleaning, and budgeting, individuals with ID gain the ability to manage daily tasks and responsibilities effectively. These skills are foundational for self-sufficiency and contribute to a higher quality of life [1]. Life skills training typically includes practical instruction in areas such as meal preparation, household maintenance, and financial management. For instance, cooking classes might cover topics such as meal planning, safe food handling, and using kitchen appliances. Cleaning training might involve teaching organization, hygiene practices, and proper use of cleaning products. Budgeting education often includes understanding financial concepts, managing expenses, and planning for future needs [102].

7.3 Behavioral interventions

Behavioral interventions grounded in cognitive behavioral therapy (CBT) and applied behavioral analysis (ABA) are essential for fostering independence among NDDs. ABA, in particular, provides a structured, evidence-based approach that is highly effective in promoting the development of skills necessary for independent living, such as self-care, social interaction, and adaptive functioning. This approach utilizes systematic, data-driven methods to modify behavior and teach new skills, making it a cornerstone of effective behavioral interventions. ABA operates on the principles of behaviorism, which emphasizes the role of reinforcement and environmental factors in shaping behavior. This approach is distinguished by its focus on measurable outcomes and individualized interventions, ensuring that strategies are tailored to meet the specific needs of each individual [103]. Central to ABA is the concept of using empirical data to guide the development and implementation of behavior change programs. This involves conducting thorough assessments to identify the antecedents and consequences of behaviors, which informs the creation of individualized behavior plans aimed at promoting positive outcomes and reducing maladaptive behaviors. One of the significant strengths of ABA is its ability to provide detailed, personalized support that enhances the individual's capacity for independent living. Various evidence-based strategies have been identified for improving adaptive behaviors, including daily living skills (DLS). These strategies involve behavioral techniques like direct instruction, reinforcement, chaining, task analysis, and prompting, along with the use of technology, visual aids, and video modeling. Interventions incorporate a variety of these approaches to help adolescents learn and refine DLS during sessions, and then generalize these skills to their home and community environments. Research has shown these methods to be effective in teaching adaptive behavior skills to individuals with ASD [73]. For example, ABA can help individuals develop essential life skills, such as managing personal finances, maintaining a household, and navigating social interactions. Through systematic instruction and reinforcement, individuals learn how to perform daily tasks independently and efficiently. The approach is highly structured, often involving the breakdown of complex tasks into smaller, more manageable steps. This method not only facilitates learning but also ensures that individuals can gradually build confidence and competence in their abilities. In addition to its practical applications, ABA emphasizes the importance of creating supportive and adaptive environments that minimize triggers for challenging behaviors. This involves making modifications to the individual's surroundings and daily routines to reduce stressors and promote positive interactions. For instance, adjustments might include organizing a living space to minimize distractions or establishing consistent routines to provide stability and predictability. By focusing on environmental factors and behavioral triggers, ABA helps create conditions that support successful independent living. Furthermore, ABA incorporates ongoing data collection and analysis to monitor progress and make necessary adjustments to interventions. This continuous feedback loop ensures that interventions remain effective and responsive to the individual's evolving needs. Regular assessment of behavioral outcomes allows practitioners to refine strategies, reinforce successful behaviors, and address any emerging challenges. Positive behavior support (PBS) complements ABA by providing a broader framework for understanding and addressing behavior. PBS focuses on identifying the underlying causes of challenging behaviors and developing comprehensive behavior support plans that incorporate proactive strategies. These plans often include teaching new skills, modifying the environment to reduce behavioral triggers, and applying positive reinforcement to encourage desired behaviors [104, 105]. PBS is designed to be both proactive and preventive, aiming to enhance the individual's quality of life by promoting positive behavior and reducing the occurrence of challenging behaviors. Research has demonstrated the effectiveness of PBS in improving behavior and engagement among individuals with ID, underscoring its value in promoting independent living [104]. By integrating PBS principles with ABA techniques, practitioners can provide a holistic approach that addresses both immediate behavioral concerns and long-term goals for independence. The application of ABA and PBS in promoting independent living has far-reaching implications. These behavioral interventions support individuals in developing the skills necessary to manage their daily lives effectively, participate in social and occupational activities, and achieve greater autonomy. By providing tailored support and addressing both behavioral and environmental factors, ABA and PBS create a robust framework for enhancing independence and improving overall quality of life.

As the field continues to evolve, ongoing research and advancements in behavioral science will further refine these approaches, ensuring that they remain effective and responsive to the needs of NDDs. The commitment to evidence-based practices and individualized support will be crucial in advancing the goals of independent living and ensuring that all individuals have the opportunity to lead fulfilling and autonomous lives.

7.4 Social skills development

Developing social skills is vital for independent living. Individuals with neurodevelopmental disabilities (DNS) often face challenges in social skills, such as maintaining eye contact, initiating and sustaining conversations, and engaging appropriately with others. As they mature and seek more independent experiences like employment, higher education, and living on their own, it becomes crucial for them to develop these skills. Programs designed to enhance social interaction focus on teaching effective communication, relationship-building, and social problem-solving skills. There are various methods for teaching social skills, including task analysis, social stories, script fading, and prompting. These programs often use structured teaching methods, role-playing, and social stories to facilitate skill development [106]. The effectiveness of social skill development is enhanced when practiced in natural settings, as some of these techniques facilitate interactions in real-world environments [107]. Social skills training may cover areas such as initiating and maintaining conversations, understanding social cues, and managing interpersonal conflicts.

Evidence suggests that such training improves social interactions, reduces isolation, and enhances the quality of life for individuals with ID [108]. By participating in these programs, individuals with ID gain the skills necessary for forming and maintaining meaningful relationships. Building and maintaining relationships involves teaching individuals how to navigate social interactions effectively. Strategies include practicing conversation skills, expressing emotions appropriately, and engaging in reciprocal interactions [109]. Creating opportunities for social participation, such as joining community groups or recreational activities, is also crucial. Encouraging individuals to pursue shared interests can help them develop social connections and friendships. Additionally, providing ongoing support and guidance in social situations helps individuals manage challenges and strengthen their relationships over time [65].

7.5 Employment and vocational training

Employment is a key factor in achieving independent living. Meaningful employment provides not only financial stability but also a sense of purpose and social inclusion. Research highlights the positive impact of employment on quality of life, community integration, and personal satisfaction for individuals with ID [81].

Existing research typically emphasizes the customization of job opportunities through approaches like customized employment (CE). CE is a person-centered method that involves two main stages: (1) discovery, where an individual's skills, goals, and potential job opportunities are explored and (2) job carving, in which individuals or professionals collaborate with employers to identify and negotiate appropriate open or competitive job opportunities that align with the needs and support requirements of both the employer and employee [110].

Programs that match individuals with ID to suitable job opportunities based on their skills and interests are crucial for ensuring meaningful employment. Such programs often involve collaboration with employers, job coaches, and support staff to secure appropriate job placements [75]. Job coaching and supported employment models are effective strategies for facilitating successful employment outcomes. Job coaching provides individualized support to employees with ID, including assistance with job tasks, workplace interactions, and adaptation to the work environment [111]. Job coaches work closely with both the employee and the employer to ensure that the individual's needs are met and that they can perform their job effectively. Supported employment models, such as the individual placement and support (IPS) model, emphasize finding competitive jobs in the open labor market and providing ongoing support to ensure job retention [112]. These models have been shown to improve employment outcomes and job satisfaction for individuals with ID, supporting their ability to live independently and participate fully in the workforce [84].

7.6 Housing options

Selecting appropriate housing is a crucial aspect of promoting independent living for individuals with ID; however, many adults with intellectual and developmental disabilities (IDD) face challenges in finding and maintaining housing that meets their behavioral support needs. Adequate housing for adults with IDD typically includes features like good lighting, ventilation, durability, cleanliness, safety, and a balance between privacy and communal spaces. Effective supported housing also incorporates universal design principles, appropriate fixtures and appliances (e.g., lever handles instead of doorknobs), personalized touches (e.g., choosing paint colors), access to meaningful activities (e.g., visual and physical access to outdoor areas), and a home-like feel with a variety of private and shared spaces. Adults with IDD have expressed a desire for housing that promotes independence and privacy while allowing access to social networks and community involvement [113].

Various housing models offer different levels of support and independence. Group homes provide a shared living environment with on-site support staff who assist with daily activities and care. This model is suitable for individuals who require moderate support while benefiting from a communal living arrangement [114]. Independent apartments offer greater autonomy, allowing individuals to manage their own living space while having access to external support services as needed. This model is ideal for those who are capable of handling daily living tasks independently but may still require occasional assistance [45]. Regardless of the housing model, ensuring that the living environment is safe and supportive is paramount. Safe housing features include accessibility, security, and emergency preparedness. Supportive environments offer necessary services such as personal care assistance, social support, and access to community resources. Creating a supportive housing environment enhances the individual's ability to live independently and contributes to their overall well-being and quality of life [115, 116].

8. Policy and advocacy

The policy landscape supporting independent living for individuals with ID is shaped by several critical laws and regulations designed to enhance accessibility, equity, and opportunities for this population. Prominent among these is the Americans with Disabilities Act (ADA) [13], enacted in 1990, which provides comprehensive protections against discrimination for individuals with disabilities. This landmark legislation ensures equal access to public services, employment, and accommodations, and mandates that government entities and private businesses make reasonable modifications to facilitate the participation of individuals with disabilities in all aspects of public life [13]. Similarly, the Individuals with Disabilities Education Act (IDEA), first passed in 1975 and reauthorized in 2004, guarantees students with disabilities access to a free and appropriate public education. IDEA emphasizes the importance of individualized education programs (IEPs) tailored to each student's unique needs, which include transitional services aimed at preparing students for adulthood and independent living (Individuals with Disabilities Education Act, 2004). Both pieces of legislation are instrumental in setting a framework for support and inclusion but require effective implementation to realize their full potential. Government and non-governmental organizations (NGOs) play pivotal roles in both enacting and enforcing these policies. Federal agencies, such as the U.S. Department of Education and the Administration for Community Living [117], oversee compliance and provide guidance to ensure that educational and community services adhere to legal standards [117, 118]. NGOs, including the National Disability Rights Network [119] and The Arc [120], advocate for the rights of individuals with ID by engaging in policy advocacy, providing resources and support, and ensuring that the needs of this population are addressed at both state and federal levels [119, 120]. These organizations also play a crucial role in bridging gaps between legislative intent and real-world practice by offering training, resources, and advocacy to support the effective implementation of policies. Advocacy for independent living is further reinforced by the promotion of self-advocacy and the efforts of advocacy groups. Self-advocacy, where individuals with ID learn to express their own needs and preferences, is a fundamental aspect of promoting autonomy and independence. Empowering individuals to advocate for themselves helps them gain greater control over their lives and decisions, thereby enhancing their quality of life [121]. Advocacy groups and organizations, such as The Arc and the National Association of Councils on Developmental Disabilities, are vital in this context. They work tirelessly to influence policy, raise awareness, and provide resources that support independent living for individuals with ID [120]. These groups also engage in lobbying efforts, participate in policy formulation, and offer support services that help individuals navigate the complexities of their rights and available resources. Despite these efforts, significant challenges remain in the implementation of policies designed to support independent living. One major issue is the gap between policy and practice. While laws like the ADA and IDEA establish high standards, discrepancies often arise in how these laws are applied across different regions and service providers. Variations in local resources, training, and enforcement can lead to uneven access to services and support [122]. To address these issues, several recommendations have been proposed. These include increasing funding for support services, enhancing training for service providers to ensure they are well-equipped to meet the needs of individuals with ID, and establishing more robust mechanisms for monitoring and enforcing compliance with existing laws [60]. Additionally, efforts to streamline and standardize policy implementation across different jurisdictions can help mitigate these gaps and ensure that the benefits of legislative frameworks are realized more consistently.

9. Case studies and real-life examples

9.1 Case study 1: Independent living for an individual with autism

Giovanni, a 24-year-old diagnosed with ASD, faced numerous obstacles in his pursuit of independent living. His primary challenges included sensory sensitivities, difficulties with executive functioning, and struggles with social interactions. Sensory overload from everyday stimuli, such as bright lights and loud noises, often caused Giovanni considerable distress. Additionally, his executive functioning difficulties made it challenging for him to plan, organize, and execute daily tasks, such as managing household chores and personal finances. Socially, Giovanni found it hard to navigate complex social environments, which affected his ability to build and maintain relationships. To address these challenges, a comprehensive support plan was developed. The plan began with modifying Giovanni's living environment to reduce sensory triggers. This included installing dimmable lights, using noise-canceling headphones, and creating a quiet space where Giovanni could retreat when overwhelmed. A structured daily routine was introduced, incorporating visual schedules and reminders to help Giovanni stay organized and manage his time effectively. Occupational therapy focused on developing coping strategies for sensory processing issues and improving daily living skills. Social skills training was provided to enhance Giovanni's ability to engage in social interactions, and cognitive behavioral therapy (CBT) was employed to address anxiety and build resilience. Additionally, a personal care assistant was hired to help with essential tasks such as grocery shopping and meal preparation. This support was crucial in helping Giovanni maintain a clean and organized living space while also alleviating some of the stress associated with daily responsibilities. Giovanni's journey toward independent living saw notable improvements as a result of the implemented strategies. He reported a significant reduction in sensory-related distress, better management of daily tasks, and increased confidence in social situations. The personalized environment adjustments proved essential in creating a comfortable living space tailored to his sensory needs. One critical lesson learned was the importance of flexibility and ongoing assessment in support plans; Giovanni's needs evolved over time, necessitating regular adjustments to his support strategies. The case underscores the value of a multifaceted approach that combines environmental modifications, therapeutic interventions, and practical assistance to achieve successful independent living outcomes for individuals with autism.

9.2 Case study 2: Vocational training and employment for an individual with ID and ADHD

Sara, a 30-year-old woman with ID and ADHD, encountered significant difficulties in maintaining stable employment due to her symptoms, including inattention, impulsivity, and difficulties with time management. Sara's previous employment history was marked by frequent job changes, driven by performance challenges related to her ADHD. Her struggle to stay organized and manage time effectively often resulted in missed deadlines and incomplete tasks, contributing to a cycle of job instability. To improve Sara's employment prospects, a tailored vocational support plan was established. This plan included vocational training that focused on building specific skills relevant to her strengths and areas of difficulty. Workshops on time management, organizational skills, and effective strategies for maintaining focus were integral components of the training. Additionally, Sara was paired with a job coach who provided ongoing support and practical strategies to help her manage her ADHD symptoms in the workplace. The job coach worked with Sara to develop customized organizational tools, such as digital reminders and task management apps, and provided coaching on techniques for sustaining attention during work tasks. Sara was placed in a job that offered flexible scheduling and the option to work remotely, which helped accommodate her need for a less structured work environment. Regular check-ins with a career counselor ensured that any emerging issues were addressed promptly, and adjustments to her work plan were made as needed. The interventions led to substantial improvements in Sara's employment situation and overall quality of life. She successfully secured a stable position that matched her skills and allowed for flexibility, which was critical in managing her ADHD symptoms. The vocational training and job coaching significantly enhanced her ability to perform effectively at work, resulting in improved job satisfaction and reduced job turnover. Sara's increased job stability not only boosted her self-esteem but also contributed to her overall sense of independence and well-being. This case highlights the importance of tailored vocational support and flexible work arrangements in achieving employment success for individuals with ADHD.

9.3 Case study 3: Life skills training for an individual with an intellectual disability

Michele, a 28-year-old with an intellectual disability, experienced considerable difficulties with daily living skills, including cooking, budgeting, and personal hygiene. These challenges often resulted in a disorganized living environment and financial mismanagement, which impacted his independence and overall quality of life. Michele's difficulty with these tasks stemmed from his intellectual disability, which affected his ability to understand and manage complex processes. To address these challenges, a comprehensive life skills training program was implemented. This program included practical exercises and role-playing activities to teach Michele essential skills, such as meal preparation, budgeting, and personal care. Family members played a crucial role in supporting Michele by providing guidance and encouragement during the learning process. They were actively involved in setting up a structured routine and creating a supportive home environment conducive to learning. Community resources also played a significant role. Michele participated in local life skills workshops and supported employment programs designed to enhance daily living skills and foster greater independence. These programs provided hands-on training and opportunities for Michele to practice skills in real-life settings. Community support networks, such as local disability advocacy organizations, offered additional resources and guidance to ensure that Michele had access to the necessary support services. Michele's progress was notable in several areas. He became more proficient in managing his daily routines and demonstrated improved financial management skills. His living environment became more organized, and he was able to maintain personal hygiene more effectively. However, challenges remained, particularly in maintaining consistency and managing unexpected changes to his routine. Continued support from his family, community programs, and ongoing life skills training were essential in addressing these areas of improvement. The case emphasizes the importance of a collaborative approach involving family, community resources, and structured training to support the development of independent living skills for individuals with ID.

10. Conclusions

Independent living is a fundamental objective for NDDs. It encompasses more than merely residing in one's own space; it involves the ability to manage daily life effectively, engage in meaningful social and occupational activities, and lead a fulfilling life with autonomy and dignity. The pursuit of independent living is critical as it empowers individuals to develop self-reliance, participate fully in society, and experience an enhanced quality of life [121]. However, achieving independent living for NDDs presents several challenges. These challenges include cognitive and learning difficulties that impact decision-making and problem-solving, social and communication barriers that hinder interaction and integration, and sensory processing issues that affect daily activities [122]. Addressing these challenges requires a multifaceted approach that involves robust support systems. Family support structures, individualized education programs (IEPs), vocational training, and community-based services are vital components of this approach. For instance, individualized support plans and life skills training help individuals manage daily tasks and navigate social environments, while vocational training provides essential skills for employment. Looking ahead, several emerging trends and research directions promise to further enhance independent living for NDDs. Technological advancements play a pivotal role in this area. Innovations such as smart home technologies, assistive communication devices, and adaptive software are transforming how individuals manage daily activities and interact with their environment [100]. These technologies offer personalized solutions that cater to individual needs, making independent living more accessible and manageable. Additionally, ongoing research into personalized and evidence-based practices is crucial for developing effective interventions and supports. Continued advocacy and policy development are equally important. Advocacy groups and policymakers must work together to address the gaps between policy and practice, ensuring that NDDs receive the resources and support they need. This includes pushing for legislation that accommodates evolving needs and addresses disparities in service availability [120]. Advocates also play a critical role in raising awareness and driving systemic change to create inclusive environments that support independent living. Promoting independence for NDDs has broader societal benefits. It not only enhances the lives of individuals but also contributes to a more inclusive and equitable society. By supporting the independence of all individuals, regardless of their abilities, society benefits from diverse perspectives, increased participation in community life, and the fulfillment of human potential. As we move forward, it is imperative that we continue to invest in research, support systems, and policy enhancements to ensure that every individual has the opportunity to live independently and achieve their full potential.

Acknowledgements

We extend our sincere thanks to all those who have supported our research and development, particularly acknowledging the late Prof. Gilberto Marzano for his inspiring guidance throughout our scientific journey. The authors acknowledge the use of DeepL Write for language polishing of the manuscript.

Conflict of interest

The authors declare no conflict of interest.

Author details

Simone Zorzi[1,2]* and Laura Berteotti[3]

1 Azienda Sanitaria Universitaria Friuli Centrale, Italy Rezekne Academy of Technologies, Rezekne, Latvia

2 Ecoisitituto del Friuli Venezia Giulia, Italy

3 Pyramid Educational Consultants, Udine, Italy

*Address all correspondence to: simone.zorzi@asufc.sanita.fvg.it

References

[1] Bouck EC. Life skills instruction for students with severe intellectual disabilities. Teaching Exceptional Children. 2010;**43**(6):32-40

[2] World Health Organization. International Classification of Functioning, Disability, and Health: ICF. Geneva: World Health Organization; 2001

[3] Wehmeyer ML, Bolding N. Enhanced self-determination of adults with intellectual disabilities as an outcome of moving to community-based work or living environments. Journal of Intellectual Disability Research. 2001;**45**(5):371-383

[4] Zambri IM, Amin AS, Kamil NKM, Akhir NM, Sutan R, Khairuddin KF, et al. Factor affecting independent living of persons with intellectual disabilities: A systematic review. International Journal of Academic Research in Progressive Education and Development. 2023;**12**(1):623-644

[5] Jeste SS. Neurodevelopmental behavioral and cognitive disorders. Continuum: Lifelong Learning in Neurology. 2015;**21**(3):690-714

[6] Ellenkamp JJ, Brouwers EP, Embregts PJ, Joosen MC, van Weeghel J. Work environment-related factors in obtaining and maintaining work in a competitive employment setting for employees with intellectual disabilities: A systematic review. Journal of Occupational Rehabilitation. 2016;**26**:56-69

[7] Johansson M, Björne P, Runesson I, Ahlström G. Healthy ageing in people with intellectual disabilities from managers' perspective: A qualitative study. In: Healthcare; Vol. 5(3). MDPI; 2017. p. 45. DOI: 10.3390/healthcare5030047

[8] American Psychiatric Association. Diagnostic and Statistical Manual of Mental Disorders. 5th ed. Arlington, VA: American Psychiatric Publishing; 2013

[9] Roos E, Søndenaa E. Improving the transition process to independent living for adolescents with profound intellectual disabilities. Experiences of parents and employees. BMC Health Services Research. 2020;**20**:1-12

[10] Agarwal R, Heron L, Burke SL. Evaluating a postsecondary education program for students with intellectual disabilities: Leveraging the parent perspective. Journal of Autism and Developmental Disorders. 2021;**51**:2229-2240

[11] Chan W, Smith LE, Hong J, Greenberg JS, Lounds Taylor J, Mailick MR. Factors associated with sustained community employment among adults with autism and co-occurring intellectual disability. Autism. 2018;**22**(7):794-803

[12] Holburn S, Vietze PM. Person-centered planning: A focus on outcomes. Journal of Applied Research in Intellectual Disabilities. 2002;**15**(3):238-250

[13] Americans with Disabilities Act. Public Law 101-336. 1990. Available from: https://www.ada.gov/pubs/ada.htm

[14] Schalock RL, Verdugo MA, Bonham GS, Fantova F, Van Loon J. The conceptualization and measurement of quality of life: Implications for program

planning and evaluation in the field of intellectual disabilities. Evaluation and Program Planning. 2002;**25**(3):229-238

[15] Buescher AV, Cidav Z, Knapp M, Mandell DS. Costs of autism spectrum disorders in the United Kingdom and the United States. JAMA Pediatrics. 2014;**168**(8):721-728

[16] Schalock RL. Quality of life and support needs: Bridging the gap between policy and practice. Journal of Intellectual Disability Research. 2017;**61**(3):279-288. DOI: 10.1111/jir.12345

[17] Carter EW, Lane KL, Pierson MR, Stang KK. Promoting self-determination for transition-age youth: Views of high school general and special educators. Exceptional Children. 2012;**78**(3):334-349

[18] Terras MM, Boyle EA, Ramsay J, Jarrett D. The opportunities and challenges of serious games for people with an intellectual disability. British Journal of Educational Technology. 2018;**49**(4):690-700

[19] Bryant BR, Seay PC. The role of assistive technology in supporting the independence of individuals with disabilities. Disability and Rehabilitation: Assistive Technology. 2017;**12**(1):1-10

[20] Cullen JM, Simmons-Reed EA, Weaver L. Using 21st century video prompting technology to facilitate the independence of individuals with intellectual and developmental disabilities. Psychology in the Schools. 2017;**54**(9):965-978

[21] Bennett R, Vijaygopal R, Kottasz R. Willingness of people with mental health disabilities to travel in driverless vehicles. Journal of Transport & Health. 2019;**12**:1-12

[22] Morris-Rosendahl DJ, Crocq MA. Neurodevelopmental disorders—The history and future of a diagnostic concept. Dialogues in Clinical Neuroscience. 2020;**22**(1):65-72

[23] Parenti I, Rabaneda LG, Schoen H, Novarino G. Neurodevelopmental disorders: From genetics to functional pathways. Trends in Neurosciences. 2020;**43**(8):608-621

[24] Lichtenstein P, Carlström E, Råstam M, Gillberg C, Anckarsäter H. The genetics of autism spectrum disorders and related neuropsychiatric disorders in childhood. American Journal of Psychiatry. 2010;**167**(11):1357-1363

[25] Thapar A, Rutter M. Neurodevelopment mental disorders. In: Rutter's child. Adolescent Psychiatry; 2015. pp. 31-40. DOI: 10.1002/9781118381953.ch3

[26] Schalock RL, Borthwick-Duffy SA, Bradley VJ, Buntinx WHE, Coulter DL, Craig EM, et al. Intellectual Disability: Definition, Classification, and Systems of Supports. 11th ed. Washington, DC: American Association on Intellectual and Developmental Disabilities; 2010

[27] Antolini G, Colizzi M. Where do neurodevelopmental disorders go? Casting the eye away from childhood towards adulthood. In: Healthcare. Vol. 11(7). MDPI; 2023, April. p. 1015

[28] Lord C, Elsabbagh M, Baird G, Veenstra-VanderWeele J. Autism spectrum disorder. The Lancet. 2020;**392**(10146):508-520

[29] Hyman SL, Levy SE, Myers SM. Identification, evaluation, and management of children with autism spectrum disorder. Pediatrics. 2020;**145**(1):e20193447

[30] Maenner MJ, Shaw KA, Baio J, Washington A, Patrick M, DiRienzo M, et al. Prevalence of autism spectrum disorder among children aged 8 years—Autism and developmental disabilities monitoring network, 11 sites, United States, 2016. MMWR Surveillance Summaries. 2020;**69**(4):1

[31] Polanczyk G, de Lima MS, Horta BL, Biederman J, Rohde LA. The worldwide prevalence of ADHD: A systematic review and metaregression analysis. American Journal of Psychiatry. 2007;**164**(6):942-948

[32] Maulik PK, Mascarenhas MN, Mathers CD, Dua T, Saxena S. Prevalence of intellectual disability: A meta-analysis of population-based studies. Research in Developmental Disabilities. 2011;**32**(2):419-436

[33] Robinson KE, Kaizar E, Catroppa C, Godfrey C, Yeates KO. Systematic review and meta-analysis of cognitive interventions for children with central nervous system disorders and neurodevelopmental disorders. Journal of Pediatric Psychology. 2014;**39**(8):846-865

[34] Barkley RA. Attention-Deficit Hyperactivity Disorder: A Handbook for Diagnosis and Treatment. 4th ed. The Guilford Press; 2015

[35] Matson JL, Neal D. Seemingly meaningless behaviors in children with autism: Pica and other disorders. Research in Autism Spectrum Disorders. 2009;**3**(3):423-431. DOI: 10.1016/j.rasd.2008.09.003

[36] Lai MC, Lombardo MV, Baron-Cohen S. Autism. The Lancet. 2014;**383**(9920):896-910. DOI: 10.1016/S0140-6736(13)61539-1

[37] Howlin P, Moss P. Adults with autism spectrum disorders. Canadian Journal of Psychiatry. 2012;**57**(5):275-283. DOI: 10.1177/070674371205700502

[38] Baranek GT. Efficacy of sensory and motor interventions for children with autism. Journal of Autism and Developmental Disorders. 2002;**32**(5):397-422. DOI: 10.1023/A:1020541906063

[39] Dunn W. Supporting children to participate successfully in everyday life by using sensory processing knowledge. Infants & Young Children. 2007;**20**(2):84-101. DOI: 10.1097/01.IYC.0000264477.05076.5d

[40] Gilissen C, Hehir-Kwa JY, Thung DT, Van De Vorst M, Van Bon BW, Willemsen MH, et al. Genome sequencing identifies major causes of severe intellectual disability. Nature. 2014;**511**(7509):344-347

[41] Collier M, Griffin MM, Wei Y. Learning from students about transition needs: Identifying gaps in knowledge and experience. Journal of Vocational Rehabilitation. 2017;**46**(1):1-10

[42] Ioanna D. Independent living of individuals with intellectual disability: A combined study of the opinions of parents, educational staff, and individuals with intellectual disability in Greece. International Journal of Developmental Disabilities. 2020;**66**(2):153-159

[43] Sandjojo J, Gebhardt WA, Zedlitz AM, Hoekman J, den Haan JA, Evers AW. Promoting independence of people with intellectual disabilities: A focus group study perspectives from people with intellectual disabilities, legal representatives, and support staff. Journal of Policy and Practice in Intellectual Disabilities. 2019;**16**(1):37-52

[44] Shakespeare T. Disability Rights and Wrongs. London: Routledge; 2006

[45] Mansell J. Supporting people with intellectual disabilities: Options and approaches. Journal of Intellectual Disabilities. 2010;**14**(4):321-336

[46] Stancliffe RJ, Lakin KC. Costs and Outcomes of Community Services for People with Intellectual Disabilities. Brookes Publishing; 2005

[47] Wehmeyer ML, Patton JR. The Praeger International Handbook of Special Education. ABC-CLIO; 2017

[48] Racino JA. Center for Independent Living (CIL): Disabled People Take the Lead for Full Community Lives. Syracuse Univ., NY: Center on Human Policy; 1991

[49] United Nations. Convention on the Rights of Persons with Disabilities. New York: United Nations; 2006

[50] Fullana J, Pallisera M, Vila M, Valls MJ, Díaz-Garolera G. Intellectual disability and independent living: Professionals' views via a Delphi study. Journal of Intellectual Disabilities. 2020;**24**(4):433-447

[51] Šiška J, Beadle-Brown J. Report on the transition from institutional care to community-based services in 27 EU member states. European Expert Group on Transition from Institutional to Community-Based Care. 2020

[52] Kozma A, Mansell J, Beadle-Brown J. Outcomes in different residential settings for people with intellectual disability: A systematic review. American Journal on Intellectual and Developmental Disabilities. 2009;**114**(3):193-222

[53] van Dam K, Gielissen M, Bles R, van der Poel A, Boon B. The impact of assistive living technology on perceived independence of people with a physical disability in executing daily activities: A systematic literature review. Disability and Rehabilitation: Assistive Technology. 2024;**19**(4):1262-1271

[54] Carter EW. Research on disability and congregational inclusion: What we know and where we might go. Journal of Disability & Religion. 2023;**27**(2):179-209

[55] Zorzi S, Strods G. Overcoming social inclusion barriers for people with intellectual disability. In: Society. Integration. Education. Proceedings of the International Scientific Conference. Vol. IV. Special Pedagogy, Social Pedagogy, Information Technologies In Education; 22-23 May 2020. pp. 187-195. DOI: 10.17770/sie2020vol4.5176

[56] Cannella-Malone H, Sigafoos J, O'Reilly M, de la Cruz B, Edrisinha C, Lancioni GE. Comparing video prompting to video modeling for teaching daily living skills to six adults with developmental disabilities. Education and Training in Developmental Disabilities. 2006:344-356

[57] Krell K, Haugen K, Torres A, Santoro SL. Description of daily living skills and independence: A cohort from a multidisciplinary down syndrome clinic. Brain Sciences. 2021;**11**(8):1012

[58] Puyaltó C, Pallisera M. Living independently in Spain: Barriers and supports from the views of people with intellectual disabilities. International Journal of Disability, Development and Education. 2020;**67**(3):306-319

[59] Harrison P, Oakland T. Adaptive Behavior Assessment System. 2nd ed. Harcourt Assessment; 2003

[60] Schalock RL et al. Intellectual Disability: Definition, Diagnosis, Classification, and Systems of Supports. AAIDD; 2021. DOI: 10.1352/1944-7558-126.6.439

[61] Switzky HN. Cognitive functioning and cognitive therapy in individuals with intellectual disabilities. In: Jacobson W, Mulick JA, editors. Handbook of Intellectual and Developmental Disabilities. Springer; 2006. pp. 355-372

[62] Shogren KA, Wehmeyer ML, Martinis J, Blanck P. Supported Decision-Making: Theory, Research, and Practice to Enhance Self-Determination and Quality of Life. Cambridge University Press; 2018. DOI: 10.1017/9781108633314

[63] Matson JL, Sturmey P, editors. International Handbook of Autism and Pervasive Developmental Disorders. New York, Dordrecht, Heidelberg, London: Springer; 2011. DOI: DOI 10.1007/978-1-4419-8065-6

[64] Emerson E, Hatton C. People with intellectual disabilities: Self-report on life experiences. Advances in Mental Health and Intellectual Disabilities. 2008;**2**(1):3-14

[65] Guralnick MJ. Early intervention for children with intellectual disabilities: A review. Journal of Intellectual Disability Research. 2005;**49**(3):205-217

[66] Barkley RA. Attention-Deficit Hyperactivity Disorder: A Handbook for Diagnosis and Treatment. Guilford Publications; 2014

[67] Dunn W. The Sensory Profile: User's Manual. Psychological Corporation; 2001

[68] Yell ML, Collins J, Kumpiene G, Bateman D. The individualized education program: Procedural and substantive requirements. Teaching Exceptional Children. 2020;**52**(5):304-318

[69] Bateman BD, Linden MA. Better IEPs: How to Develop Legally Correct and Educationally Useful Programs. Attainment Company; 2012

[70] Turnbull HR, Turnbull AP, Wehmeyer ML. Exceptional Lives: Special Education in today's Schools. Merrill/Prentice Hall; 2010

[71] Cattane N, Richetto J, Cattaneo A. Prenatal exposure to environmental insults and enhanced risk of developing schizophrenia and autism Spectrum disorder: Focus on biological pathways and epigenetic mechanisms. Neuroscience & Biobehavioral Reviews. 2020;**117**:253-278

[72] Sparrow S, Cicchetti D, Balla D, Saulnier C. Vineland Adaptive Behavior Scales, (VABS 3). San Antonio, TX: NCS Pearson INC; 2016

[73] Duncan A, Liddle M, Stark LJ. Iterative development of a daily living skills intervention for adolescents with autism without an intellectual disability. Clinical Child and Family Psychology Review. 2021;**24**(4):744-764

[74] Brown L, Percy M. Practical exercises in life skills training: A review. Journal of Special Education. 2007;**41**(1):56-65

[75] Wehman P. In: Paul H, editor. Life beyond the Classroom: Transition Strategies for Young People with Disabilities. Baltimore, Maryland: Brookes Publishing; 2013

[76] Laragy C. Self-determination within Australian school transition programs for students with a disability. Journal of Intellectual and Developmental Disability. 2004;**29**(4):393-402

[77] Francescutti C, Fusaro G, Leonardi M, Martinuzzi A, Sala M, Russo E, et al. Italian ICF training programs: Describing and promoting human functioning and research. Disability and Rehabilitation. 2009;**31**(Suppl. 1):S46-S49

[78] Lemay R. Deinstitutionalization of people with developmental disabilities: A review of the literature. Canadian Journal of Community Mental Health. 2009;**28**(1):181-194

[79] Verdonschot MM, De Witte LP, Reichrath E, Buntinx WH, Curfs LM. Community participation of people with an intellectual disability: A review of empirical findings. Journal of Intellectual Disability Research. 2009;**53**(4):303-318

[80] O'Brien J, O'Brien CL. The principles of person-centered planning. Journal of Applied Research in Intellectual Disabilities. 2002;**15**(2):92-101

[81] Cimera RE. The employment outcomes of individuals with intellectual disabilities: A review. Journal of Vocational Rehabilitation. 2011;**34**(2):95-105

[82] Lysaght R, Kranenburg R, Armstrong C, Krupa T. Participant recruitment for studies on disability and work: Challenges and solutions. Disability and Work. 2015;**26**(2):125-140

[83] Hedley D, Uljarević M, Cameron L, Halder S, Richdale A, Dissanayake C. Employment programmes and interventions targeting adults with autism spectrum disorder: A systematic review of the literature. Autism: The International Journal of Research and Practice. 2017;**21**(8):929-941

[84] Francescutti C, Diminutto M, Zorzi S. Work and occupation. In: Bertelli MO, Deb Ss, Munir K, Hassiotis A, Salvador-Carulla L, editors. Textbook of Psychiatry for Intellectual Disability and Autism Spectrum Disorder. Switzerland AG: Springer Nature; 2022. pp. 941-968

[85] Zwicker J, Zaresani A, Herb Emery JC. Describing heterogeneity of unmet needs among adults with a developmental disability: An examination of the 2012 Canadian survey on disability. Research in Developmental Disabilities. 2017;**65**:1-11

[86] Dempsey I, Keen D. A review of processes and outcomes in family-centered services for children with a disability. Topics in Early Childhood Special Education. 2008;**28**(1):42-52

[87] Dufresne P, Légaré F. Transition planning for youth with intellectual disabilities: An analysis of policies and practices. Journal of Policy and Practice in Intellectual Disabilities. 2012;**9**(4):248-258

[88] Neufeld A, Harrison MJ, Stewart MJ, Hughes KD. Advocacy of marginalized populations: Nursing perspectives on health policy and social justice. Policy, Politics, & Nursing Practice. 2002;**3**(3):240-248

[89] Mansell J, Beadle-Brown J. Active Support: Enabling and Empowering People with Intellectual Disabilities. Jessica Kingsley Publishers; 2012

[90] Bigby C. Social inclusion and people with intellectual disability and challenging behaviour: A systematic review. Journal of Intellectual and Developmental Disability. 2012;**37**(3):1-11

[91] Perry J, Felce D, Kerr M. Outcomes for people with intellectual disabilities in supported accommodation in the community: A systematic review. Journal of Policy and Practice in Intellectual Disabilities. 2013;**10**(1):1-14

[92] Hawkins R, Redley M, Holland AJ. Duty of care and autonomy: How support workers managed the tension between protecting service users from risk and promoting their independence

in a specialist group home. Journal of Intellectual Disability Research. 2011;**55**(9):873-884

[93] Tassé MJ, Wagner JB, Kim M. Using technology and remote support services to promote independent living of adults with intellectual disability and related developmental disabilities. Journal of Applied Research in Intellectual Disabilities. 2020;**33**(3):640-647

[94] Alper S, Raharinirina S. Assistive technology for individuals with disabilities: A review and synthesis of the literature. Journal of Special Education Technology. 2006;**21**(2):47-64

[95] Light J. Shattering the silence: Development of communicative competence by individuals who use AAC. In: Communicative Competence for Individuals Who Use AAC. Brookes Publishing; 2003. pp. 1-38

[96] Martin LJ, Nagalakshmi M. Bridging the social & technical divide in augmentative and alternative communication (AAC) applications for autistic adults. arXiv preprint arXiv:2404.17730. 2024

[97] Edyburn DL. Critical Issues in Special Education Technology Research and Practice. Springer; 2013

[98] Cook AM, Polgar JM. Assistive Technologies: Principles and Practice. Elsevier Health Sciences; 2015

[99] Claes C et al. Person-centered planning for people with intellectual disabilities: An overview. Journal of Applied Research in Intellectual Disabilities. 2010;**23**(3):242-252

[100] Zorzi S, Dalmonego C, De Vreese LP, Gomiero T. Adult Independence living measurement scale: Psychometric validation of a scale to estimate personal skills for independent living in people with intellectual and developmental disabilities. Journal of Intellectual Disability Research. 2023;**67**(6):560-572

[101] Donnellan AM, Leary MR, Schopler E. Goal setting and progress monitoring in the development of independent living skills. Research in Developmental Disabilities. 1985;**6**(1):67-80

[102] Lefebvre H et al. Training life skills: Evidence and practice. Journal of Developmental and Physical Disabilities. 2008;**20**(3):223-239

[103] Cooper JO, Heron TE, Heward WL. Applied Behavior Analysis. 2nd ed. Ohio: Pearson Merrill Prentice Hall; 2007

[104] Carr EG et al. Positive behavior support: Evolution of an applied science. Journal of Positive Behavior Interventions. 2002;**4**(1):4-16

[105] Horner RH et al. Toward a technology of "positive behavior support". Journal of Positive Behavior Interventions. 2002;**4**(2):76-82

[106] Gray C. Social stories: Improving social skills in individuals with autism spectrum disorders. Autism. 2000;**4**(1):71-84

[107] Tomlinson C. Effective Supports Used to Increase Independence in Individuals with Autism Spectrum Disorder. Culminating Projects in Special Education; 2023. p. 156. Available from: https://repository.stcloudstate.edu/sped_etds/156

[108] Lundqvist LO. Social skills training for individuals with intellectual disabilities: An overview. Research in Developmental Disabilities. 2002;**23**(1):1-11

[109] McVilly KR et al. Improving social skills for individuals with intellectual disabilities. Journal of Applied Research in Intellectual Disabilities. 2006;**19**(1):1-14

[110] Weld-Blundell I, Shields M, Devine A, Dickinson H, Kavanagh A, Marck C. Vocational interventions to improve employment participation of people with psychosocial disability, autism and/or intellectual disability: A systematic review. International Journal of Environmental Research and Public Health. 2021;**18**(22):12083

[111] Luecking RG. The role of job coaching in supported employment. Journal of Vocational Rehabilitation. 2009;**31**(2):97-106

[112] Bond GR, Drake RE, Becker DR. An update on supported employment for people with severe mental illness. Psychiatric Services. 2008;**59**(5):518-528

[113] McConkey R, Sowney M, Milligan V, Barr O. Views of people with intellectual disabilities of their present and future living arrangements. Journal of Policy and Practice in Intellectual disabilities. 2004;**1**(3-4):115-125

[114] McCallion P et al. Group homes and community-based living: A review. Journal of Intellectual Disability Research. 2014;**58**(9):832-844

[115] Brodsky G, Marx K. Safe and supportive housing: Concepts and practices. Housing and Society. 2001;**28**(1):24-32

[116] Friedman C. The influence of residence type on personal outcomes. Intellectual and Developmental Disabilities. 2019;**57**:112-126. DOI: 10.1352/1934-9556-57.2.112

[117] Administration for Community Living. About ACL. 2020. Available from: https://www.acl.gov/about-acl

[118] U.S. Department of Education. Office of Special Education Programs. 2020. Available from: https://www2.ed.gov/about/offices/list/osers/osep/index.html

[119] National Disability Rights Network. Annual report 2020. 2020. Available from: https://www.ndrn.org/annual-reports/

[120] The Arc. Advocacy and policy. 2021. Available from: https://thearc.org/advocacy-policy/

[121] Simplican SC, Leader G, Kosciulek J, Leahy M. Self-advocacy and independent living: Key components for achieving independence. Journal of Applied Research in Intellectual Disabilities. 2015;**28**(6):538-550. DOI: 10.1111/jar.12178

[122] Harris J, McBride K. Discrepancies between policy and practice: Implementing the ADA and IDEA. Journal of Disability Policy Studies. 2020;**31**(1):12-24. DOI: 10.1177/1044207319890995

Chapter 4

Lysine Acetyltransferase 6A and Its Paralog: From Biological Functions to Neurodevelopmental Disorders, Cancer and New Therapeutics

Arezousadat Razavi and Xiang-Jiao Yang

Abstract

Post-translational modifications of histones, such as lysine acetylation and methylation, significantly influence chromatin structure in the eukaryotic nucleus. Lysine acetyltransferase 6A (KAT6A) and its paralog, KAT6B, participate in a variety of cellular processes crucial for normal development by influencing cell cycle progression, cell differentiation, signal transduction and responses to cellular stress. Studies using knockout mouse models have revealed the important effects of KAT6A and KAT6B on development, with the absence of the former resulting in embryonic lethality and the loss of the latter causing brain anomalies. Moreover, both KAT6A and KAT6B are implicated in hematopoiesis, including regulation of hematopoietic stem cells and development of various blood cells. These two enzymes also play important roles in neurodevelopment, heart formation, body segment identity, skeletogenesis and craniofacial development. This review is aimed to provide a brief overview of research on KAT6A and KAT6B, especially about their molecular structure and biological functions. Also explored are the latest findings on involvement of KAT6A and KAT6B in governing chromatin functions, gene expression and cellular processes, including roles in histone acetylation and their interaction with other epigenetic regulators. Furthermore, emerging evidence links KAT6A and KAT6B dysfunction to human diseases, with a particular focus on neurodevelopmental disorders and cancer, which has also led to novel therapeutic strategies.

Keywords: ClinVar variant, germline mutation, somatic mutation, neurodevelopmental disorder, cancer, histone acetylation, acylation

1. Introduction

Composed of DNA and histones, chromatin in unique to the eucaryotic nucleus. Post-translational modifications (PTMs) of histones are highly important for regulating chromatin structure [1]. In higher organisms, there are three major groups of histone acetyltransferases (HATs), including the GNAT (Gcn5-related N-acetyltransferase), MYST (MOZ- and p300/CBP families [2–4]. The MYST family of histone acetyltransferases plays a crucial role in chromatin modifications [3]. Initially, the first three founding members of the MYST family were initially identified in the budding yeast and from leukemia human patients [5, 6]. This family is composed of five members, including Tip60 (HIV Tat-interactive protein of 60 kDa), MOZ (monocytic leukemia zinc finger protein), MORF (MOZ-related factor), HBO1 (histone acetyltransferase binding to ORC1), and MOF (male-specific lethal on the first), which have been formally renamed as KAT5, KAT6A, KAT6B, KAT7 and KAT8, respectively, due to their ability to acetylate many non-histone proteins [3]. A notable characteristic of the MYST family members is the highly conserved MYST domain, which comprises an acetyl-CoA binding motif and a zinc finger. This domain serves as the catalytic core and enables the five HATs to acetylate histone proteins, affecting chromatin accessibility and regulating transcriptional activity [2, 7].

The MYST family of HATs has homologs in eukaryotic organisms, including yeasts and plants [8]. These HATs form multisubunit complexes, with those by KAT5 conserved from yeasts to mammal species, whereas those by the remaining KATs are only conserved from worms to humans [4, 8]. Dysfunction of these HATs is linked to many human diseases, including cancer, in agreement with the notion that they participate in many important nuclear processes like DNA repair, transcriptional activation, and cell cycle regulation [9].

KAT6A and KAT6B are involved in a range of developmental processes from embryonic development to organ formation. Notably, they contribute to neural development through controlling neural progenitor proliferation and differentiation and regulating neural stem cell maintenance [10, 11]. This review aims to provide an overview of KAT6A and KAT6B about their molecular and biological functions, as well as their direct links to diseases. We will also describe therapeutic strategies targeting KAT6A and KAT6B [12].

2. Domain organization of KAT6A and KAT6B

KAT6A and KAT6B function in multiunit complexes sharing the trimeric BRPF1-ING5 (or ING4)-EAF6 subcomplex [13, 14]. KAT6A, KAT6B, BRPF1, ING4 and ING5 contain chromatin reader domains for recognizing and binding to specific PTMs on histone tails, and consequently stabilizing the HAT complex on specific regions of chromatin for further chromatin modification and gene regulation [13, 14]. This epigenetic complex contributes to various cellular mechanisms from cell cycle regulation and apoptosis to hematopoiesis, embryonic development, skeletal patterning and neurodevelopment [13–16]. In this section, we discuss domain composition of MOZ and MORF, and emphasize their roles in catalyzing histone acetylation and recognizing histone modifications, for consequently understanding the functioning at the chromatin level.

The NEMM domain (N-terminal part of Enok, MOZ/MORF) is located at the N-terminus of KAT6A and KAT6B [8]. It has sequence homology to the N-terminal regions of the Drosophila Enok protein and the human MOZ and MORF proteins. Some similarities have been found between the C-terminal part of NEMM domain and Histones H1 and H5; however, the exact function remains unclear [8]. There is an H-15 like domain within this region which promotes nuclear targeting [8].This domain has been proposed to have a role in transcriptional regulation [17].

The double PHD fingers (PHD1 and PHD2) are tandem plant homeodomains within KAT6A/KAT6B [8]. The double PHD fingers are capable of recognizing histone H3 tails, particularly acetylated H3K14 and H3K9 [18, 19]. This interaction may facilitate the recruitment of KAT6A/B to specific chromatin regions and promote acetylation of nearby histone H3 tails [20].

The MYST catalytic domain is responsible for the histone acetyltransferase activity of KAT6A and KAT6B [8]. The MYST domain transfers an acetyl group from acetyl-CoA to the ε-amino group of lysine residues on histone tails [21]. Studies on recombinant MORF indicate that the full-length protein shows higher activity than the MYST domain in isolation. This suggests that other domains or interactions with additional proteins might regulate the HAT activity of the MYST domain [8]. Mutations in this domain have shown to affect the catalytic activity of the protein and protein stability [8].

The acidic domain is located in the C-terminal region of KAT6A or KAT6B and is rich in two negatively charged amino acid residues, glutamate and aspartate [8]. In KAT6B, most mutations in this domain are related to Genitopatellar syndrome [10], a rare genetic disorder characterized by lower extremities, genitals, and brain abnormalities. This domain might have transcriptional activation activity, and its overall negative charge might facilitate protein-protein interactions [22].

The serine- and methionine-rich (SM) domain is located at the C-terminus of KAT6A and KAT6B, and as the name indicates, is enriched in serine and methionine residues [8]. While both MOZ and MORF contain SM domains, there is a notable difference in their composition. The SM domain of MOZ contains an insertion of a proline/glutamine-rich (PQ) stretch absent in the SM domain of MORF. Interestingly, the presence of this PQ stretch in MOZ appears to reduce its activation potential compared to the SM domain of MORF [19]. The SM domain has been implicated in transcriptional activation, possibly through interactions with other transcriptional regulators [17]. The SM domain can significantly enhance transcriptional activity when fused to DNA-binding domains like Gal4 or LexA. This activation function has been observed in both mammalian cells and yeast, suggesting a conserved mechanism across species [19].These domains work together to regulate the chromatin targeting, histone acetylation, and transcriptional functions of the KAT6A/KAT6B-containing complexes. Mutations affecting these domains can disrupt the normal functions of these complexes and lead to developmental disorders and cancers (**Figures 1** and **2**).

3. Molecular and cellular functions of KAT6A and KAT6B

3.1 Role in regulating gene expression

KAT6A and KAT6B contribute to gene regulation by acetylating histone H3 at different lysine residues *in vitro*, but mainly lysine 23 *in vivo* [23, 24]. KAT6A and KAT6B function as key regulators of gene expression. They achieve this through their HAT activity, which modifies histones, the proteins responsible for packaging DNA. This modification, known as acetylation, affects DNA accessibility to transcription factors, hence influencing gene expression levels. KAT6A primarily acetylates H3K9 and H3K23, while KAT6B focuses on H3K23 acetylation, although it can also acetylate H3K9 and H3K14 [25].

MOZ and MORF contain several distinct domains. These include the NEMM domain, a double plant homeodomain (PHD) finger, the MYST domain, and regions rich in glutamate/aspartate and serine/methionine [15]. The glutamate/aspartate-rich and serine/methionine-rich domains are located in the C-terminal portion of MOZ/MORF proteins. Research has shown that these domains play a role in activating

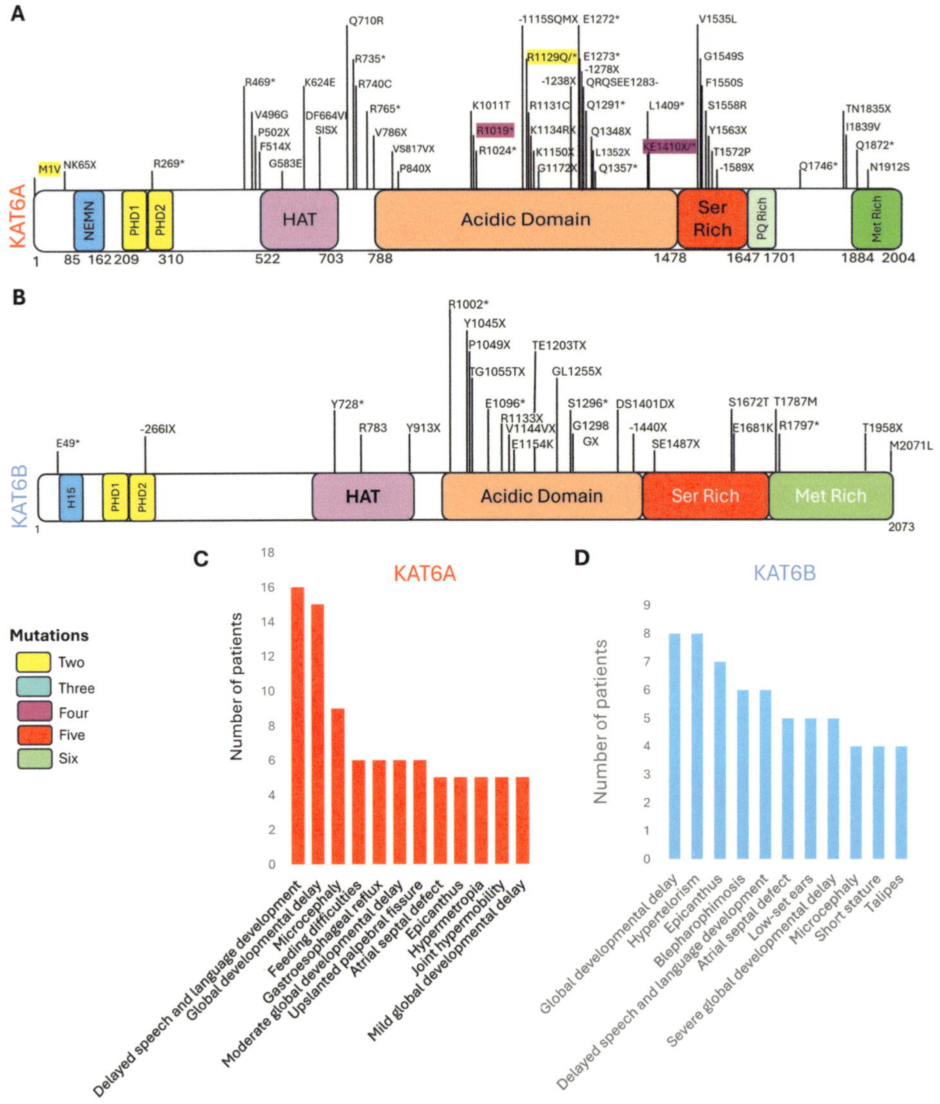

Figure 1.

Mutation profile of KAT6A and KAT6B in neurodevelopmental disorders. (A-B) Mutations in KAT6A (A) and KAT6B (B) are associated with different phenotypes. Mutations are visualized across the KAT6A (A) and KAT6B (B) proteins and their domains. Yellow, blue, purple, red, and green reflect two, three, four, five, and six mutations in specific amino acids of the proteins, respectively. (C-D) Phenotype present in patients with the KAT6A (C) and KAT6B (D) mutations. Delayed speech and language development are the most common phenotype across the samples with KAT6A mutations. Y-axis indicates the number of patients, and X-axis shows phenotypes. All analyses and visualizations in all panels were done based on data downloaded from DECIPHER v11.27.

transcription [17, 19]. Research findings provide evidence for this role, demonstrating that the serine/methionine-rich domain can interact with and stimulate the activity of several transcription factors, including RUNX1, RUNX2, and TP53 [26, 27]. Additionally, chromosomal translocations frequently result in leukemic protein fusions involving MOZ/MORF. In these fusion proteins, the glutamate/aspartate-rich and serine/methionine-rich domains are typically missing. This loss may interfere with the usual MOZ-regulated gene expression patterns, which could lead to cancer

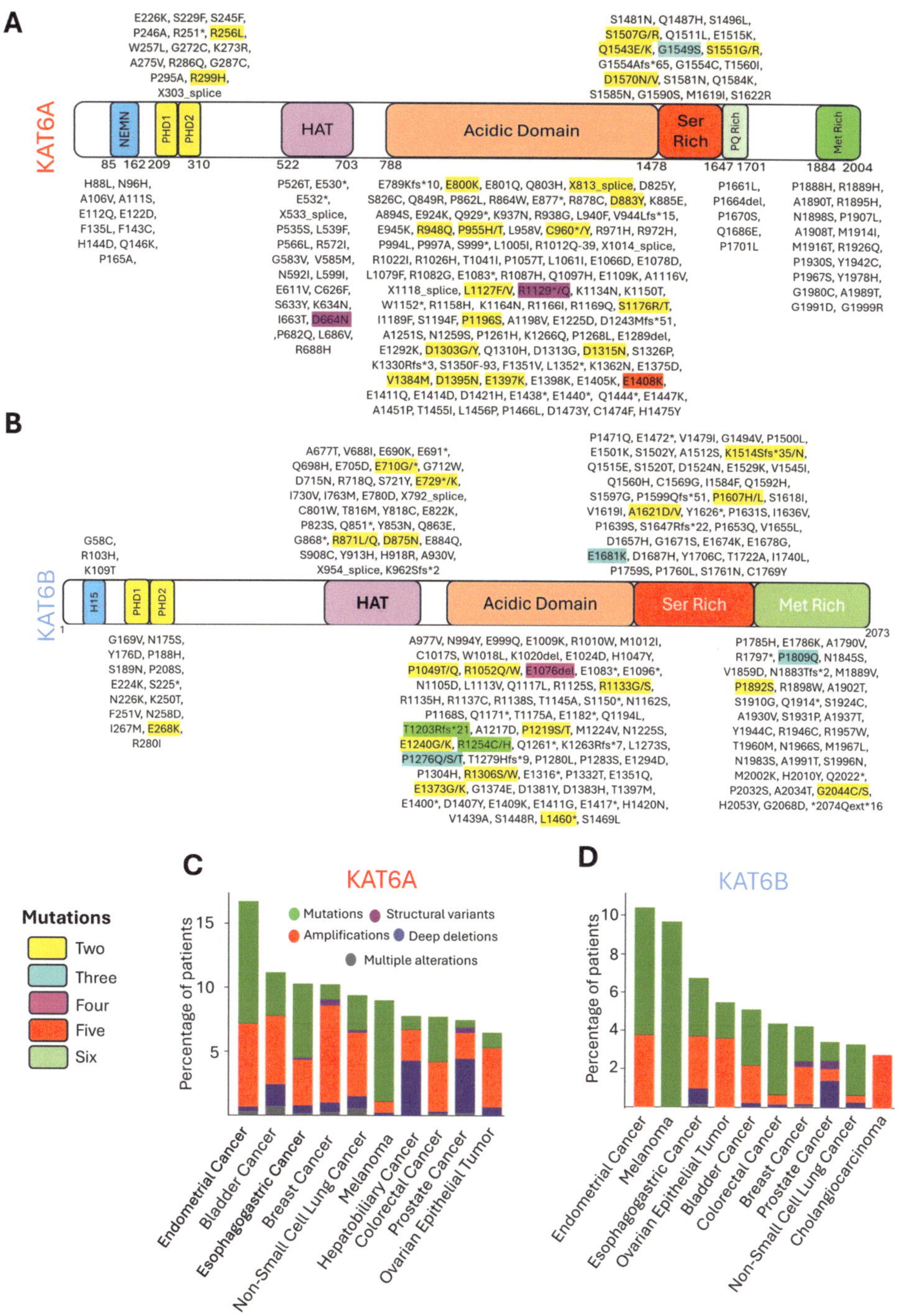

Figure 2.
Mutation profile of KAT6A and KAT6B in different types of cancer. (A-B) Mutations present in different protein domains of KAT6A (A) and KAT6B (B) across 33 cancer types are visualized. Mutations are profiled and visualized based on the domain and their location in the KAT6A and KAT6B proteins. Yellow, blue, purple, red, and green reflect two, three, four, five, and six mutations in specific amino acids of the proteins, respectively. (C-D) Presence of different genetic abnormalities in the KAT6A *(A) and* KAT6B *(B) genes in different types of cancers. Data for all genetic abnormalities for different cancers are downloaded from cBioPortal. The top 10 cancer types based on the percentage of patients (Y-axis) carrying KAT6A and KAT6B genetic abnormalities are visualized. Color key highlights the type of genetic abnormalities in each cancer type.*

development [28]. RNA polymerase 2 may interact with N-terminal region (1–84) of MOZ, likely playing a role in gene regulation [29]. Furthermore, this N-terminal region may identify unmethylated CPG islands on DNA both *in vivo* and in *vitro*. This recognition is essential for guiding MOZ/MORF and its histone acetyltransferase (HAT) activity to specific genomic locations [29]. The winged helix 1 (WH1) domain plays a crucial role in identifying unmethylated CpG sites. It works in conjunction with the winged helix 2 (WH2) domain to attach to nucleosomes [29, 30].

The N-terminal region of MOZ or MORF protein contains the double PHD finger (DPF) and MYST domains, which have been extensively investigated. Initial studies revealed that the DPF domain interacts with the N-terminal portion of the histone H3 tail, facilitating the protein's association with chromatin. Interestingly, this interaction is enhanced when either lysine 9 or 14 on histone H3 (H3K9 or H3K14) is acetylated. However, modification or methylation of lysine 4 on histone H3 (H3K4) significantly weakens this interaction [31]. Recent biochemical, structural, and chromatin immunoprecipitation (ChIP) studies have revealed a specific *in vivo* communication mechanism involving the DPF domain [32]. This domain recognizes acetylated lysine 14 on histone H3 (H3K14ac), which is deposited by another histone acetyltransferase, HBO1/KAT7. This recognition then prompts MOZ/MORF to acetylate lysine 23 on histone H3 (H3K23) in the surrounding area [33].

Initial laboratory experiments examining the histone acetyltransferase activity of MOZ's MYST domain demonstrated its ability to acetylate isolated histones H3, H4, and H2A. However, the domain alone was insufficient to acetylate histones within nucleosomes [14, 19, 27]. A small region in the MYST domain's C-terminal part is responsible for interaction with BRPF1 [14]. This interaction allows MOZ to acetylate histone H3 tails within nucleosomal structures efficiently. Furthermore, BRPF1 augments MOZ's ability to coactivate transcription, suggesting that the formation of this complex aids MOZ in targeting specific genomic regions to stimulate gene expression.

The MOZ-BRPF1 acetyltransferase complex possesses multiple chromatin-interacting domains, leading to various proposed mechanisms for its chromatin recruitment. For instance, ING4/5 and BRPF1 appear to guide the complex to active transcription sites through their affinity for H3K4me3 [34] or H3K36me3 [35]. Additionally, MOZ's C-terminal region has been shown to interact with various transcription factors [26, 27, 36, 37], potentially directing the complex to specific gene subsets. The complex's ability to recognize particular histone post-translational modifications suggests that its positioning is influenced by other histone-modifying complexes, such as the recognition of HBO1-deposited H3K14ac by the MOZ DPF reader domain [33].

3.2 Role in DNA damage response and cellular senescence

MOZ/KAT6A plays a crucial role in DNA repair by recognizing and responding to DNA double-strand breaks (DSBs). When a DSB occurs, the surrounding chromatin is modified, notably through the phosphorylation of histone H2AX to form γ-H2AX, which signals the recruitment of repair proteins, including KAT6A. It interacts with γ-H2AX and other DNA damage response proteins, facilitating its localization to the DSBs. Once at the break site, MOZ promotes chromatin remodeling, making the DNA more accessible to other repair proteins. The recruitment of MOZ to DSBs is facilitated by its interaction with the DNA damage response protein 53BP1. At these sites, MOZ acetylates histone H4 on lysine 16 (H4K16), which is crucial for the accessibility of chromatin structure and the subsequent recruitment of DNA repair factors [38].

This process is essential for homologous recombination (HR), an error-free repair pathway that uses a homologous sequence as a template to accurately repair the break, thereby maintaining genomic stability and preventing mutations that could lead to cancer [38–41].

Furthermore, the involvement of BRPF1 in this process has also been demonstrated. BRPF1 depletion leads to a decrease in H3 acetylation levels in response to DNA damage, suggesting that BRPF1 is important for MOZ-mediated histone acetylation during the DNA repair process [42].

KAT6A is a key factor in the DNA damage response and premature cellular senescence pathways. It directly interacts with p53, a key tumor suppressor protein, and is essential for p53-dependent regulation of p21 expression in response to DNA damage. Upon cellular stress such as UV irradiation, MOZ is recruited to promyelocytic leukemia nuclear bodies (PML-NBs), also known as nuclear domain, and plays a crucial role in cellular stress responses and apoptosis, where it forms a ternary complex with PML and p53. This interaction enhances MOZ's ability to acetylate p53 at lysine residues K120 and K382, which in turn promotes p53-dependent p21 expression. The acetylation of p53 by MOZ appears to play a role in selective gene regulation, particularly favoring p21 expression over other p53 target genes like Bax [43].

The importance of MOZ in the DNA damage response is further emphasized by experiments with MOZ knockout mouse embryonic fibroblasts (MEFs). These MOZ-deficient cells show impaired p21 expression and fail to arrest in G1 phase in response to DNA damage [32]. Moreover, loss of MOZ contributes to resistance to PML-induced premature senescence, suggesting its crucial role in the DNA damage-induced senescence pathway. The study also reveals an interesting regulatory mechanism involving Akt kinase. Akt-mediated phosphorylation of MOZ at T369 inhibits its interaction with PML, thereby suppressing p53 acetylation and p21 expression, and consequently preventing premature cell senescence. However, in cellular stress situations like arsenic exposure, hypoxia and UV radiation, PML suppresses Akt activity, leading to increased PML-MOZ interaction, enhanced p21 expression, and p53-dependent premature senescence. This provides a novel link between the PI3K-Akt signaling pathway and p53-mediated cellular responses to DNA damage [43].

Moreover, the researchers found that a leukemia-associated MOZ-CBP fusion protein inhibits p53-mediated transcription, suggesting that disruption of normal MOZ function might contribute to leukemogenesis [43]. Interestingly, p53 has been shown to regulate the expression of MOZ itself, creating a feedback loop. Under normal conditions, p53 represses MOZ expression, but this repression is relieved under stress conditions, allowing for increased MOZ-mediated acetylation of p53 and other targets [44].

While BRPF1's direct involvement in p53 acetylation is less clear, its role as a scaffold protein in the MOZ complex suggests that it likely facilitates MOZ's interaction with and acetylation of p53. BRPF1 depletion has been shown to affect cellular responses to stress, including DNA damage responses [42].

3.3 Roles in pathological processes

Mutations in *KAT6A* and *KAT6B* genes can lead to developmental disorders collectively termed as KAT6 syndromes. These syndromes are characterized by intellectual disability, developmental delay, and various neurological and physical abnormalities [10]. The specific characteristics and severity of these syndromes vary depending on the location and type of mutation. Missense mutations often affect highly conserved residues within the MYST domain or other functionally important regions, potentially altering protein function [22].

Both KAT6A and KAT6B exhibit complex and context-dependent roles in cancer development. They can function as oncogenes, promoting tumor growth, or as tumor suppressors, inhibiting cancer progression. This duality is evident in their involvement in different types of cancer [10].

KAT6A is frequently involved in chromosomal translocations in acute myeloid leukemia (AML), leading to the formation of fusion proteins with altered functionality that contribute to leukemogenesis [10, 45]. For instance, KAT6A fusion with CREB-binding protein (CBP) disrupts normal gene regulation, affecting cell differentiation and proliferation, ultimately driving the development of AML [10, 45–47].

In solid tumors like glioblastoma (GBM), *KAT6A* overexpression contributes to tumor growth by activating the PI3K/AKT signaling pathway, a pathway crucial for cell growth and proliferation [25]. KAT6A achieves this by upregulating the expression of *PIK3CA*, a gene encoding a subunit of the PI3K enzyme. Notably, the sources demonstrate that silencing *KAT6A* in GBM cells suppresses their proliferation, migration, and colony formation, suggesting a potential therapeutic target [25].

KAT6B is also implicated in solid tumors, with its overexpression observed in ovarian high-grade serous carcinomas (HGSCs). This overexpression is associated with poor patient prognosis, highlighting its potential as a prognostic marker. The sources, however, primarily focus on KAT6B's role in ovarian cancer and do not provide direct evidence for KAT6A's involvement [48].

KAT6B proteins exhibit a variety of roles in other cancers. For example, *KAT6B* overexpression is linked to poor prognosis in ovarian, breast, and hepatocellular carcinomas, while its downregulation inhibits cell cycle progression and reduces tumor cell proliferation and migration. Conversely, KAT6B acts as a tumor suppressor in small cell lung cancer and gastric cancer, where its low expression correlates with diminished patient survival [10].

MicroRNAs (miRNAs) are small non-coding RNA molecules that regulate gene expression, including the expression of *KAT6A* and *KAT6B*. These miRNAs can fine-tune KAT6 protein levels, influencing cancer development and response to therapy. For instance, KAT6A is both a target and a repressor of miR-223, creating a feedback loop. Dysregulation of miR-223 expression can affect KAT6A levels, contributing to AML development and potentially influencing treatment response [10].

4. Roles of KAT6A and KAT6B in animal development

4.1 KAT6A in mouse embryonic development

MOZ forms a multi-subunit complex that exhibits acetylation activity towards free histones H3, H4, H2A, and H2B *in vitro* [14, 19, 49–51]. This enzymatic function has significant implications for gene regulation, as histone acetylation in the vicinity of gene promoters is correlated with transcriptional upregulation. Notably, the acetylation activity of the MOZ complex has been demonstrated to modulate the expression of *HOX* genes, which are critical regulators of embryonic development [52].

MOZ's histone acetylation activity plays a crucial role in *HOX* gene regulation. These genes are essential for determining the anterior-posterior (head-to-tail) axis during embryonic development. They control the identity of body segments and the development of limbs and organs. This is evidenced by the fact that inhibiting histone deacetylases (HDACs) rescues the phenotypic effects of MOZ depletion in zebrafish, particularly the reduced expression of *HOXB* genes essential for head formation [53, 54].

Mechanistic studies have shown that MOZ is vital for skeletal development in the head region of zebrafish [54]. Interestingly, *BRPF1* knockout studies in zebrafish produce similar effects to *MOZ* knockout, suggesting that BRPF1 does not have MOZ-independent functions in skeletal development [49, 50]. This mechanism appears to be evolutionarily conserved, as MOZ knockout mice also exhibit defects in craniofacial and caudal skeletons [49]. MOZ has an important impact on *HOX* genes, specifically affecting the anterior expression boundary of *HOX* genes (*Hoxc8/9*) [55].

Moreover, MOZ plays a crucial role in embryonic development by regulating the expression of several essential transcription factor families, including homeobox (*HOX*), T-box (*TBX*), and distal-less homeobox (*DLX*) genes. Studies in zebrafish and mice have demonstrated MOZ's importance in regulating developmental *HOX* genes [53–55]. Knockout experiments have revealed that *MOZ* deletion decreases H3K9 acetylation marks at specific Hox genes, without affecting global H3K9ac levels, as shown by chromatin immunoprecipitation (ChIP) assays [55]. This suggests that the MOZ-BRPF1 complex specifically regulates H3K9ac at developmental genes during embryogenesis. The complex's role in histone acetylation is further supported by *BRPF1* knockout studies in zebrafish, which produce effects similar to *MOZ knockout* [49].

4.2 Role of KAT6A in hematopoiesis

KAT6A exhibits a direct and crucial function in the process of hematopoiesis [45]. It functions as a potent co-activator of the RUNX1 transcription factor, which is widely recognized as the master regulator of hematopoiesis. This co-activator role suggests a mechanistic explanation for MOZ's critical involvement in hematopoietic processes [27, 56]. *MOZ* deletion in mice negatively affects hematopoiesis and leads to embryonic lethality [57, 58]. The acetyltransferase activity of MOZ is essential for proper hematopoiesis, as demonstrated by studies on mice with mutations in MOZ's catalytic site [45]. Moreover, BRPF1 has been reported to be important for MOZ-mediated acetylation in hematopoietic stem cells (HSCs) and its depletion could significantly reduce H3 acetylation in bone marrow [42].

MOZ and MLL (mixed-lineage leukemia) cooperate in regulating HSCs maintenance and differentiation. They co-regulate several genes crucial for hematopoiesis, including *HOX* genes [27, 57]. MOZ regulates the expression of key hematopoietic transcription factors. For instance, it's involved in the regulation of RUNX1, a crucial factor in definitive hematopoiesis [27]. As well, MOZ and MLL are involved in repressing the *INK4A-ARF* locus in HSCs. This locus encodes for p16INK4A and p14ARF (p19ARF in mice), key regulators of cellular senescence [59]. By repressing the *INK4A-ARF* locus, MOZ and MLL contribute to decreased cellular senescence in HSCs, which is crucial for maintaining their self-renewal capacity [59]. Chromosomal translocations involving MOZ or MLL can lead to leukemogenesis. For example, the MOZ-TIF2 fusion protein, resulting from t (8;16) translocation, has been associated with AML [27].

4.3 Roles of KAT6A and KAT6B in neurodevelopment

KAT6A and KAT6B play crucial roles in neurodevelopment. These proteins acetylate histones and non-histone proteins, influencing gene expression and various cellular processes vital for nervous system development. KAT6A, particularly, has been identified as a regulator of *HOX* genes, which are critical for patterning the body during development, including the nervous system. *HOX* genes ensure the proper organization and differentiation of cells along the anterior-posterior axis, impacting brain segmentation and the formation of neural circuits. In zebrafish, loss of KAT6A function leads to defects in hindbrain development, consistent with its role in maintaining *HOX* gene expression [10].

Both KAT6A and KAT6B have been implicated in craniofacial development, a process intimately linked to the development of the peripheral nervous system. Cranial neural crest cells, which contribute to the formation of facial structures, cranial nerves, and ganglia, are particularly sensitive to disruptions in KAT6A/B function. Research indicates that KAT6A is required for the proper migration and differentiation of neural crest cells, impacting the formation of cranial ganglia and the development of cranial nerves [53]. In mice, loss of KAT6A function can result in craniofacial abnormalities, including cleft palate, highlighting its importance in coordinating these developmental processes [10].

KAT6B, has been directly linked to neurogenesis, the process of generating new neurons. Studies in mice have shown that *Kat6b* is essential for the development of the cerebral cortex. Loss of *Kat6b* function disrupts cortical development, impacting the production and migration of neurons. This finding suggests that KAT6B is crucial for maintaining the neural stem cell pool and regulating their differentiation into mature neurons [8, 45].

Since BRPF1 is a key subunit of the MOZ histone acetyltransferase complex, BRPF1 has also implicated in neurodevelopment. BRPF1 knockout in mice leads to multiple defects in brain development, including reduced forebrain size, corpus callosum agenesis, and impaired learning and memory. This study highlighted the importance of BRPF1 in neurodevelopment [60].

The MOZ complex, including BRPF1, is responsible for acetylation of histone H3 at lysine 23 (H3K23ac). This specific histone modification is associated with active gene expression. H3K23ac is enriched at promoters and enhancers of genes involved in neural development. It has been reported that MOZ and its paralog MORF (KAT6B) are the primary acetyltransferases responsible for H3K23ac in neural progenitor cells [24].

Furthermore, MOZ and BRPF1 regulate the expression of key neurodevelopmental genes. MOZ acetylates and activates the transcription factor Neurogenic 2 (Ngn2), a key regulator of neuronal differentiation. This acetylation is crucial for Ngn2's ability to promote neurogenesis [61]. Moreover, KAT6A/B interact with transcription factors crucial for neurodevelopment, such as RUNX1, which is essential for proper development of the central nervous system and hematopoiesis [10].

4.4 Role of KAT6A in controlling immunity and regulating $CD8^+$ T cell responses

KAT6A is crucial for the long-term repopulation of hematopoietic stem cells, which are the precursors of all immune cells, including T cells [58]. KAT6A, is shown to maintain the transcriptional activity of the *CD8* gene locus by acetylating histones (specifically at the promoter and E8I enhancer regions). An important part of this process is maintaining CD8 co-receptor expression, and thereby, strong TCR signaling during T cell activation. In KAT6A-deficient CD8+ T cells, the surface expression of the CD8 co-receptor is significantly reduced during clonal expansion, leading to impaired TCR signaling. This reduction is linked to decreased histone H3 lysine 9 acetylation (H3K9ac) at the Cd8 locus and diminished transcription of the *CD8a* gene.

The absence of KAT6A results in a marked decrease in the number of effector-like memory CD8⁺ T cells, which are critical for the immediate immune response.

In contrast, the formation of long-lived memory T cells (which are crucial for lasting immunity) is less affected. This selective impact on T cell subsets suggests that KAT6A-mediated histone acetylation at the Cd8 locus is particularly important for sustaining effector-like memory T cells while having a minimal effect on long-lived memory T cells. Moreover, removing the CD8 E8I enhancer, a regulatory element essential for maintaining *CD8a* expression, phenocopies the loss of *KAT6A*. Both conditions result in downregulated *CD8* expression and similar defects in T cell function and memory formation, reinforcing the idea that histone acetylation at the *CD8* locus by KAT6A is crucial for regulating T cell fate. The lack of KAT6A-mediated acetylation diminishes *CD8* expression, destabilizes the CD8-TCR complex, and leads to weakened antigen-specific signaling, compromising the generation and maintenance of effector-like memory T cells [62].

4.5 Role of KAT6A in regulating B cell development

KAT6A was found to be crucial for optimal germinal center (GC) responses. In secondary lymphoid organs, germinal centers are specialized areas where B cells proliferate, undergo somatic hypermutation, and change antibody classes. KAT6A-deficient mice showed a reduction in the size and number of germinal centers following immunization. In the absence of KAT6A, there was a decrease in the quantity of Ki67+ (a marker of cell proliferation) B cells, which supported this [63].

Interestingly, despite the impaired germinal center response, the formation of short-lived plasma cells was not significantly affected in KAT6A-deficient mice. This indicates that KAT6A has a distinct function in the germinal center reaction rather than in all aspects of B cell differentiation [63] One of the most striking findings was the severe impairment in the generation of antigen-specific memory B cells in KAT6A-deficient mice compared to wild-type controls, potentially leading to reduced long-term antibody responses and highlighting the importance of KAT6A in maintaining long-lasting immunity [63].

5. KAT6A and KAT6B in neurodevelopmental disorders

As stated before, mutations in MOZ have been associated with neurodevelopmental disorders [22]. *KAT6A* mutations cause KAT6A syndrome (also known as Arboleda-Tham syndrome), a neurodevelopmental disorder characterized by intellectual disability, global developmental delay, microcephaly, hypotonia, and distinctive facial features, arises from pathogenic variants in the *KAT6A* gene (**Figure 1D**) [64]. A majority of reported KAT6A syndrome cases involves *de novo* heterozygous truncating mutations in the *KAT6A* gene, often leading to the loss of the C-terminal transactivation domain. These mutations lead to the production of truncated KAT6A proteins. Truncating mutations in *KAT6A* result in haploinsufficiency, where only one copy of the gene is functional, leading to reduction in the wild-type KAT6A protein level and impaired histone acetylation [22]. The severity of the phenotype may be influenced by the location of the truncating mutation. For example, late-truncating mutations (exons 16-17) in *KAT6A* are associated with more severe intellectual disability and a higher prevalence of certain syndromic features, such as microcephaly, neonatal hypotonia, and gastrointestinal complications, compared to early-truncating mutations [64]. While truncating mutations are more common, missense mutations in *KAT6A* have also been reported. These mutations, which alter a single amino acid in the protein, can have variable effects on KAT6A function and contribute to a broader phenotypic spectrum [65]. The clinical presentation of KAT6A syndrome is diverse, reflecting the widespread impact of KAT6A on neurodevelopment. Key features include intellectual disability and global developmental delay, which are hallmark features of KAT6A syndrome. The severity can range from mild to profound, with individuals often exhibiting significant delays in motor, language, and cognitive milestones [64, 65]. *KAT6A* mutations could affect neural stem cell proliferation and differentiation, leading to a reduced number of neurons and ultimately contributing to microcephaly [11]. Hypotonia is commonly present in KAT6A syndrome, often manifesting as delayed motor development and difficulty with feeding. While the specific mechanisms remain unclear, it's possible that *KAT6A* mutations affect genes involved in neuromuscular junction formation or muscle fiber development [10]. Individuals with KAT6A syndrome often share certain facial characteristics, including a broad nasal tip, thin upper lip, bitemporal narrowing, and low-set or posteriorly rotated ears [65]. Neurobehavioral and psychiatric features are not common among individuals with KAT6A syndrome, but they can exhibit various neurobehavioral and psychiatric features, including autism spectrum disorder-like behaviors, attention deficits, anxiety, and aggression [64]. One study observed decreased expression of schizophrenia-related genes in the prefrontal cortex, accompanied by reduced levels of H3K9ac and H3K14ac at their promoters. This suggests a potential role for reduced histone acetylation in the dysregulation of neurotransmission-related genes, which is often observed in schizophrenia [11, 65].

KAT6B mutations lead to two main syndromes: Say-Barber-Biesecker-Young-Simpson variant of Ohdo syndrome (SBBYSS) and genitopatellar syndrome (GPS). These syndromes share common features like developmental delay, intellectual disability, hypotonia, and distinctive facial features, but also have distinct clinical presentations (**Figure 1E**) [10].

The clinical presentation of KAT6B disorders is highly variable, even among individuals with the same *KAT6B* mutation [66]. Mutations in the proximal part of exon 18 of *KAT6B* are often associated with the more severe GPS phenotype. These mutations may lead to the production of a truncated protein with altered functionality, potentially resulting in a dominant-negative or gain-of-function effect [65, 66]. Mutations located more proximally in the gene or in the distal part of exon 18 are typically associated with SBBYSS or an intermediate phenotype. These mutations are thought to primarily result in *KAT6B* haploinsufficiency, where the reduced amount of functional KAT6B protein leads to a milder phenotype [66]. Most *KAT6B* mutations are *de novo*; however, a few cases of familial inheritance have been reported (**Figure 1E**) [10, 66].

6. KAT6A and KAT6B in cancer

KAT6A and KAT6B can function as both oncogenes and tumor suppressors, depending on the specific cancer type and context. Chromosomal translocations in KAT6A which are leading to fusion proteins and *KAT6A* overexpression in ER+ and GBM are examples of oncogenic activity [10]. As an example of tumor suppressor activity, KAT6B acts as a tumor suppressor in small cell lung cancer and gastric cancer [10]. Low KAT6B expression in these cancers correlates with a diminished patient survival.

In small cell lung cancer, KAT6B downregulation is thought to promote tumor growth by reducing the expression of BRM, a catalytic subunit of the SWI/SNF chromatin remodeling complex [10].

6.1 KAT6A in development of acute myeloid leukemia (AML)

In AML, specific chromosomal translocations involving the *MOZ* gene lead to the formation of fusion proteins that combine MOZ with other proteins such as CBP, p300, or TIF2. These fusion proteins retain the acetyltransferase activity of MOZ, but also gain new functions or lose regulatory controls, contributing to leukemia [45]. MOZ-CBP, resulting from the chromosomal translocation t(8;16) (p11; p13)), is one of the most well-characterized. It combines MOZ with CBP, another acetyltransferase. The MOZ-CBP fusion protein has enhanced transcriptional activity and can aberrantly activate genes that should remain silent, leading to uncontrolled cell proliferation [46, 47]. MOZ-p300, resulting from chromosomal translocation t(8;22) (p11;q13), fuses the N-terminal part of MOZ to the C-terminal part of p300. The resulting fusion protein can recruit other transcriptional regulators, which will further disrupt typical gene expression [19, 47]. While MOZ-CBP affects CBP, MOZ-P300 involves the p300 acetyltransferase. The fusion protein can disrupt normal acetylation patterns, leading to the activation of oncogenes or repression of tumor suppressor genes [47].

MOZ-TIF2 fusion protein, resulting from the chromosomal inversion inv. (8) (p11q13), has been implicated in the pathogenesis of acute myeloid leukemia (AML). This chimeric protein combines elements from two distinct functional entities: MOZ, a member of the MYST family of histone acetyltransferases (HATs), and TIF2, a nuclear receptor coactivator known to interact with CREB binding protein (CBP) [67]. Mechanistic investigations have revealed critical structural requirements for the leukemogenic activity of MOZ-TIF2. The C2HC nucleosome recognition motif of MOZ is essential for cellular transformation, suggesting the importance of chromatin targeting in the oncogenic process. The histone acetyltransferase activity of MOZ is dispensable for the transforming capacity of the fusion protein [67]. This mechanistic insight suggests that the MOZ-TIF2 fusion results in a gain of function for MOZ, contributing to leukemogenesis through altered chromatin interactions and aberrant recruitment of transcriptional coactivators.

6.2 KAT6B in ovarian cancer

MYST4(KAT6B) is overexpressed in ovarian high-grade serous carcinomas (HGSCs) and this overexpression has been linked to decreased patient survival in advanced-stage HGSCs. *MYST4* is significantly overexpressed in HGSCs compared to other ovarian cancer types, like endometrioid carcinomas and clear cell carcinomas [68]. This overexpression is correlated with diminished patient survival, particularly in advanced-stage HGSCs (FIGO stage III/IV). This observation suggests that MYST4 could serve as a potential prognostic marker for HGSC patients (**Figure 2D-E**) [68]. As it is indicated in the graphs, we could see that most ovarian cancers related to KAT6A/B are due to amplifications.

Knockdown of MYST4 in three different cell lines [A2780 (ovarian cancer), SKBR3 (breast cancer) and Huh7 (hepatocellular carcinoma)] significantly reduced cellular proliferation, migration, and cell cycle progression, suggesting that MYST4 promotes tumor growth and progression [68]. *In vivo* studies using Huh7 cells in a mouse xenograft model further confirmed these findings. Mice injected with MYST4-knockdown

Huh7 cells developed significantly smaller tumors compared to those injected with control Huh7 cells, providing strong evidence for MYST4's role in tumor growth [68]. Based on these findings, the study suggests that targeting MYST4 could be a potential therapeutic strategy for treating advanced solid tumors, including HGSCs, that overexpress *MYST* [68]. Moreover, MYST4's role in tumorigenesis might involve regulating the RAS/MAPK signaling pathway via histone H3 acetylation, further supporting its connection to epigenetic modifications and cancer development [68].

6.3 KAT6A in glioblastoma multiforme

Glioblastoma multiforme (GBM) is the most common and aggressive primary brain cancer. One study, using U87 GBM cells, found that *KAT6A* expression is correlated with *PIK3CA* expression [25]. KAT6A upregulates *PIK3CA* expression to activate the PI3K/AKT signaling pathway (crucial pathway involved in regulating a variety of cellular functions, including growth, proliferation, survival, and metabolism), contributing to glioma tumorigenesis. Inhibiting KAT6A suppressed cell proliferation, migration, colony formation, and tumor development in an orthotopic mouse xenograft model [25]. KAT6A acetylates lysine 23 of histone H3 (H3K23), which then recruits TRIM24, a nuclear receptor binding protein. TRIM24 activates *PIK3CA* transcription, enhancing PI3K/AKT signaling. Overexpressing activated *AKT* or *PIK3CA* rescued the growth inhibition caused by *KAT6A* silencing, while the pan-PI3K inhibitor LY294002 counteracted KAT6A's growth-promoting effect [25]. The study concluded that KAT6A plays a crucial role in glioma formation and could be a potential therapeutic target for GBM treatment [25].

6.4 KAT6A in endometrial serous sarcinoma (ESC)

KAT6A and *MYC* amplifications are associated with Endometrial Serous Carcinoma (ESC) worse clinical outcomes [69]. *KAT6A* amplifications correlated with shorter progression-free survival and overall survival, while *MYC* amplifications were linked to advanced disease stage [69]. KAT6A is newly identified as a potential driver in ESC pathogenesis, suggesting new therapeutic targets for this aggressive cancer type (**Figure 2D-E**). As it is indicated in the graphs, endometrial cancer is the most common cancer related to KAT6A/B mutations.

7. Therapeutic strategies targeting KAT6A and KAT6B

7.1 KAT6A/B inhibitors as therapeutics against leukemia

KAT6A is frequently found to be chromosomally translocated in various hematological malignancies, leading to the formation of fusion genes like *KAT6A-CBP* and *KAT6A-TIF2*. These fusion genes contribute to the development of acute myeloid leukemia. Similarly, chromosomal translocations in *KAT6B* have also been identified in various cancers [12]. Inhibiting KAT6A and KAT6B can suppress tumor growth and induce cellular senescence. These altered KATs are important for maintaining the proliferative capacity of cancer cells and they could be a potential target for cancer therapies. WM-8014 and WM-1119 are identified as competitive inhibitors of KAT6A [70]. Crystal structure analysis revealed these compounds compete directly with acetyl-CoA in the binding site, leading to reduced H3K14 acetylation globally and H3K9 acetylation at specific gene loci. The compounds trigger cell cycle arrest in G0/G1 phase and cellular senescence through the p16INK4A-p19ARF pathway, as demonstrated in mouse embryonic fibroblasts. It has been found that WM-8014 led to a concentration-dependent reduction in the level of *E2f2* mRNA and *Cdc6* mRNA which play an important role in cell cycle progression and DNA replication, accompanied by an upregulation of both splice products of the *Cdkn2a* locus, *Ink4a* (inhibits CDK4 and CDK6) and *Arf* (stabilizes p53 by inhibiting its degradation, also functioning as a tumor suppressor) [12].

7.2 KAT6A/B inhibitors as therapeutics for treating ER^+ breast cancer

KAT6 operates through complex epigenetic and hormonal regulatory pathways in ER+ breast cancers. As histone lysine acetyltransferases, KAT6A and its paralog KAT6B specifically catalyze H3K23 acetylation (H3K23ac), which is crucial for lineage-specific gene transcription. In ER+ breast cancer, KAT6A appears to function as an epigenetic activator of ERα, thereby influencing estrogen receptor signaling pathways and hormone-dependent breast cancer growth [71]. KAT6A critical role in Erα (estrogen receptor alpha protein) signaling is conducted through both direct and indirect mechanisms, directly by regulating ERα gene (*ESR1*) expression and protein levels, and indirectly by modulating pioneering transcription factors like FOXA1 and GATA3, while also affecting ER target genes such as *TFF1* (Trefoil Factor 1), which are crucial for estrogen-responsive cellular processes. KAT6A inhibition triggers various cellular effects, including cell cycle arrest in G1 phase, increased apoptosis through enhanced caspase 3/7 activity, and modulation of multiple signaling cascades including glucose metabolism, VEGF signaling, *TP53* transcription, DNA repair, and PIK/AKT pathways.

The amplification of KAT6A is one of the most notable amplifications on 8p11-p12, and its strategic location in this 12–15% breast cancer amplicon implicates it as a potential driver oncogene. Its impact on cell cycle regulation and ability to influence tumor cell proliferation is evidenced by the observation that its inhibition induces cell senescence [71]. The clinical significance of KAT6A in breast cancer is evaluated by the effectiveness of its inhibitor, PF-07248144. Particularly in ER+ breast cancer, it has been demonstrated that after administration of this drug, a median reduction of at least 70% from baseline in H3K23Ac levels in peripheral blood mononuclear cells was achieved. This evidence suggests a potent KAT6 target inhibitor effect, as H3K23Ac is a marker of KAT6A and KAT6B activity [71]. Moreover, there is a reduction in H3K23Ac levels in tumor biopsies from patients, indicating the inhibitory effect on H3K23ac extends to the tumor microenvironment [71].

CTx-648 (PF-9363) is another newly discovered KAT6A/B inhibitor. This selective KAT6A/B inhibitor is a benzisoxazole compound and has shown efficacy against KAT6A-high ER+ breast cancer leading to a decrease in H3K23 acetylation. This decrease in H3K23ac contributes to chromatin remodeling and limits the accessibility of crucial regulatory regions, including the ESR1 promoter. This reduced accessibility leads to the downregulation of ER expression and the disruption of estrogen signaling, ultimately hindering the growth of ER^+ breast cancer cells [72].

8. Conclusion

The KAT6A/KAT6B-BRPF1 complexes constitute a sophisticated epigenetic regulatory system with crucial roles in development, cellular homeostasis and human diseases. BRPF1 functions as a scaffold protein within the tetrameric complexes [14, 34], containing multiple functional domains [15]. The domains work in concert with KAT6A and KAT6B, each of which contains an NEMM domain, two PHD fingers, a MYST catalytic domain and a serine/methionine-rich domains [17], to regulate histone acetylation and propionylation at lysine 23 of histone H3 [23, 24, 73]. The complexes are essential for embryonic development, hematopoiesis, neurogenesis, and skeletal formation [49, 53, 54], while also regulating critical cellular processes including cell cycle progression, DNA damage response, and cellular senescence [39, 41]. Mutations and dysregulation of the complexes lead to various pathological conditions: *KAT6A* and *KAT6B* germline mutations lead to two different developmental disorders [22, 64–66]; *BRPF1* mutations cause Intellectual Developmental Disorder with Dysmorphic Facies and Ptosis (BRPF1 syndrome) [23, 74, 75], characterized by developmental delays and distinct facial features; KAT6A translocations are implicated in acute myeloid leukemia through fusion proteins like MOZ-CBP and MOZ-TIF2 [45–47]; KAT6A drives glioblastoma progression through PI3K/AKT pathway activation [25]; and *KAT6B* overexpression is associated with poor prognosis ovarian cancer [68]. The complexes also play significant roles in immune regulation, particularly in CD^+ T cell responses [62] and B cell function through germinal center reactions [63]. Therapeutic targeting of these complexes is promising, with inhibitors like WM-8014 and WM-1119 demonstrating effectiveness in cancer treatment by inducing cellular senescence [12], while BRPF1 inhibitors show potential in treating ER^+ breast cancer [76] and liver cancer [77]. Recent research has also revealed the complexes' involvement in DNA damage response pathways, where they interact with p53 and contribute to cellular stress responses [43, 44]. Therefore, since their initial identification almost three decades ago [5, 6, 17], KAT6A and KAT6B are known to play important roles in diverse cellular process and have become valuable new drug targets.

Acknowledgements

We thank Miss Paulina Varela-Castillo for carefully editing the manuscript. This work was supported by funds from Canadian Institutes of Health Research (CIHR), Natural Sciences and Engineering Research Council of Canada (NSERC) and Compute Canada (to X.J.Y.).

Author details

Arezousadat Razavi[1,2*] and Xiang-Jiao Yang[1,2,3,4*]

1 Rosalind and Morris Goodman Cancer Institute, McGill University, Montreal, Quebec, Canada

2 Department of Medicine, McGill University, Montreal, Quebec, Canada

3 Department of Biochemistry, McGill University, Montreal, Quebec, Canada

4 McGill University Health Center, Montreal, Quebec, Canada

*Address all correspondence to: arezousadat.razavi@mail.mcgill.ca and xiang-jiao.yang@mcgill.ca

References

[1] Wolffe A. Chapter two - Chromatin structure. In: Wolffe A, editor. Chromatin. 3rd ed. London: Academic Press; 2000. pp. 7-172

[2] Yang XJ. The diverse superfamily of lysine acetyltransferases and their roles in leukemia and other diseases. Nucleic Acids Research. 2004;**32**:959-976

[3] Allis CD, Berger SL, Cote J, et al. New nomenclature for chromatin-modifying enzymes. Cell. 2007;**131**:633-636. DOI: 10.1016/j.cell.2007.10.039

[4] Lee KK, Workman JL. Histone acetyltransferase complexes: One size doesn't fit all. Nature Reviews. Molecular Cell Biology. 2007;**8**:284-295

[5] Borrow J, Stanton VP, Andresen JM, et al. The translocation t(8;16)(p11;p13) of acute myeloid leukaemia fuses a putative acetyltransferase to the CREB–binding protein. Nature Genetics. 1996;**14**:33-41. DOI: 10.1038/ng0996-33

[6] Reifsnyder C, Lowell J, Clarke A, Pillus L. Yeast SAS silencing genes and human genes associated with AML and HIV–1 tat interactions are homologous with acetyltransferases. Nature Genetics. 1996;**14**:42-49. DOI: 10.1038/ng0996-42

[7] Utley RT, Côté J. The MYST family of histone Acetyltransferases. In: Workman JL, editor. Protein Complexes that Modify Chromatin. Berlin Heidelberg, Berlin, Heidelberg: Springer; 2003. pp. 203-236

[8] Yang XJ, Ullah M. MOZ and MORF, two large MYSTic HATs in normal and cancer stem cells. Oncogene. 2007;**26**:5408-5419

[9] Avvakumov N, Côté J. The MYST family of histone acetyltransferases and their intimate links to cancer. Oncogene. 2007;**26**:5395-5407

[10] Wiesel-Motiuk N, Assaraf YG. The key roles of the lysine acetyltransferases KAT6A and KAT6B in physiology and pathology. Drug Resistance Updates. 2020;**53**:100729. DOI: 10.1016/j.drup.2020.100729

[11] Park J, Lee K, Kim K, Yi S-J. The role of histone modifications: From neurodevelopment to neurodiseases. Signal Transduction and Targeted Therapy. 2022;**7**:217. DOI: 10.1038/s41392-022-01078-9

[12] Baell JB, Leaver DJ, Hermans SJ, et al. Inhibitors of histone acetyltransferases KAT6A/B induce senescence and arrest tumour growth. Nature. 2018;**560**:253-257. DOI: 10.1038/s41586-018-0387-5

[13] Doyon Y, Cayrou C, Ullah M, et al. ING tumor suppressor proteins are critical regulators of chromatin acetylation required for genome expression and perpetuation. Molecular Cell. 2006;**21**:51-64. DOI: 10.1016/j.molcel.2005.12.007

[14] Ullah M, Pelletier N, Xiao L, et al. Molecular architecture of quartet MOZ/MORF histone Acetyltransferase complexes. Molecular and Cellular Biology. 2008;**28**:6828-6843. DOI: 10.1128/mcb.01297-08

[15] Zu G, Liu Y, Cao J, et al. BRPF1-KAT6A/KAT6B complex: Molecular structure, biological function and human disease. Cancers (Basel). 2022;**14**:1-18

[16] Carlson S, Glass KC. The MOZ histone Acetyltransferase in epigenetic

signaling and disease. Journal of Cellular Physiology. 2014;**229**:1571-1574. DOI: 10.1002/jcp.24617

[17] Champagne N, Bertos NR, Pelletier N, et al. Identification of a human histone Acetyltransferase related to Monocytic leukemia zinc finger protein*. Journal of Biological Chemistry. 1999;**274**:28528-28536. DOI: 10.1074/jbc.274.40.28528

[18] Qiu Y, Liu L, Zhao C, et al. Combinatorial readout of unmodified H3R2 and acetylated H3K14 by the tandem PHD finger of MOZ reveals a regulatory mechanism for HOXA9 transcription. Genes and Development. 2012;**26**:1376-1391. DOI: 10.1101/gad.188359.112

[19] Champagne N, Pelletier N, Yang X-J. The monocytic leukemia zinc finger protein MOZ is a histone acetyltransferase. Oncogene. 2001;**20**:404-409. DOI: 10.1038/sj.onc.1204114

[20] Dreveny I, Deeves SE, Fulton J, et al. The double PHD finger domain of MOZ/MYST3 induces α-helical structure of the histone H3 tail to facilitate acetylation and methylation sampling and modification. Nucleic Acids Research. 2014;**42**:822-835. DOI: 10.1093/nar/gkt931

[21] Huang F, Paulson A, Dutta A, et al. Histone acetyltransferase enok regulates oocyte polarization by promoting expression of the actin nucleation factor spire. Genes & Development. 2014;**28**(24):2750-2763. DOI: 10.1101/gad.249730.114

[22] Tham E, Lindstrand A, Santani A, et al. Dominant mutations in KAT6A cause intellectual disability with recognizable syndromic features. American Journal of Human Genetics. 2015;**96**:507-513. DOI: 10.1016/j.ajhg.2015.01.016

[23] Yan K, Rousseau J, Littlejohn RO, et al. Mutations in the chromatin regulator gene BRPF1 cause Syndromic intellectual disability and deficient histone acetylation. American Journal of Human Genetics. 2017;**100**:91-104. DOI: 10.1016/j.ajhg.2016.11.011

[24] Yan K, Rousseau J, Machol K, et al. Deficient histone H3 propionylation by BRPF1-KAT6 complexes in neurodevelopmental disorders and cancer. Science Advances. 2020;**6**:eaax0021. DOI: 10.1126/sciadv.aax0021

[25] Lv D, Jia F, Hou Y, et al. Histone acetyltransferase KAT6A upregulates PI3K/AKT signaling through TRIM24 binding. Cancer Research. 2017;**77**:6190-6201. DOI: 10.1158/0008-5472.CAN-17-1388

[26] Pelletier N, Champagne N, Stifani S, Yang X-J. MOZ and MORF histone acetyltransferases interact with the runt-domain transcription factor Runx2. Oncogene. 2002;**21**:2729-2740. DOI: 10.1038/sj/onc/1205367

[27] Kitabayashi I, Aikawa Y, Yokoyama A, et al. Fusion of MOZ and p300 histone acetyltransferases in acute monocytic leukemia with a t(8;22)(p11;q13) chromosome translocation. Leukemia. 2001;**15**:89-94. DOI: 10.1038/sj.leu.2401983

[28] Chaffanet M, Gressin L, Preudhomme C, et al. MOZ is fused to p300 in an acute monocytic leukemia with t(8;22). Genes, Chromosomes and Cancer. 2000;**28**:138-144. DOI: 10.1002/(SICI)1098-2264(200006)28:2<138::AID-GCC2>3.0.CO;2-2

[29] Becht DC, Klein BJ, Kanai A, et al. MORF and MOZ acetyltransferases

target unmethylated CpG islands through the winged helix domain. Nature Communications. 2023;**14**:1-20. DOI: 10.1038/s41467-023-36368-5

[30] Weber LM, Jia Y, Stielow B, et al. The histone acetyltransferase KAT6A is recruited to unmethylated CpG islands via a DNA binding winged helix domain. Nucleic Acids Research. 2023;**51**:574-594. DOI: 10.1093/nar/gkac1188

[31] Ali M, Yan K, Lalonde ME, et al. Tandem PHD aingers of MORF/MOZ acetyltransferases display selectivity for acetylated histone H3 and are required for the association with chromatin. Journal of Molecular Biology. 2012;**424**:328-338. DOI: 10.1016/j.jmb.2012.10.004

[32] Viita T, Côté J. The MOZ-BRPF1 acetyltransferase complex in epigenetic crosstalk linked to gene regulation, development, and human diseases. Front Cell Developmental Biology. 2023;**10**:1-14

[33] Klein BJ, Jang SM, Lachance C, et al. Histone H3K23-specific acetylation by MORF is coupled to H3K14 acylation. Nature Communications. 2019;**10**:1-13. DOI: 10.1038/s41467-019-12551-5

[34] Lalonde ME, Avvakumov N, Glass KC, et al. Exchange of associated factors directs a switch in HBO1 acetyltransferase histone tail specificity. Genes & Development. 2013;**27**:2009-2024. DOI: 10.1101/gad.223396.113

[35] Vezzoli A, Bonadies N, Allen MD, et al. Molecular basis of histone H3K36me3 recognition by the PWWP domain of Brpf1. Nature Structural and Molecular Biology. 2010;**17**:617-619. DOI: 10.1038/nsmb.1797

[36] Rokudai S, Aikawa Y, Tagata Y, et al. Monocytic leukemia zinc finger (MOZ) interacts with p53 to induce p21 expression and cell-cycle arrest. Journal of Biological Chemistry. 2009;**284**:237-244. DOI: 10.1074/jbc.M805101200

[37] Aikawa Y, Katsumoto T, Zhang P, et al. PU.1-mediated upregulation of CSF1R is crucial for leukemia stem cell potential induced by MOZ-TIF2. Nature Medicine. 2010;**16**:580-585. DOI: 10.1038/nm.2122

[38] Gursoy-Yuzugullu O, Ayrapetov MK, Price BD. Histone chaperone Anp32e removes H2A.Z from DNA double-strand breaks and promotes nucleosome reorganization and DNA repair. Proceedings of the National Academy of Sciences of the United States of America. 2015;**112**:7507-7512. DOI: 10.1073/pnas.1504868112

[39] Modesti M, Kanaar R. Homologous recombination: From model organisms to human disease. Genome Biology. 2001;**2**:1-5

[40] Ito M, Shinohara A. Chromosome architecture and homologous recombination in meiosis. Frontiers in Cell and Development Biology. 2023;**10**:1-11

[41] Kowalczykowski SC. An overview of the molecular mechanismsof recombinational DNA repair. Cold Spring Harbor Perspectives in Biology. 2015;**7**:1-36

[42] You L, Li L, Zou J, et al. BRPF1 is essential for development of fetal hematopoietic stem cells. Journal of Clinical Investigation. 2016;**126**:3247-3262. DOI: 10.1172/JCI80711

[43] Rokudai S, Laptenko O, Arnal SM, et al. MOZ increases p53 acetylation and premature senescence through its complex formation with PML. Proceedings of the National Academy of Sciences of the United States of America.

2013;**110**:3895-3900. DOI: 10.1073/pnas.1300490110

[44] Sykes SM, Mellert HS, Holbert MA, et al. Acetylation of the p53 DNA-binding domain regulates apoptosis induction. Molecular Cell. 2006;**24**:841-851. DOI: 10.1016/j.molcel.2006.11.026

[45] Perez-Campo FM, Borrow J, Kouskoff V, Lacaud G. The histone acetyl transferase activity of monocytic leukemia zinc finger is critical for the proliferation of hematopoietic precursors. Blood. 2009;**113**:4866-4874. DOI: 10.1182/blood-2008-04-152017

[46] Rozman M, Camós M, Colomer D, et al. Type I MOZ/CBP (MYST3/CREBBP) is the Most common chimeric transcript in acute myeloid leukemia with t(8;16)(p11;p13) translocation. Genes, Chromosomes and Cancer. 2004;**40**:140-145. DOI: 10.1002/gcc.20022

[47] Sun XJ, Man N, Tan Y, et al. The role of histone acetyltransferases in normal and malignant hematopoiesis. Frontiers in Oncology. 2015;**5**:1-11

[48] Sheikh BN, Phipson B, El-Saafin F, et al. MOZ (MYST3, KAT6A) inhibits senescence via the INK4A-ARF pathway. Oncogene. 2015;**34**:5807-5820. DOI: 10.1038/onc.2015.33

[49] Hibiya K, Katsumoto T, Kondo T, et al. Brpf1, a subunit of the MOZ histone acetyl transferase complex, maintains expression of anterior and posterior Hox genes for proper patterning of craniofacial and caudal skeletons. Developmental Biology. 2009;**329**:176-190. DOI: 10.1016/j.ydbio.2009.02.021

[50] Laue K, Daujat S, Crump JG, et al. The multidomain protein Brpf1 binds histones and is required for hox gene expression and segmental identity. Development. 2008;**135**:1935-1946. DOI: 10.1242/dev.017160

[51] Holbert MA, Sikorski T, Carten J, et al. The human monocytic leukemia zinc finger histone acetyltransferase domain contains DNA-binding activity implicated in chromatin targeting. Journal of Biological Chemistry. 2007;**282**:36603-36613. DOI: 10.1074/jbc.M705812200

[52] Camós M, Esteve J, Jares P, et al. Gene expression profiling of acute myeloid leukemia with translocation t(8;16)(p11;p13) and MYST3-CREBBP rearrangement reveals a distinctive signature with a specific pattern of HOX gene expression. Cancer Research. 2006;**66**:6947-6954. DOI: 10.1158/0008-5472.CAN-05-4601

[53] Miller CT, Maves L, Kimmel CB. Moz regulates Hox expression and pharyngeal segmental identity in zebrafish. Development. 2004;**131**:2443-2461. DOI: 10.1242/dev.01134

[54] Crump JG, Swartz ME, Eberhart JK, Kimmel CB. Moz-dependent Hox expression controls segment-specific fate maps of skeletal precursors in the face. Development. 2006;**133**:2661-2669. DOI: 10.1242/dev.02435

[55] Voss AK, Collin C, Dixon MP, Thomas T. Moz and retinoic acid coordinately regulate H3K9 acetylation, Hox gene expression, and segment identity. Developmental Cell. 2009;**17**:674-686. DOI: 10.1016/j.devcel.2009.10.006

[56] Bristow CAP, Shore P. Transcriptional regulation of the human MIP-1α promoter by RUNX1 and MOZ. Nucleic Acids Research. 2003;**31**:2735-2744. DOI: 10.1093/nar/gkg401

[57] Katsumoto T, Aikawa Y, Iwama A, et al. MOZ is essential for maintenance

of hematopoietic stem cells. Genes & Development. 2006;**20**:1321-1330. DOI: 10.1101/gad.1393106

[58] Thomas T, Corcoran LM, Gugasyan R, et al. Monocytic leukemia zinc finger protein is essential for the development of long-term reconstituting hematopoietic stem cells. Genes & Development. 2006;**20**:1175-1186. DOI: 10.1101/gad.1382606

[59] Perez-Campo FM, Costa G, Lie-A-Ling M, et al. MOZ-mediated repression of p16INK4a is critical for the self-renewal of neural and hematopoietic stem cells. Stem Cells. 2014;**32**:1591-1601. DOI: 10.1002/stem.1606

[60] You L, Zou J, Zhao H, et al. Deficiency of the chromatin regulator Brpf1 causes abnormal brain development. Journal of Biological Chemistry. 2015;**290**(11):7114-7129. DOI: 10.1074/jbc.M114.635250

[61] Feng Y, Vlassis A, Roques C, et al. BRPF 3- HBO 1 regulates replication origin activation and histone H3K14 acetylation. The EMBO Journal. 2016;**35**:176-192. DOI: 10.15252/embj.201591293

[62] Newman DM, Sakaguchi S, Lun A, et al. Acetylation of the Cd8 locus by KAT6A determines memory T cell diversity. Cell Reports. 2016;**16**:3311-3321. DOI: 10.1016/j.celrep.2016.08.056

[63] Good-Jacobson KL, Chen Y, Voss AK, et al. Regulation of germinal center responses and B-cell memory by the chromatin modifier MOZ. Proceedings of the National Academy of Sciences of the United States of America. 2014;**111**:9585-9590. DOI: 10.1073/pnas.1402485111

[64] Ng R, Kalinousky AJ, Harris J. Neuropsychological profile associated with KAT6A syndrome: Emergent genotype-phenotype trends. Orphanet Journal of Rare Diseases. 2024;**19**:1-11. DOI: 10.1186/s13023-024-03175-0

[65] Kennedy J, Goudie D, Blair E, et al. KAT6A syndrome: Genotype–phenotype correlation in 76 patients with pathogenic KAT6A variants. Genetics in Medicine. 2019;**21**:850-860. DOI: 10.1038/s41436-018-0259-2

[66] Zhang LX, Lemire G, Gonzaga-Jauregui C, et al. Further delineation of the clinical spectrum of KAT6B disorders and allelic series of pathogenic variants. Genetics in Medicine. 2020;**22**:1338-1347. DOI: 10.1038/s41436-020-0811-8

[67] Deguchi K, Ayton PM, Carapeti M, et al. MOZ-TIF2-Induced Acute Myeloid Leukemia Requires the MOZ Nucleosome Binding Motif and TIF2-Mediated Recruitment of CBP. Cancer Cell. 2003;**3**(3):259-271

[68] Liu C-L, Jinn-Chyuan Sheu J, Lin H-P, et al. The overexpression of MYST4 in human solid tumors is associated with increased aggressiveness and decreased overall survival. International Journal of Clinical and Experimental Pathology. 2019;**12**(2):431-442

[69] Saglam O, Tang Z, Tang G, et al. KAT6A amplifications are associated with shorter progression-free survival and overall survival in patients with endometrial serous carcinoma. PLoS One. 2020;**15**:1-15. DOI: 10.1371/journal.pone.0238477

[70] Huang F. New KAT6 inhibitors induce senescence and arrest cancer growth. Synthetic and Systems Biotechnology. 2018;**3**:244-245. DOI: 10.1016/j.synbio.2018.10.006

[71] Mukohara T, Park YH, Sommerhalder D, et al. Inhibition of lysine acetyltransferase KAT6 in

ER+HER2– metastatic breast cancer: A phase 1 trial. Nature Medicine. 2024;**30**:2242-2250. DOI: 10.1038/s41591-024-03060-0

[72] Jeselsohn R, Polyak K. HATS off to KAT6A/B inhibitors: A new way to target estrogen-receptor-positive breast cancer. Cell Chemical Biology. 2023;**30**:1183-1185

[73] Smolko AE, Sullivan DW, Olsen SN, et al. A MOZ-TIF2 leukemia mouse model displays KAT6-dependent H3K23 propionylation and overexpression of a set of active developmental genes. Proceedings of the National Academy of Sciences of the United States of America. 2024;**121**:1-11. DOI: 10.1073/pnas.2405905121

[74] Pode-Shakked N, Barel O, Pode-Shakked B, et al. BRPF1-associated intellectual disability, ptosis, and facial dysmorphism in a multiplex family. Molecular Genetics & Genomic Medicine. 2019;7:1-5. DOI: 10.1002/mgg3.665

[75] Abarca-Barriga HH, Chavesta Velásquez F, Punil Luciano R. Intellectual developmental disorder with dysmorphic facies and ptosis caused by copy number variation including the BRPF1 gene in Peruvian patient. Egyptian Journal of Medical Human Genetics. 2022;**23**:1-6. DOI: 10.1186/s43042-022-00356-z

[76] Salvati A, Giurato G, Lamberti J, et al. Essential gene screening identifies the bromodomain-containing protein BRPF1 as a new actionable target for endocrine therapy-resistant breast cancers. Molecular Cancer. 2024;**23**:1-11

[77] Cheng CLH, Tsang FHC, Wei L, et al. Bromodomain-containing protein BRPF1 is a therapeutic target for liver cancer. Communications Biology. 2021;**4**:1-14. DOI: 10.1038/s42003-021-02405-6

Chapter 5

Neuromuscular Adaptations to Exercise Training in People with Intellectual Disabilities

Hojjatollah Siavoshy

Abstract

Based on the principle features compatibility exercise, many neuromuscular responses to exercise training occur based on the type, intensity, duration, and volume adjustment training. Several occurring join the four major categories, include aerobic exercise (endurance), anaerobic exercise, strength training, and training speed and power, each compatibility related to the demand. In this review, we summarize compatibility by neuromuscular in response to each of these exercises that take place joins the presentation and then also with a new search, the studies and research tips were also undertaken regarding the compatibility in the brain and central nervous system that occur in response to exercise training the material also offers.

Keywords: neurological adaptation, brain adaptation, resistance training, strength training, aerobic training, endurance training, anaerobic training, speed training

1. Introduction

Exceptional children need special education and services to flourish their potential talents. These people themselves are divided into seven categories of people with visual disabilities, hearing disabilities, physical and movement disabilities, behavioral disorders, learning disorders, multiple disabilities, and intellectual disabilities [1]. Various definitions have been used for intellectual disabilities, but the definition that most experts have accepted is the definition of "The American Association on Intellectual and Developmental Disabilities (AAIDD)," which is the most specialized organization in the field of intellectual disabilities. Based on this definition, "intellectual disabilities refers to the general performance of intelligence, which is significantly two standard deviations lower than the average of common intelligence tests, that is, Stanford-Binet and Wechsler tests, and at the same time, it is accompanied by deficits in adaptive behavior during the development and growth period [2]." After many years, the theories of intellectual disabilities are now focused on an approach called the "whole child approach" [3], which emphasize all the factors that characterize abnormal development and provide a complete description of development in people with intellectual disabilities. In line with this perspective, there is a good consensus among theorists that sports and free time can play an essential role among children and adolescents with intellectual disabilities and functional deficiencies [4, 5]. Recent studies have confirmed this hypothesis that regular physical activity is closely related to improved reaction time [6] and better working memory [7] in children with intellectual disabilities. The background of research up to now has confirmed a causal relationship between regular physical activity and brain development, especially in the prefrontal area of the cerebral cortex [8, 9]. Movement problems are commonly reported in intellectual disabilities people, among the symptoms of intellectual disabilities are defects in cognitive and motor functions [10]. Intellectual disabilities hurt people with disabilities by reducing motor activities, which is revealed by defects in vision and motor coordination, limited motor accuracy, prevention of emotions, and problems in learning new activities [11, 12]. Due to defects in cognitive and motor functions in people with intellectual disabilities, these people engage in less activity during life or are even inactive throughout the stages of life [10, 13]. People with intellectual disabilities are much weaker in performing tasks that include a combination of two activities; they also significantly have problems with static and dynamic balances, so this weakness is manifested by unbalanced movements and an increased probability of falling [14]. Falls that lead to injury is very common in intellectual disabilities people [15]. A relationship between balance and gait in falls has been well demonstrated [16]. Some research has shown that people with intellectual disabilities have a relatively high rate of falls and face an increased risk of fall injuries [17, 18]. Children with intellectual disabilities are less active during puberty [19]. This is especially important for intellectually disabled teenagers because of their lower cardiovascular fitness compared to their healthy peers [20]. The reason for their lower readiness is not known, but part of it can be due to their lower maximum heart rate (HRPeak) (about 30% lower than expected), which may cause a decrease in physical activity level, respiratory problems, and muscle strength [20, 21]. Individuals with intellectual disabilities are also more prone to developing cardiovascular diseases [22], diabetes [23], osteoporosis, and obesity and, therefore, are more prone to a significant and early decline in performance compared to their age [24]. Research has also shown that, except for flexibility, there is a significant relationship between the levels of intelligence and other factors of physical fitness in intellectually disabilities students. This means that students who have a higher level of intelligence have better balance, muscular endurance, strength, speed, and cardiorespiratory endurance, and in other words, the lower the level of intelligence, the lower the physical fitness factors [25]. However, although it is agreed among theorists that children with intellectual disability can enjoy the benefits of sports training, people with intellectual disabilities face many obstacles to participating in sports programs, such as the need for someone to exercise with them [26], and the need a suitable program [27]. Sports adjustments for this group include the need for close supervision, motivational support, and the need to gain assurance of doing sports at the appropriate intensity [28, 29] and improving social interactions [27]. It seems that one of the most important obstacles is a sedentary lifestyle with a lack of motivation and difficulty in maintaining a planned sports activity protocol for sufficient periods [30]. On the other hand, the participation and involvement of people with intellectual disabilities in organized sports activities are limited by environmental factors such as access to gyms, lack of an expert teacher or coach, and limited access to exercises [31]. These factors are often closely related to known barriers, ranging from dependence on others in moving to beliefs about limiting medical conditions related to special disabilities or prejudices about reducing physical and behavioral skills. All these factors in the long run can cause some families to overprotect their disabled children and reduce or limit the participation of these people in sports activities [32]. It also seems that the degree of influence of sports programs is influenced by personality characteristics, such as age and degree of intellectual disability. Thus, younger people and those who are on the border of intellectual disability show more improvement after specific movement exercises than people who have a higher level of intellectual disability [29]. In 1965, the American Association for Health, Physical Education, and Recreation (AAHPER) started implementing a project that was active in the fields of recreation and preparation for people with intellectual disabilities, and its goal was to increase the amount of recreation and preparation body skills of the people with intellectual disabilities [33, 34]. Later, this project expanded its scope of action to all cases of disabilities, including intellectual disabilities, and after that, the levels of research in the field of movement needs of the disabled and norm-making and the standardization of physical fitness tests for people with intellectual disability increased; for example, the set of Eurofit Special Tests, the Brockport Physical Fitness Test, and the Canadian Standardized Test of Fitness can be mentioned, which are used to measure physical fitness factors in people with intellectual disabilities have been exposed. It may be possible to consider physical fitness as qualitative efficiency in activities while performing assigned duties without feeling excessive and abnormal fatigue, as well as recovery and returning to a suitable initial state after hard physical work by using reasonable rest and preparation to participate in subsequent activities; which is a general term consisting of a combination of physical fitness factors such as cardiovascular capacity, muscular strength, muscular endurance, and flexibility [35]. Through some tests, it is possible to detect the level of these factors in people, and in case of a significant decrease in the scores of these physical factors, can be taken to improve these factors, because, for example, reducing the levels of cardiorespiratory endurance in people exposes them to the risk of many health problems such as obesity, cardiovascular diseases, and diabetes [36].

Improving the life expectancy of people with intellectual disabilities and people with Down syndrome requires knowing the conditions that frequently occur in adults in these communities, and health workers should be aware of it because this group of people is especially susceptible to infections of the urinary tract, respiratory and gastrointestinal tract; at least part of which may be explained due to the severe disturbance in the secretion of some biomarkers of the immune system [37].

Good muscle strength is especially important for people with intellectual disabilities and people with Down syndrome because the workplace activities of these people emphasize physical skills rather than cognitive and mental skills, and muscle weakness, as an effective physical component in doing things, can be a serious problem in these people [29]. Also, muscle weakness can affect the ability of these people to perform daily life activities, such as walking, and strength improvement can be accompanied by positive changes in functional activities and work-related skills in individuals with intellectual disability [29]. Destruction, atrophy, and loss of muscle cells are associated with decrease in muscle strength [38].

The excessive obsession of parents and guardians of people with intellectual disabilities in taking care of these people and the fear of getting injured during sports programs prevent this group of people from participating in sports programs, and such phenomena strengthen the hypothesis that these people from In terms of physical fitness profile and physiological and anthropometric variables, they have a lower status compared to their healthy peers without intellectual disability [39]. Also, on the other hand, it can be said that people with intellectual disabilities may not be able to participate in sports programs due to some restrictions or that these people cannot follow the instructions and learn sports compared to healthy people without intellectual disabilities, that this phenomenon can reduce the benefits they get from these sports programs [29, 40]. It seems that the special conditions of these people and separating them from the communities without an intellectual disability can be a major reason for not participating in sports programs and consequently having a sedentary life [41]. The evidence shows that the chronic conditions of people with intellectual disabilities, apart from the limitations it creates for them, also affect their families in financial, social, emotional, behavioral, and cognitive abilities, and families with children with intellectual disabilities are under a lot of psychological pressure [42]. It seems that people with intellectual disabilities have a more or equal need for physical fitness and health of the cardiovascular and musculoskeletal systems to live a healthy life with health and prevent diseases and premature death compared to healthy people [43]. On the other hand, due to intellectual disabilities, they cannot engage in jobs that require mental and cognitive skills and work in environments with mental busyness, and the activities entrusted to them emphasize physical skills more than mental and cognitive skills [29, 40]. Apart from this, as people with intellectual disabilities get older, they need more strength and physical fitness to gain independence in doing personal work and daily life activities, and the ability to have an independent life is a key factor for people with intellectual disabilities; therefore, In this group of people, having muscle strength, general and special endurance, flexibility and other physical fitness factors is a key factor to ensure the quality of life and independence in performing assigned tasks and personal tasks [29]. Due to a sedentary lifestyle and reduction of physical activities, with increasing age, the condition of physical fitness worsens and this phenomenon increases dependence on others in doing personal work and tasks assigned to them [44].

Therefore, based on the materials and points that have been said, people with intellectual disabilities have a lower level of physical fitness compared to people without intellectual disabilities [29]. Reducing physical fitness due to its effects on overweight and obesity leads to some risks related to inactivity, and this problem shows itself more in people with intellectual disabilities [45]. For this reason, it is necessary to provide opportunities for people with intellectual disabilities to be more involved in physical activities, so that, as a result, they can have a healthy lifestyle along with the health and wellness benefits of physical activities and reduce the death rate and increase life expectancy and health, to be able to achieve improvements in doing personal work and living an independent life; in this regard, people with intellectual disabilities or their parents and guardians, teachers and sports coaches, health workers, or anyone who is in some way connected with these people should be responsible for intelligent and efficient planning and designing and compiling activities. Sports for this group of people should have the tools and equipment to be able to measure and evaluate the level of physical fitness of people with intellectual disabilities so that using these data and also using the principles of training and exercise science, determine the intensity, duration, and number of sessions of sports training programs and also consider the progress of training programs and possible changes during the periods of exercise programs by measuring and monitoring the level of physical fitness achieved. Also, in the prescription of any activity or exercise program, the individual abilities of each person should be taken into account to avoid health risks that may arise due to incorrect and inappropriate prescription of an activity or exercise program. Therefore, measuring and evaluating physical fitness levels in people with intellectual disability is especially important [34]. Despite this, most of the sports and exercise tests have been standardized for people without intellectual disability and healthy societies, and the generalization of these tests and norms to people with intellectual disability is not reasonable and logical due to their little physical activity. Therefore, according to the above, determining the physical fitness normative data for this group of people in society is an undeniable fact because if there are such suitable and appropriate tools for people with intellectual disabilities, it is better to plan for their design and activities and sports exercises, and by measuring and monitoring the level of physical fitness of these people, it is possible to determine the level of progress and improvement, efficiency and ensure the effectiveness of exercise training programs. And also, it is better to recognize the problems of motor development and physical fitness of these people and plan to solve them in training sessions. To achieve this goal, a suitable measurement tool is needed that can be implemented easily and at the lowest cost without using complex sports equipment anywhere.

The exercise tests that are used to measure physical fitness factors in special schools are the tests that are often normalized and standardized on people without intellectual disabilities, while, as mentioned before, the level of physical fitness of people with intellectual disabilities is often lower than their peers without intellectual disabilities [29, 40]. Therefore, these tools that have been standardized and normalized (normative data) in societies without intellectual disability are not suitable tools for measuring the physical fitness factors of people with intellectual disabilities. In this regard, a series of special exercise tests have been prepared and compiled for these people, for example, the Eurofit Special Test (EST), the Brockport Physical Fitness Test (BPFT), and the Canadian Standardized Test of Fitness (CSTF). The CSTF was first designed and standardized in Canada in 1981 on communities without intellectual disabilities and then standardized and normalized (normative data) on people with intellectual disabilities in Canada [46, 47] and Iran [39]. However, each of these tests has its disadvantages; for example, the Brockport physical fitness test set requires special complex sports equipment to be implemented, and most special schools do not have equipment and facilities to measure such physical fitness factors. Therefore, it is not possible to do it in most of these special schools, and no matter how accurate and reliable these tests are, if they are not implemented everywhere, they will not have good generalizability.

2. Neural and muscular adaptations to sports training

Although the structure and metabolic and physiological characteristics of athletes have been studied over the years, the physiological mechanisms that support the effectiveness and effect of exercise programs on neuromuscular adaptations remain unclear. Available scientific information mainly focuses on observations and comparisons.

Many adaptations occur in the nerve and muscle department in response to physical activities. The four main categories include aerobic (endurance) exercises, anaerobic exercises, strength exercises, and speed and strength exercises.

High levels of athletic performance result from years of rigorous, consistent training combined with excellent planning. During these years, athletes try to adapt their bodies and functions to the specific needs of that sport. The level of compatibility can be determined using functional capabilities; or in better words, it can be expressed as: "More compatibility, better performance."

Training adaptation is the result of changes that result from regular repetition of sports. Such structural and physiological changes are the result of special pressures that athletes put on their bodies with continuous and non-stop activity, which depends on the volume, intensity, and repetition of sports exercises. Physical exercises are beneficial only if they lead to adaptation to the force due to the pressure applied to the body during the activity, and if these pressures are not enough, no adaptation will happen. On the other hand, if these pressures are unbearable and beyond a person's ability, there is a possibility that they will cause injury or overtraining. The time required to achieve high levels of adaptation depends on the complexity of the skill and the physiological and psychological difficulties of that sport or activity; so, more difficult and complex sports require a longer time for neuromuscular and functional adaptation.

Regular and organized training programs create many changes in the body; although researchers have reported more functional and physical changes in endurance athletes [48, 49], most athletes witness neuromuscular, biochemical, and cardiopulmonary changes in their bodies, and of course, psychological improvements and improvements also occur after physical training.

The studies conducted on anatomical adaptations also indicate that intense sports activities reduce the strength of bone constituents. On the other hand, it can be safely said that the mechanical properties and characteristics of bones do not depend on the chronological age of people but are caused by the mechanical pressures applied to the athlete. For this reason, low-intensity sports training at early ages may stimulate the longitudinal growth and thickness of long bones, while high-intensity and intense training may stop bone growth [50].

However, researchers believe that bone adaptations due to exercise are a function of people's age. So, the bones of immature people are more sensitive to periodic changes in exercise load compared to the bones of adults. However, doing strength training at a young age accelerates the maturation process and leads to permanent retardation of bone growth [50]. Therefore, sports exercises should be performed with the aim that the pressure applied to the body is such that it causes adaptation responses of the body and not worsening the body condition.

In athletes who perform strength and power exercises with an intensity close to the maximum muscle contraction, the cross-sectional area of their muscle fibers increases, which is called muscle hypertrophy. Most muscle growth and muscle weight increase are caused by hypertrophy, but sometimes muscle growth can be caused by increasing the amount of proteins in muscles or the longitudinal division of muscle fibers, which is called muscle hyperplasia.

Usually, researchers attribute superior performance in strength and speed events to genetic factors and dominant muscle fiber type. However, Simoneau et al. [51] stated that muscle fiber type composition cannot be determined by genetics alone. Researchers have seen conflicting results when converting fast-twitch to slow-twitch muscle fiber types. Some results have confirmed that when the stimulation is appropriate, there is a capacity to convert one type of muscle fiber to another; therefore, the adaptation of the muscle fiber type can depend on the nature and duration of the appropriate training program and the pre-training conditions of the athlete; therefore, it is not considered a genetic factor alone.

We can fully understand the explosive power performance enhancement and biocompatibility of specific training stimuli. Gravity naturally provides most of the mechanical stimuli that drive structural muscle growth in everyday life and exercise; therefore, it seems reasonable to imagine that higher gravity conditions could affect the muscle mechanics of highly trained athletes. Researchers have reported improvements due to rapid adaptation to higher simulated gravity fields. They postulated that adaptation occurs in both muscle function and metabolic processes [52].

Improved performance is also associated with changes in the neuromuscular system. During maximal or submaximal sustained activities, the average firing rate of a motor unit increases over time. This neuromuscular strategy can increase the length of time athletes can sustain a contraction. During prolonged submaximal activity, as fatigue develops in active motor units, the recruitment of new motor units also maintains force output. However, when maximal voluntary contractions continue, units with the highest initial frequency show the greatest reduction.

Short-duration activities and high-speed activities cause low enzyme adaptations (protein substances that cause chemical reactions) and increased creatine phosphate (CP). More intense activity causes faster functioning of this enzyme and more metabolism of oxidative glycolysis. It can be mentioned that hypertrophy increases the activity of oxidative enzymes. Aerobic activity is not enough to change the processes of glycolysis. Consequently, the more an athlete participates in training, the more hypertrophied his slow-twitch fibers will be [53].

Moderate-intensity and long-duration endurance exercise increases aerobic capacity, mostly due to increased myoglobin (the part that binds and releases oxygen), mitochondrial enzymes (both in number and size), glycogen stores, and oxidative capacity. The main adaptations to long-term activities include increased respiratory capacity and respiratory rate, increased oxygen transport, increased cardiac output, and structural changes in the volume and number of muscle mitochondria; therefore, the increase in maximum oxygen consumption indicates an increase in aerobic capacity in long-term activities and an increase in enzyme activity in active muscles. An important benefit of increasing enzyme levels is the oxidation of fatty acids, which improves the body's ability to use fats as an energy source. Researchers believe that the increase in mitochondria and muscle myoglobin explains about 50% of the increase in maximal oxygen consumption. The other 50% is probably explained by better oxygen transport through the cardiovascular system [54]. Also, dominant aerobic exercises significantly increase anaerobic capacity.

Many adaptations occur in the nerve and muscle department in response to physical activities. The four main categories include aerobic (endurance) exercises, anaerobic exercises, strength exercises, and speed and power exercises. They are explained about them, and then we discuss the adaptations of the brain and central nervous system and the events that happen to these organs during physical activities.

2.1 Neural and muscular adaptations to aerobic (endurance) exercises

A possible benefit of neuromuscular adaptations to slow, long-distance exercise is the development of neuromuscular patterns. It should be noted that the strengthening of neuromuscular patterns during low-intensity sports activity does not necessarily reflect the neuromuscular demands of the competition. Therefore, endurance athletes must train at a high-intensity range to facilitate the neuromuscular adaptations employed in the activity rhythm.

In recent years, other complementary strength training methods, such as plyometric exercises, have been developed. Plyometric training is a form of strength training that is increasingly advocated by strength and conditioning coaches in elite endurance athletes. In a recent paper, the same group examined several athletic factors including 5 km sprint time, running economy, 20 m sprint maximum speed, vo2max, and maximum running speed before and after 9 weeks of explosive strength training in 22 elite male cross-country runners [55]. Athletes were divided into a control group and an experimental group, and each group replaced 3 and 32% of their normal training volume with explosive training, respectively. Explosive exercises included basic speed exercises and various plyometric exercises. After 9 weeks of training program in the experimental group, a significant improvement in the performance of two 5 km was observed, but this was not observed in the control group. It has previously been suggested that the observed improvements in performance may be due to an increase in Vo2max or lactate threshold (LT). However, no changes in Vo2max and lactate threshold were observed in most phases of the study. Correlation of the data showed that the improvement in the performance of two 5 km was the result of the increase in running economy and muscle power, which is defined as the ability of the neuromuscular system to produce power during maximal exercise when glycolytic or oxidative energy production is high and muscle contraction is possible limited. The authors of this paper went on to show that running economy is likely to be affected by explosive strength training through increased neuromuscular properties, leading to greater stiffness and efficiency of the muscle structure. Support for this theory was provided by additional data obtained by examining cross-country skiers. The effect of strength training in increasing aerobic endurance performance when evaluated on an ergometer for cross-country skiing was investigated by Hoff et al. [56]. Elite athletes were studied for 8 weeks with resistance training (three times per week, three sets of six repetitions, 3–4 minutes rest between sets at a workload of 85% of one-repetition maximum). With more emphasis on summoning maximum force in concentric movements suggested by researchers, especially neuromuscular adaptation is targeted. Following the training program, several positive results were observed, which include the power evaluated by a maximum repetition, the time to reach the peak of the force, the time of relaxation, and the economy of activity, which were all increased.

2.1.1 Local muscular endurance

Local muscle endurance is the extent to which specific muscle groups can continue to contract against a certain load for a period or a certain number of repetitions, which is determined by the type of muscle contraction, the rate of contraction, the rate of repetition, and the amount of resistance. The limiting factors of muscle endurance are the amount of exercise of muscle groups and their neuromuscular control, and it has nothing to do with cardiorespiratory or cardiovascular factors [57].

2.2 Adaptations to anaerobic endurance training

Unlike aerobic endurance adaptation exercises that occur both centrally and peripherally, anaerobic capacity adaptation occurs peripherally and often within muscle cells. Unfortunately, limited well-controlled scientific studies are measuring physiological adaptations to high-intensity exercise; however, a summary of key findings regarding neuromuscular adaptation to anaerobic exercise is shown in **Table 1**.

The major adaptations that enhance ATP-CP capacity and, therefore, lead to increased short-term anaerobic endurance include:

- Intramuscular CP and ATP reserves.

- Intramuscular free creatine stores.

- Concentration and activity of key enzymes (creatin-kinase and myo-kinase).

Duration	Type of activity	Adaptations	Non-adaptations	Reference
6 weeks	Intermittent hill running	↑ 17% maximum treadmill test ↑ 14% peak blood lactate ↑ 15% high-energy phosphates	VO2max anaerobic power Composition of muscle fibers	Houston and Thomson [58]
8 weeks	Sprint training	↑ 20% peak muscle lactate ↔ intramuscular pH* ↑ 46% PFK activity		Sharp et al. [59]
6 weeks	Speed ergometer bike, two to three times a week 2 × 15 seconds and 2 × 30 seconds in week 1 Increase to 15 × 6 seconds and 30 × 6 seconds	↑ Peak blood lactate ↑ % of all muscle fibers ↑ PFK activity ↓ Mb	Wingate performance	Jacobs et al. [60]
6 weeks	Running on a treadmill three times a week. Or: 3 × 2 minutes, 8 minutes rest Or: 8 × 20 seconds, with about 5 minutes of rest	↑ 10% MAOD in both groups	Peak blood lactate	Medbo and Burgers [61]
3 weeks	Bike ergometer at full speed 6 × 10 seconds of speed, 24 seconds of rest A total of 10 sessions	↑ Mean power at 2 out of 10 speeds ↑ Peak power in three out of four speeds ↑ Peak blood lactate ↔ PH post-exercise*	VO2max Plasma volume blood sugar	Jenkins et al. [62]
8 weeks	Running on a treadmill, three to four times a week Maximum 30 seconds × 2, 10 minutes rest Maximum 6 × 10–6 seconds, 54 seconds rest 2 × 5–2 minutes at 110% VO2max, 5 minutes rest	↑ 120% peak power in 30-second speed test ↑6% mean power in 30-second speed test ↑ muscle lactate post-exercise ↓ blood pH post-exercise	Muscle buffering capacity (*in vitro*) Metabolic responses to a 2 minutes test at 110% VO2max	Nevill et al. [63]

**The lack of change in muscle and blood pH after passive exercise indicates an increase in buffering capacity. ↑ increase, ↓ decrease, ↔ unchanged.*

Table 1.
Findings and research about adaptations to anaerobic exercises.

The major adaptations that develop the capacity of the glycolytic system and consequently improve long-term anaerobic endurance include:

- Glycolytic enzymes (e.g., PFK and phosphorylase).
- Intracellular and extracellular buffer capacity.

These and other adaptations to vigorous exercise are discussed below.

2.2.1 Capacity of ATP-CP

Short-term anaerobic endurance training increases resting intramuscular CP and ATP. An increase in free creatine, which is used to regenerate CP, is often observed following exercise. When substrate stores are upgraded, the time of this pathway and its contribution to ATP-PC depletion during maximal activity seem to be similar for trained and untrained subjects. It has been shown that anaerobic exercises increase the concentration of creatine kinase and myo-kinase in fast-twitch muscle fibers [64]. However, there is little evidence for such adaptations in response to other forms of anaerobic exercise.

2.2.2 Glycolytic capacity

Long-term anaerobic endurance training has been shown to increase glycogen metabolism during high-intensity activity and to increase post-exercise muscle acidity and blood lactate, indicating a high or low level of anaerobic glycolysis. Blood lactate concentration after exercise has a direct relationship with performance in short-term intense sports. As a result, sports scientists often use blood lactate concentration after exercise to show the anaerobic contribution of activity. The concentration of lactate in the blood is usually at its peak after a few minutes of intense exercise, and the highest concentration is observed in a maximum exercise of 2–3 minutes. This increase in anaerobic glycolysis may be in response to increasing the activity of special enzymes or increasing the buffer capacity to overcome metabolic acidosis. An increase in glycolytic enzymes improves the rate of ATP regeneration in glycolysis. As a result, the intensity of activity will be available in short-term activities. Sharp et al. [59] and Jenkins et al. [62] showed that the increase in muscle buffering capacity due to exercise leads to an increase in blood lactate with no change in blood and muscle pH (**Table 1**). This is due to the increase in the buffer capacity that cleans the hydrogen ions produced by lactic acid catabolism, and as a result, the amount of glycolysis and the intensity of exercise remain constant, and therefore, the concentration of blood lactate increases.

2.2.3 Other adaptations

2.2.3.1 Performance

Performance tests are often used in sports science laboratories to assess the anaerobic capacity of specific sports in a controlled environment. These tests may be used to evaluate the effectiveness of anaerobic exercise in increasing anaerobic endurance. Perhaps the reason for this is due to the non-specialization of some specific methods used in determining anaerobic capacity; however, some research has shown consistency in several physiological measurements in the absence of continuous improvement in laboratory functional tests. For example, Jacobs et al. [60] found that 6 weeks of training resulted in several adaptations that were not associated with development in the Wingate functional test (**Table 1**). These results suggest that cellular adaptations are not required in the development and improvement of performance, or the Wingate test is not sensitive for assessing anaerobic capacity.

2.2.3.2 Muscle fiber composition

The question of whether people's muscle fiber composition is determined by genetics or is the result of athletes' long training has been debated for many years.

The first study that showed that athletes in different disciplines are characterized by a different share of fiber types was published in 1972 [65]. The next work of the same group showed that endurance training can increase the percentage of slow-twitch fibers by 36% [66]. These results were supported by Tesch and Karlsson [67], who reported that long-distance runners had more slow-twitch fibers in the latissimus dorsi and deltoid medius, 60% and 49%, respectively, compared to marathon kayakers, who showed the opposite profile that the slow-twitch fibers in the middle deltoid and the broad outer deltoid were 71% and 41%, respectively. The difference in fiber composition between trained and untrained people, and actually between trained and untrained muscles, is evidence that long-term training and not heredity alone determines muscle fiber characteristics. Major changes in slow-twitch fibers have been less demonstrated by anaerobic exercise; however, muscle variability may allow adaptations in short-duration, high-intensity athletes. The selective hypertrophy of muscle fibers by exercise is evidence for this claim. Gollnick et al. [65] pointed out the high hypertrophy of slow-twitch fibers in endurance athletes, while Klarsson et al. [68] showed that although there is no difference between the percentage of muscle fiber composition in the brachial and latissimus dorsi in speed kayakers, the fast-twitch muscle fibers The biceps brachii had hypertrophy and a larger cross-sectional area than the vastus externus muscle (following opposite numbers). Therefore, both this muscle fiber composition and selective hypertrophy are the result of special physical exercises. Contemporary understanding of skeletal muscle suggests that classifying fibers into three distinct types is probably too simplistic, but rather, there is a continuum of fiber types based on biochemical characteristics, all of which show adaptations to physical activity [40].

2.2.3.3 Aerobics

Anaerobic endurance exercises should be performed at high intensities to obtain the required training adaptations. As previously emphasized, aerobic fitness is high for short bursts of intense activity, especially during a full training session. In addition, recent research has shown that the effective way to develop aerobic power (VO2max) is to perform repetitions of short-term intense activities with an active rest period, for example, a 30-second burst at 100% VO2max with 30 seconds of recovery at 50% VO2max is suitable [69]. Therefore, it is possible that training for anaerobic endurance has some effect on VO2max, which is especially important for athletes participating in semi-endurance disciplines that require a large share of aerobic and anaerobic energy and whose performance depends on both aerobic and anaerobic endurance.

2.2.3.4 Nervous

It is thought that anaerobic endurance training may be the result of an increase in the athlete's mental toughness or pain tolerance. This may occur when the individual's performance may not be the only factor in the development of untrained individuals. However, the high-intensity nature of anaerobic training probably requires high levels of mental strength and coordination. Short-term anaerobic endurance exercises with maximum speed-power output can be the result of more and simultaneous use of movement units. As a result, the production capacity of muscle power increases. Such neural adaptations occur relatively quickly in response to exercise. This is demonstrated by the innate response to resistance training and when strength gains are achieved without any concomitant hypertrophy.

By knowing the physiological needs and performance limitations in sports events, training programs can be designed based on scientific principles. Special exercises aimed at the required physiological adaptations reduce the functional limitations of people and, as a result, increase the athlete's performance.

2.3 Strength

In general, the initial improvement in strength is often due to neuromuscular changes. The reason for the initial increase in strength is often achieved by neuromuscular adaptations that do not require an increase in protein synthesis, while subsequent increases in strength are related to muscle hypertrophy [70]. The response to strength training is very specific depending on the type of light combinations and training loads used in the neuromuscular system; that is, different training methods cause a certain type of adaptation. However, it is necessary to pay attention to the effects of various exercises and their general transfer to sports movements [64].

However, muscle force production is determined not only by muscle cross-sectional area and contractile fiber type density but also by neuromuscular conduction generated by the nervous system. The main factor determining the pattern of using motor units is determined by the amount of force used in the motor activity. The size of the muscle is the main factor suggested for the use of motor units [71]. When the intensity of contractions increases from close to the rest state, the involvement of the motor unit is contracted according to the size of the contraction in order of character and hierarchy, so the force generation potential is also such that the smallest motor units during low force contractions are employed, that is, slow oxidative fibers (type I) followed by fast oxidative fibers (type IIa), then fast glycolytic fibers (type IIb) (with low threshold) and finally fast glycolytic fibers (type IIb) (with high threshold) are used to produce the maximum force of muscle contractions. For the fast-twitch fibers to be recruited and therefore receive the training effects, the exercise must be intense. Also, if the position of the body changes, even if the muscle acts at the same intensity, the order of recruitment can change [72]. For example, the recruitment of movement units of the pectoralis major muscle during the flat bench press movement is selected differently than the incline bench press movement.

Also, the production of new force in motor units or muscles can be modified and adjusted by transmitting the frequency of nerve impulses on the motor end plate, which is known as the firing rate. Therefore, type (IIb) twitch fibers are used when a very high amount of neuro-motor impulses are available. The force generation capability of a single motor unit can change up to 10 times depending on the stimulation of nerve stimuli; therefore, the maximum force production in compliant muscles is determined by the highest possible number of used motor units and the highest amount of neuro-motor stimulation.

For the unconscious coordination of body movements and muscle activity to approach the maximum level, the production of maximum force must be done voluntarily. Inherently, the neural program to produce maximum force from the motor cortex or cortex is received and controlled by the stimulation of the upper levels of the brain; thus, maximal strength efforts are responded to by maximal motor arousal or motivation.

The action of the antagonist's muscles provides a supportive space during the activity of the agonist's muscles following a strong contraction to prevent damage to the active joints. Antagonist muscle activity in stabilizing and supporting by slowing the rate of contraction is a proposed mechanism for muscle contractions to prevent injury. The torque of the opposing muscles is about 10% of the torque of the sympathetic muscles, but it inherently acts as an inhibitor that is the main torque reducer in voluntary movements.

2.3.1 Neurological changes

People who have never done strength training cannot initially use all the motor units up to the maximum stimulation threshold to perform their maximum effort. As a result, the person cannot provide the necessary potential to produce force in the involved muscles. During the first stage of preparation for resistance exercises, adaptation in neural control is the factor of using motor units up to the maximum stimulation threshold. The production of greater force is created by adaptation in motor units, and the use of new motor units, as well as the ability to produce force to integration and unity, are dependent on all motor units. Also, increasing muscle activity through exercises may create more nerve excitation in individual units, which causes more force to be provided through the uniform use of all muscle fibers.

Electromyography (EMG) is one of the methods of recording the conduction and transmission of electric current in a muscle. Although it is difficult to fully explain the true shape of neural adaptations from EMG data, the sum of integrated electromyography (IEMG) signals recorded from a working muscle that increases following strength training can provide information about whether more motor units are being recruited or motor units are stimulated with a higher intensity. The ratio of EMG activity in terms of muscle force can provide information about the sequence of movement units used during an activity. Moritani and DeVries [73] noted that following 8 weeks of resistance training, a decrease in EMG activity was observed for greater force production. Therefore, the reduction in the force EMG ratio has made researchers believe more in the selectivity and sequential recall factor of the company of motor units for contraction, which is determined by the increase in force production due to exercise. A large number of studies have also demonstrated that an overall increase in neural excitability is associated with an increase in strength levels. Häkkinen and Komi [74] reported an immediate and observable increase of 34–35% in IEMG activity within the first few weeks of quadriceps training. It has been reported that increasing efferent nerve stimulation, increasing motor neuron excitability, and reducing nerve messages in inhibitory pathways such as muscle spindles help to stimulate the active muscle.

It has also been proven that when an agonist muscle is trained, the EMG activity in the antagonist muscle decreases. Hakkinen et al. [75] demonstrated a sustained 5–10% decrease in biceps EMG activity during maximal forward movement exercises when leg extensor strength increased by approximately 20–30% following 6 months of strength training in leg press was observed in elderly people. Researchers have stated that non-training of the antagonist's muscle following training in the agonist's muscle causes a reduction in the opposition of the traction force of the extrinsic contraction by collective action in the muscle fibers of the antagonist's muscle. The independent activity of the antagonist muscle is not eliminated during the contraction of the agonist muscle, as it is necessary to help stabilize the joint during exercise and acts as a support mechanism. However, the inactivation of the antagonist muscle increases the tension ability of the agonist muscle as a special effect. In addition, Lee et al. [76] proved that more activity in the synergistic muscles of the arm improves wrist stability and exercise performance. In addition, for the ability to produce more force in the agonist muscles, it should be accompanied by less inhibition of the activity of the antagonist muscles because for more stability in the execution of the correct form of movement, more action is needed in the activity of the assisting muscles in active muscle.

2.3.2 Time of nerve and muscle adaptation

The creation of maximum force is the result of the amount of nerve conduction and the use of muscle and the type of contraction fibers through training [64]. However, the contribution of neural changes and increase in muscle volume to increase in maximal force production does not occur simultaneously. Hakkinen et al. [75] proved that the increase in force production at the end of the first 8 weeks of introvert and extravert exercises equals an increase in IEMG. In addition, when athletes without strength training begin resistance training, a weak relationship between increases in strength and increases in muscle fiber cross-sectional areas [77] or muscle diameter [73] is obtained. It has been proven that an increase in the amount of neural excitation and the use of motor units above the threshold have the largest contribution to the increase in force production; also, the aforementioned issue and its importance in participation for force production is greater than muscle volume [70]. It has been shown that during the early stages of strength training (first 2–8 weeks), the musculoskeletal system "learns" how to apply force. Changes in the type of contractile proteins, as shown by the change in the type of myosin heavy chains and the type of myosin ATPase enzymes, can be seen from the beginning of resistance training programs.

2.3.3 Kinaesthetic stability and control

It is common for experienced athletes to experience a lack of motor control when performing a dumbbell chest press when all previous training has been barbell chest press. In addition, there is a high dependence between exercises that exclusively involve movements in the sagittal and frontal planes, while there is little dependence in both the transverse planes and the combination of one or more parts of the movements.

2.3.4 Activity speed

Exercising at low speeds may cause inhibition of nerve impulse activity because the speed reduction is in the direction of contractile excitation; therefore, it has been proven that low-speed training is more suitable for muscle hypertrophy, and high-speed training causes neural adaptations of strength.

Table 2 shows a general plan that follows the most common methods in training repetitions. In a resistance training session that tends to be 'neurologically' heavy, during the handling of such heavy loads, the neuromuscular system endures severe fatigue as measured by a reduction in maximal voluntary neural activity, that is, a reduction in the ability to produce maximal force and a reduction In the force-time characteristic of force application, to perform a small number of maximum repetitions, it is necessary to produce maximum muscle forces, and as a result, maximum motivation should be created in the athlete. Maximum force execution takes more time than power-oriented movements during execution. Power development during efforts cannot produce maximal adaptation in power due to spending more time to develop maximal power. Maximal force development during efforts may not result

Type of activity	Neurological adaptations	Muscle adaptations (hypertrophy)
One to three maximum repetitions, strength/power	High	Moderate
Three to six maximum repetitions, strength/power	High	Moderate to high
Six to twelve maximum repetitions, moderate to high strength gains	Moderate	High
More than 12 repetitions maximum, high increase endurance	Low	Moderate

Table 2.
Differentiation in neural adaptations and muscular adaptations in the range of training repetitions [78].

in the ability to produce absolute maximal force because movement velocity plateaus when high resistances are used. This method, that is, the implementation of high resistances with the ability to produce absolute maximum force during a training session, in addition to neural changes, should be considered as a primary stimulus for strength adaptation.

However, when an athlete trains with heavy resistance, or trains with high acceleration and low mass, or trains with moderate mass and acceleration, they experience very distinct and important physical and performance adaptations and responses because the load components and acceleration act in the direction of high force production and it has been proven that they are special and important stimuli for neuromuscular and metabolic adaptations [79].

The combination of metabolic factors and mechanical loads experienced by a muscle means that the muscle has acquired the first stimulus to adapt the muscle fibers and the genetic expression of their phenotype. As muscle fibers do not exist in separate types, but as it was said, they are placed in a hierarchy from slow to fast-twitch characteristics that determine the motor units of the muscle fiber type and innervate them, and phenotypic, genetic expression in the characteristic of the type of contraction fibers as an adaptation factor is expressed [64].

2.4 Neuromuscular adaptations to speed and strength training

Neural adaptations to speed training have been widely reviewed throughout [80]; however, most of them were carried out by Hakkinen [78] which can be summarized as follows: (1) increasing the activity of agonist's muscles in the leg, (2) decreasing the activity of antagonist's muscles in the leg, and (3) advanced activation of synergist muscles. Increases in muscle activity are commonly assessed through testing using EMG, with many exercise studies showing increases in the overall electrical activity of the exercised muscles during maximal contractions. This increase in EMG quantity suggests that the number of motor units recruited has increased or the motor units are excited at higher rates. Or a combination of the two occurs. While these adaptations will increase the maximum contraction force. Faster improvement in the amount of force increase is an additional neural adaptation that can happen, if the exercises include rapid maximal efforts or so-called ballistic contractions with submaximal loads. This adaptation returns to before and is caused by the increased level of excitation of motor units at the beginning of the movement [81]. As a result of such neural adaptations, both the maximum force increases and the power and speed increase much faster. These changes may become apparent after 2 weeks of speed training and promote hypertrophy changes in the trained muscles [70]. It has also been revealed that resistance training, which combines heavy loads with low repetitions and light loads with more repetitions at very high ballistic movement speeds, probably has maximum neural adaptations and minimum hypertrophy adaptations in trained muscles [82]. In short, such researches show that various types of resistance training can cause a specific relationship in the force-speed curve diagram. Examining the exercises that have been done to date have reported results in favor of lighter explosive resistance exercises to increase jumping power and speed [83–85].

However, Blazevitch and Jenkins [86] found no difference in the outlook for high-velocity versus low-velocity training, while Aargaard et al. [87] reported a 15% increase in strength growth after 14 weeks of heavy resistance training. In addition, it should be remembered that the so-called explosive resistance exercises are determined based on a percentage of the maximum strength. This setting is normally between 30 and 60% of a one-repetition maximum associated with a resistance that provides maximum power output for the upper and lower body [88]. Therefore, the quality of explosive resistance training is directly related to maximal reinforcement levels that enable stronger athletes to train and perform higher absolute force outputs. Resistance exercises, in any given training cycle, should probably start with a base increase in maximum strength. There is some experimental evidence to prove the usefulness of such light and heavy resistance exercises [89].

Limited experimental studies support a relationship between short-term power output (speed endurance) and maximal strength [80, 90]. The dependence of these relationships is that the actions performed at the same absolute load after the training period become less boring. This appears to be because stronger muscles require less neural activity, as shown by muscle EMG tests [70].

Unfortunately for sprinters and other strength athletes, available evidence suggests that prolonged exercise may change the profile from IIb (fast-twitch glycolytic) to IIa (fast-twitch oxidative glycolytic) and finally to type I (slow-twitch oxidative), but this transformation in the opposite direction, that is, from slow contraction to rapid contraction, is probably not possible [89, 91]. An exception to the latter claim was made by Almeida-Silveira et al. [92] using intense exercise and a stretch-shortening cycle in rats to produce a significant increase in type 2 fibers in the soleus muscle. This effect of exercise in humans is still under study, although interestingly, human muscles contract faster when exposed to long-term disuse [93]. These latter observations provide clues to the mechanisms by which muscle fibers shift from fast-twitch to slow-twitch with strenuous exercise, regardless of whether it is associated with strength, speed, or endurance exercise.

Early experiments involving surgery and changing the nerves of fast-twitch and slow-twitch muscles showed that nerves determine the contractile and metabolic properties of muscle fibers. In further investigations, it was seen that the special quality of the nerve and the total amount of electrical activity transferred to the muscle cells in contact with a certain level of mechanical tension determines whether its muscle fibers are slow-twitch or fast-twitch [93]. So the genetic change to regulate the production of the slow-twitch myosin type 1 isoform, and related proteins, appears to be through intense stimulation of the relevant nerve to the muscles being used in that state, or indeed, the muscles under heavy exercise. Similarly, type IIb tissues, which normally receive relatively few nerve impulses, do not produce slower isoforms of myosin unless they are altered by increased contractile activity and, thus, electrical activity. In this sense, genes regulate the expression of myosin twitch phenotypes, which can exist as default genes because they appear largely in the absence of vigorous activity. For example, it has been shown that the soleus muscle of the foot, when immobilized in a shortened position or exposed to hypo-gravity, expresses myosin fast-contraction genes [93].

Training for a strength event such as the high jump is characterized by dynamic explosive movements of short duration but with maximal intensity. Such activity, according to the principle of the size of motor unit recruitment, according to which motor units are used regularly and in order from smaller and slower motor units to larger and faster motor units according to the force and speed requirements of the contraction, all motor units are used regardless of the speed of contraction in a trained athlete applies [94]. Type 2 fast-twitch fibers appear to show greater hypertrophy with a variety of regular resistance exercises than type 1 fibers [95], which is probably due to the selective regulation of androgen receptors [96]. Therefore, intense high-resistance training of the type performed by high jumpers and other strength athletes may simply result in selective hypertrophy of type 2 fibers because these fibers are much more responsive to such stimulation when they are used. One proposed explanation is that the selective hypertrophy of type 2 fibers may result from the selective use of these faster motor units in dynamic and ballistic-type movements; it means the reversal of the "Size Principle." Although there is evidence that type 2 motor units may be preferentially recruited to fast eccentric and concentric contractions [97], there is also considerable evidence to support the persistence of the "size principle" [98].

3. Adaptations and responses of the brain and central nervous system to sports activities

By studying the research carried out in the field of sports activity, we can reach the important point that many adaptations caused by sports activity can take place in the central nervous system (brain and spinal cord) and ultimately lead to the improvement of sports performance.

It can point out the general point that the occurrence of physiological changes such as adaptations of the nervous system in most sports is more important than anatomical changes such as increasing muscle mass. It is worth mentioning that due to the lack of tools, there is little information available to measure the amount of changes in the nervous system compared to other factors such as anatomical changes (muscle volume).

Research background to date has confirmed the causal relationship between regular physical activity and brain development, especially in the prefrontal cortex. Regular physical activity improves neuro-trophy by controlling the maintenance, growth, and differentiation of neurons, synapses, and angiogenesis, and as a result improves cognitive functions such as processing speed, control and planning strategies, and working memory [8, 9].

In order with this perspective, there is a good consensus among theorists that sports and physical activities can play an essential role in functional adaptations among children and adolescents [4, 99] and the elderly [100, 101]. Recent studies have confirmed the hypothesis that regular physical activity is closely related to improved reaction time [6] and better working memory [102] in people.

The studies conducted on mice show that a combination of sports programs and environmental enrichment is one of the conditions that increase sensory-motor stimulation and decrease cerebral cortex inhibition through increasing cell proliferation, neurogenesis, and gliogenesis in the hippocampus [103]. Specifically, the decrease in brain volume is closely related to the hypoplasia of the hippocampus, cerebral cortex, and white matter, as well as a significant decrease in the number of nerve cells [104, 105].

Recent experiments have provided evidence of changes in electroencephalography (EEG) activity and cognitive task performance in individuals after moderate-intensity exercise, particularly in the areas of the frontal lobe, rectal gyrus, and medial gyrus [9, 102, 106].

However, little information is available about the structure of intervention programs that improve motor skills. Shin and Park [106], in a meta-analysis, researched the effects of movement programs on people with intellectual disabilities. In short, short-term interventions (31–60 minutes) and continuous programs that are repeated four times a week have the most effects. It also seems that the effectiveness of these programs is influenced by personality characteristics, such as age and the degree of intellectual disability; in other words, younger people and those who are on the border of intellectual disability after specific movement exercises compared to people who have a higher level of intellectual disability, show more improvement. It seems that the disorder in the mental functioning of children with borderline and mild mental disabilities is related to the reduction of their physical functioning [107–109]; these findings confirm the hypothesis that motor and intellectual domains are strongly related to each other in people.

4. Conclusion

Exercise as an effective physical activity can help strengthen and adapt muscles. By doing regular sports exercises, the muscles will be able to adapt to high pressures and different extreme changes. Also, exercise can increase muscle strength, flexibility, and endurance; therefore, exercising regularly can help improve the structure and function of muscles and reduce injuries caused by daily activities.

Relatively, even short-term training programs can produce many adaptations in selected neuromuscular indicators [110]. The most plausible explanation for these results is the use of different types of muscle fibers, nerve activity, and the use of different types of energy sources, which are different according to the intensity and duration of exercise. Body muscles are composed of comparable proportions of fast-twitch and slow-twitch fibers [111]. Systematic changes in training variables such as training duration, training intensity, and type of exercise in sports programs act as facilitator of adaptations needed for all types of muscle fibers and neurons that activate them [96]. In addition, these changes lead to a similar change and transformation in the used energy source, which is used again to provide energy. Another explanation may be that the groups that trained with heavier training loads and used the timed program experienced more significant adaptations and performance improvements than the control group [112].

The responsible mechanisms that cause improvements in muscle through these adaptations may be related to changes in local enzyme activity and individual muscle fiber properties, which in turn may have positive effects on neuromuscular, biomechanical, and metabolic performance [113].

Acknowledgements

We hereby acknowledge and thank the efforts of Dr. Sedigheh Sadat Hojjati (Assistant Professor, Department of Physical Education, Payam Noor University, Tehran, Iran).

Conflict of interest

There is no conflict of interest.

Author details

Hojjatollah Siavoshy
Exercise Physiology, Department of Sport Sciences, Faculty of Humanities, University College of Omran_Toseeh, Hamadan, Iran

*Address all correspondence to: seiavoshy@gmail.com

References

[1] Hallahan DP, Kauffman JM. Exceptional Children: Introduction to Special Education. 4th ed. Mashhad: Astan Qods Razavi; 2001 [Persian]

[2] Robinson NM, Robinson HB. The Mentally Retarded Children: A Psychological Approach. 5th ed. Mashhad: Astan Qods Razavi; 1998 [Persian]

[3] Zigler E. The Retarded Child as a Whole Person. The Experimental Psychology of Mental Retardation. New York: Routledge; 2017. pp. 231-322

[4] Tomporowski PD, Lambourne K, Okumura MS. Physical activity interventions and children's mental function: An introduction and overview. Preventive Medicine. 2011;**52**:S3-S9

[5] Battaglia G, Alesi M, Inguglia M, Roccella M, Caramazza G, Bellafiore M, et al. Soccer practice as an add-on treatment in the management of individuals with a diagnosis of schizophrenia. Neuropsychiatric Disease and Treatment. 2013;**9**:595

[6] Nü Y, Erbahçeci F, Ergun N, Pitetti KH, Beets MW. The effect of physical fitness training on reaction time in youth with intellectual disabilities. Perceptual and Motor Skills. 2010;**111**(1):178-186

[7] Nagamatsu LS, Chan A, Davis JC, Beattie BL, Graf P, Voss MW, et al. Physical activity improves verbal and spatial memory in older adults with probable mild cognitive impairment: A 6-month randomized controlled trial. Journal of Aging Research. 2013;**2013**

[8] Best JR. Effects of physical activity on children's executive function: Contributions of experimental research on aerobic exercise. Developmental Review. 2010;**30**(4):331-351

[9] Golubović Š, Maksimović J, Golubović B, Glumbić N. Effects of exercise on physical fitness in children with intellectual disability. Research in Developmental Disabilities. 2012;**33**(2):608-614

[10] Rintala P, Loovis EM. Measuring motor skills in Finnish children with intellectual disabilities. Perceptual and Motor Skills. 2013;**116**(1):294-303

[11] Galli M, Rigoldi C, Mainardi L, Tenore N, Onorati P, Albertini G. Postural control in patients with Down syndrome. Disability and Rehabilitation. 2008;**30**(17):1274-1278

[12] Webber A, Virji-Babul N, Edwards R, Lesperance M. Stiffness and postural stability in adults with Down syndrome. Experimental Brain Research. 2004;**155**(4):450-458

[13] Cleaver S, Hunter D, Ouellette-Kuntz H. Physical mobility limitations in adults with intellectual disabilities: A systematic review. Journal of Intellectual Disability Research. 2009;**53**(2):93-105

[14] Blomqvist S, Olsson J, Wallin L, Wester A, Rehn B. Adolescents with intellectual disability have reduced postural balance and muscle performance in trunk and lower limbs compared to peers without intellectual disability. Research in Developmental Disabilities. 2013;**34**(1):198-206

[15] Hsieh K, Rimmer J, Heller T. Prevalence of falls and risk factors in adults with intellectual disability.

American Journal on Intellectual and Developmental Disabilities. 2012;**117**(6):442-454

[16] Schmitt K, Kressig RW. Mobilität und balance. Therapeutische Umschau. 2008;**65**(8):421-426

[17] Sherrard J, Tonge BJ, Ozanne-Smith J. Injury risk in young people with intellectual disability. Journal of Intellectual Disability Research. 2002;**46**(1):6-16

[18] Wallace C, Reiber GE, LeMaster J, Smith DG, Sullivan K, Hayes S, et al. Incidence of falls, risk factors for falls, and fall-related fractures in individuals with diabetes and a prior foot ulcer. Diabetes Care. 2002;**25**(11):1983-1986

[19] Shields N, Dodd KJ, Abblitt C. Do children with Down syndrome perform sufficient physical activity to maintain good health? A pilot study. Adapted Physical Activity Quarterly. 2009;**26**(4):307-320

[20] Baynard T, Pitetti KH, Guerra M, Unnithan VB, Fernhall B. Age-related changes in aerobic capacity in individuals with mental retardation: A 20-yr review. Medicine and Science in Sports and Exercise. 2008;**40**(11):1984-1989

[21] Khalili MA, Elkins MR. Aerobic exercise improves lung function in children with intellectual disability: A randomised trial. The Australian Journal of Physiotherapy. 2009;**55**(3):171-175

[22] Hill DA, Gridley G, Cnattingius S, Mellemkjaer L, Linet M, Adami H-O, et al. Mortality and cancer incidence among individuals with Down syndrome. Archives of Internal Medicine. 2003;**163**(6):705-711

[23] Hermon C, Alberman E, Beral V, Swerdlow A. Mortality and cancer incidence in persons with Down's syndrome, their parents and siblings. Annals of Human Genetics. 2001;**65**(2):167-176

[24] Rimmer JH, Heller T, Wang E, Valerio I. Improvements in physical fitness in adults with Down syndrome. American Journal on Mental Retardation. 2004;**109**(2):165-174

[25] Mohammadi F, Rajabi R, Alizadeh MH, VaezMousavi M. Relationship between IQ levels and physical fitness factors in students with intellectual disability. Sport Psychology Studies. 2015;**3**(10):69-74. [Persian]

[26] Heller T, Hsieh K, Rimmer J. Barriers and supports for exercise participation among adults with Down syndrome. Journal of Gerontological Social Work. 2003;**38**(1-2):161-178

[27] Menear K. Parents' perceptions of health and physical activity needs of children with Down syndrome. Down Syndrome Research and Practice. 2007;**12**(1):60-68

[28] Shields N, Taylor NF, Dodd KJ. Effects of a community-based progressive resistance training program on muscle performance and physical function in adults with Down syndrome: A randomized controlled trial. Archives of Physical Medicine and Rehabilitation. 2008;**89**(7):1215-1220

[29] Siyavoshi H. Progressive tolerance exercises for young adults suffering from Down syndrome: A clinical experiment. Exceptional Education. 2013;**5**(118): 68-71. [Persian]

[30] Hutzler Y, Korsensky O. Motivational correlates of physical activity in persons with an intellectual disability: A systematic literature review. Journal of Intellectual Disability Research. 2010;**54**(9):767-786

[31] Kristén L, Patriksson G, Fridlund B. Conceptions of children and adolescents with physical disabilities about their participation in a sports programme. European Physical Education Review. 2002;**8**(2):139-156

[32] Barr M, Shields N. Identifying the barriers and facilitators to participation in physical activity for children with Down syndrome. Journal of Intellectual Disability Research. 2011;**55**(11):1020-1033

[33] AAHPER. Programing for Mentally Retarded in Physical Education and Recreation. Washington, D.C.: American Association for Health, Physical Education, and Recreation (AAHPER); 1968. 10-2 p

[34] Fait HF. Special Physical Education: Adapted, Corrective, Developmental. 3rd ed. Mashhad: Astan Qods Razavi; 1995

[35] Rahmani P, Dansehmandi H. The Study of Posture and Physical Fitness in Subjects with Down Syndrome. Guilan: University of Guilan; 2012 [Persian]

[36] Rahmani P, Shahrokhi H, Dansehmandi H. Comparative study of physical fitness factors in intellectual disability with and without Down syndrome. Studies in Sport Medicine. 2012;**4**(11):81-94. [Persian]

[37] Siavoshy H. Effects of resistance training on salivary hormone profile and immunoglobulin A in adults with Down Syndrome. Exceptional Education. 2016;**9**(137):60-64. [Persian]

[38] Siavoshi H, Agha Alinejad H, Kashi A, Samavati Sharif MA, Helalizadeh M. The relationships between some physical fitness factors and muscle damage in people with intellectual disabilities. Iranian Rehabilitation Journal. 2020;**18**(2):7

[39] Siavoshy H, Agha Alinejad H, Kashi A, Samavati Sharif MA, Helalizadeh M. Normative data for the Canadian Standardized Test of Fitness (CSTF) in intellectual disability students in middle schools and high schools of Hamadan province. Sport Physiology. 2019;**11**(42):95-112. [Persian]

[40] Siavoshy H, Bolurian F. The effects of 12 weeks of playing boccia on the social development of children with cerebral palsy and intellectual disability. Journal of Exceptional Children. 2016;**15**(4):45-51. [Persian]

[41] Mashhadi MHZ, Isa. Physical fitness in connection with and health in mentally retarded students. Exceptional Education. 2013;**4**(117):29-37. [Persian]

[42] Fathi M. The Effect of Educational Games on the Intelligence of Educable Intellectual Disability Children. Tehran: University of Tehran; 2007 [Persian]

[43] Shields N, Taylor NF. A student-led progressive resistance training program increases lower limb muscle strength in adolescents with Down syndrome: A randomised controlled trial. Journal of Physiotherapy. 2010;**56**(3):187-193

[44] Kajbaf MB, Mansuri M, Ejehei J, Dadsetan P. Investigating of diagnosis of "intellectual disability" based on Piaget's tests and Lambert's adaptive behavioral scale. The Journal of Psychology. 2000;**3**(4):341-357. [Persian]

[45] Graham A, Reid G. Physical fitness of adults with an intellectual disability: A 13-year follow-up study. Research Quarterly for Exercise and Sport. 2000;**71**(2):152-161

[46] Reid G, Montgomery DL, Seidl C. Performance of mentally retarded adults on the Canadian Standardized Test of Fitness. Canadian Journal of Public

Health = Revue Canadienne de Sante Publique. 1985;**76**(3):187-190

[47] Weller IM, Thomas SG, Gledhill N, Paterson D, Quinney A. A study to validate the modified Canadian Aerobic Fitness Test. Canadian Journal of Applied Physiology. 1995;**20**(2):211-221

[48] Astrand PORK. Textbook of Work Physiology. New York: McGraw-Hill; 1970

[49] Mathews DK, Fox EL. The Physiological Basis of Physical Education and Athletics. WB Philadelphia: Saunders Company; 1976

[50] Matsuda JJ, Zernicke RF, Vailas AC, Pedrini VA, Pedrini-Mille A, Maynard JA. Structural and mechanical adaptation of immature bone to strenuous exercise. Journal of Applied Physiology. 1986;**60**(6):2028-2034

[51] Simoneau J-A, Lortie G, Boulay M, Marcotte M, Thibault M-C, Bouchard C. Human skeletal muscle fiber type alteration with high-intensity intermittent training. European Journal of Applied Physiology and Occupational Physiology. 1985;**54**:250-253

[52] Bompa TO, Buzzichelli C. Periodization: Theory and Methodology of Training: Human Kinetics; 2019

[53] Sale D. Neural adaptation in strength and power training. Human Muscle Power. 1986;**20**(5):289-307

[54] De Vries HA, de Vries HA. Physiology of Exercise for Physical Education and Athletics. Dubuque: C. Brown; 1980

[55] Paavolainen L, Häkkinen K, Hämäläinen I, Nummela A, Rusko H. Explosive-strength training improves 5-km running time by improving running economy and muscle power. Journal of Applied Physiology. 1999;**86**(5):1527-1533

[56] Hoff J, Gran A, Helgerud J. Maximal strength training improves aerobic endurance performance. Scandinavian Journal of Medicine & Science in Sports. 2002;**12**(5):288-295

[57] Jenkins S. Sports Science Handbook. Berkshire, England: Sunningdale Publications; 1997

[58] Houston M, Thomson J. The response of endurance-adapted adults to intense anaerobic training. European Journal of Applied Physiology and Occupational Physiology. 1977;**36**(3):207-213

[59] Sharp R, Costill D, Fink W, King D. Effects of eight weeks of bicycle ergometer sprint training on human muscle buffer capacity. International Journal of Sports Medicine. 1986;**7**(01):13-17

[60] Jacobs I, Esbjörnsson M, Sylven C, Holm I, Jansson E. Sprint training effects on muscle myoglobin, enzymes, fiber types, and blood lactate. Medicine and Science in Sports and Exercise. 1987;**19**(4):368-374

[61] Medbø J, Burgers S. Effect of training on the anaerobic capacity. Medicine and Science in Sports and Exercise. 1990;**22**(4):501-507

[62] Jenkins D, Brooks S, Williams C. Improvements in sprinting with three weeks of training. New Zealand Journal of Sports Medicine. 1994;**22**:2

[63] Nevill ME, Boobis LH, Brooks S, Williams C. Effect of training on muscle metabolism during treadmill sprinting. Journal of Applied Physiology. 1989;**67**(6):2376-2382

[64] Whyte G. The physiology of training and the environment. In:

The Physiology of Training: Advances in Sport and Exercise Science Series. London: Elsevier/Churchill Livingstone; 2006. p. 191

[65] Gollnick PD, Armstrong R, Saubert C 4th, Piehl K, Saltin B. Enzyme activity and fiber composition in skeletal muscle of untrained and trained men. Journal of Applied Physiology. 1972;**33**(3):312-319

[66] Gollnick PD, Armstrong R, Saltin B, Saubert C 4th, Sembrowich WL, Shepherd RE. Effect of training on enzyme activity and fiber composition of human skeletal muscle. Journal of Applied Physiology. 1973;**34**(1):107-111

[67] Tesch P, Karlsson J. Muscle fiber types and size in trained and untrained muscles of elite athletes. Journal of Applied Physiology. 1985;**59**(6):1716-1720

[68] Clarkson PM, Kroll W, Melchionda AM. Isokinetic strength, endurance, and fiber type composition in elite American paddlers. European Journal of Applied Physiology. 1982;**48**:67-76

[69] Billat VL, Slawinski J, Bocquet V, Demarle A, Lafitte L, Chassaing P, et al. Intermittent runs at the velocity associated with maximal oxygen uptake enables subjects to remain at maximal oxygen uptake for a longer time than intense but submaximal runs. European Journal of Applied Physiology. 2000;**81**:188-196

[70] Sale DG. Neural adaptation to strength training. Strength and Power in Sport. 2003;**1**:281-314

[71] Henneman E, Somjen G, Carpenter DO. Functional significance of cell size in spinal motoneurons. Journal of Neurophysiology. 1965;**28**(3):560-580

[72] Desmedt JE, Godaux E. Ballistic contractions in man: Characteristic recruitment pattern of single motor units of the tibialis anterior muscle. The Journal of Physiology. 1977;**264**(3):673-693

[73] Moritani T, DeVries HA. Neural factors versus hypertrophy in the time course of muscle strength gain. American Journal of Physical Medicine & Rehabilitation. 1979;**58**(3):115-130

[74] Häkkinen K, Komi PV. Electromyographic changes during strength training and detraining. Medicine and Science in Sports and Exercise. 1983;**15**(6):455-460

[75] Hakkinen K. Effect of combined concentric and eccentric strength training and detraining on force-time, muscle fiber and metabolic characteristics of leg extensor muscles. Scandinavian Journal of Sports Sciences. 1981;**3**:50-58

[76] Lee J-B, Matsumoto T, Othman T, Yamauchi M, Taimura A, Kaneda E, et al. Coactivation of the flexor muscles as a synergist with the extensors during ballistic finger extension movement in trained kendo and karate athletes. International Journal of Sports Medicine. 1999;**20**(01):7-11

[77] Ploutz LL, Tesch PA, Biro RL, Dudley GA. Effect of resistance training on muscle use during exercise. Journal of Applied Physiology. 1994;**76**(4):1675-1681

[78] Hakkinen K. Training-specific characteristics of neuromuscular performance. In: Handbook of Sports Medicine and Science, Strength Training for Sport. New Jersey: Backwell Scientific Publications; 2002

[79] Siff M. Supertraining. 6th ed. Denver: Supertraining Institute; 2003. p. 290

[80] Robinson JM, Stone MH, Johnson RL, Penland CM, Warren BJ, Lewis RD. Effects of different weight training exercise/rest intervals on strength, power, and high intensity exercise endurance. The Journal of Strength & Conditioning Research. 1995;**9**(4):216-221

[81] Van Cutsem M, Duchateau J, Hainaut K. Changes in single motor unit behaviour contribute to the increase in contraction speed after dynamic training in humans. The Journal of Physiology. 1998;**513**(1):295-305

[82] Komi PV. Strength and power in sport. Medicine and Science in Sports and Exercise. 1994;**26**(11):1422

[83] Delecluse C, Van Coppenolle H, Willems E, Van Leemputte M, Diels R, Goris M. Influence of high-resistance and high-velocity training on sprint performance. Medicine and Science in Sports and Exercise. 1995;**27**(8):1203-1209

[84] Newton RU, Kraemer WJ, Haekkinen K. Effects of ballistic training on preseason preparation of elite volleyball players. Medicine and Science in Sports and Exercise. 1999;**31**:323-330

[85] Wilson GJ, Newton RU, Murphy AJ, Humphries BJ. The optimal training load for the development of dynamic athletic performance. Medicine and Science in Sports and Exercise. 1993;**25**(11):1279-1286

[86] Blazevich AJ, Jenkins DG. Effect of the movement speed of resistance training exercises on sprint and strength performance in concurrently training elite junior sprinters. Journal of Sports Sciences. 2002;**20**(12):981-990

[87] Aagaard P, Simonsen EB, Andersen JL, Magnusson P, Dyhre-Poulsen P. Increased rate of force development and neural drive of human skeletal muscle following resistance training. Journal of Applied Physiology. 2002;**93**(4):1318-1326

[88] Izquierdo M, Häkkinen K, Gonzalez-Badillo JJ, Ibanez J, Gorostiaga EM. Effects of long-term training specificity on maximal strength and power of the upper and lower extremities in athletes from different sports. European Journal of Applied Physiology. 2002;**87**:264-271

[89] Harris GR. Effects of Three Different Weight Training Programs on Measures of Athletic Performance: Maximum Strength, Power, Speed and Agility: A Thesis. North Carolina: Appalachian State University; 1996

[90] Costill D. Muscle strength: Contributions to sprint swimming. Swimmimng World. 1980;**21**:29-34

[91] Pette D. Historical perspectives: Plasticity of mammalian skeletal muscle. Journal of Applied Physiology. 2001;**90**(3):1119-1124

[92] Almeida-Silveira M, Perot C, Pousson M, Goubel F. Effects of stretch-shortening cycle training on mechanical properties and fibre type transition in the rat soleus muscle. Pflügers Archiv. 1994;**427**:289-294

[93] Goldspink G, Harridge S. Cellular and molecular aspects of adaptation in skeletal muscle. Strength and Power in Sport. 1992;**3**:231-251

[94] Moritani T. Motor unit and motoneurone excitability during explosive movement. Strength and Power in Sport. 2003;**1**:27-49

[95] Hather B, Tesch P, Buchanan P, Dudley G. Influence of eccentric actions on skeletal muscle adaptations to

resistance training. Acta Physiologica Scandinavica. 1991;**143**(2):177-185

[96] Kraemer WJ, Fleck SJ, Evans WJ. Strength and power training: Physiological mechanisms of adaptation. Exercise and Sport Sciences Reviews. 1996;**24**(1):363-398

[97] Grimby L, Hannerz J. Firing rate and recruitment order of toe extensor motor units in different modes of voluntary conraction. The Journal of Physiology. 1977;**264**(3):865-879

[98] Duchateau J, Hainaut K. Mechanisms of muscle and motor unit adaptation to explosive power training. Strength and Power in Sport. 2003;**1**:316-330

[99] Battaglia G, Alesi M, Inguglia M, Roccella M, Caramazza G, Bellafiore M, et al. Soccer practice as an add-on treatment in the management of individuals with a diagnosis of schizophrenia. Neuropsychiatric Disease and Treatment. 2013;**9**:595-603

[100] Bellafiore M, Battaglia G, Bianco A, Paoli A, Farina F, Palma A. Improved postural control after dynamic balance training in older overweight women. Aging Clinical and Experimental Research. 2011;**23**:378-385

[101] Battaglia G, Bellafiore M, Bianco A, Paoli A, Palma A. Effects of a dynamic balance training protocol on podalic support in older women. Pilot study. Aging Clinical and Experimental Research. 2010;**22**:406-411

[102] Nagamatsu LS, Chan A, Davis JC, Beattie BL, Graf P, Voss MW, et al. Physical activity improves verbal and spatial memory in older adults with probable mild cognitive impairment: A 6-month randomized controlled trial. Journal of Aging Research. 2013;**2013**(1):861893

[103] Begenisic T, Spolidoro M, Braschi C, Baroncelli L, Milanese M, Pietra G, et al. Environmental enrichment decreases GABAergic inhibition and improves cognitive abilities, synaptic plasticity, and visual functions in a mouse model of Down syndrome. Frontiers in Cellular Neuroscience. 2011;**5**:29

[104] La Grutta S, Cali A, Sarno I, Trombini E, Roccella M. People with Down's sindrome: Adolescence and the journey towards adulthood. Minerva Pediatrica. 2009;**61**(3):305-321

[105] Vecchio D, Salzano E, Vecchio A, Roccella M. A rare unbalanced translocation 1; 18 in a child with epilepsy, mild dysmorphology and mental retardation. Minerva Pediatrica. 2012;**64**(3):365-367

[106] Shin I-S, Park E-Y. Meta-analysis of the effect of exercise programs for individuals with intellectual disabilities. Research in Developmental Disabilities. 2012;**33**(6):1937-1947

[107] Hartman E, Houwen S, Scherder E, Visscher C. On the relationship between motor performance and executive functioning in children with intellectual disabilities. Journal of Intellectual Disability Research. 2010;**54**(5):468-477

[108] Bartlo P, Klein PJ. Physical activity benefits and needs in adults with intellectual disabilities: Systematic review of the literature. American Journal on Intellectual and Developmental Disabilities. 2011;**116**(3):220-232

[109] Biddle SJ, Asare M. Physical activity and mental health in children and adolescents: A review of reviews. British Journal of Sports Medicine. 2011;**45**(11):886-895

[110] Fleck SJ. Periodized strength training: A critical review. The Journal

of Strength & Conditioning Research. 1999;**13**(1):82-89

[111] McArdle W, Katch F, Katch V. Exercise Physiology: Energy, Nutrition, and Human Performance. Baltimore: Williams & Wilkins; 1996

[112] Stone M, O'bryant H, Schilling B, Johnson R, Pierce K, Haff GG, et al. Periodization: Effects of manipulating volume and intensity. Part 1. Strength & Conditioning Journal. 1999;**21**(2):56

[113] Mujika I, Padilla S, Pyne D, Busso T. Physiological changes associated with the pre-event taper in athletes. Sports Medicine. 2004;**34**:891-927

Chapter 6

Motor Developmental Delay

Daphne Golden

Abstract

During development, motor skill acquisition occurs in a relatively similar sequence and emerges at a consistent age range with a level of variability and clustering of skills. Deficits or disorders within the infant or child's movement systems or elements of motor control processing can lead to motor delays. As motor development is foundational for advanced motor skills, delays could impact function and participation throughout the lifespan. The trajectory of development in infants and children with developmental delays, including motor, can be altered with early intervention and environmental exposure. Recent research has focused on the detection through testing of infants to promptly diagnose and initiate interventions, maximizing development and lifelong success. Patterns in the development of early motor skills are studied to lead to the diagnosis and intervention of DCD and other conditions in associated developmental domains. The abnormal or delayed acquisition of movement and motor milestones can be an indicator of future developmental delays in other domains and even conditions. Thus, early intervention of motor developmental delays could be far reaching in skill acquisition in the foundational skills fundamental achieving encompassing majority of life skills.

Keywords: motor, developmental delay, movement, motor skills, intervention

1. Introduction

Movement is fundamental for environmental engagement, which is crucial for human existence. It is essential for nearly all aspects of life, including socialization, navigating the environment, dressing, and manipulation [1, 2]. Movement skills develop during infancy and continue to grow and adapt throughout life, allowing engagement within the environment. Initial typical movements and motor skills show a consistent sequential pattern of development. They act as building blocks, gradually gaining flexibility and adaptability [3], forming the bases for more complex skills [4]. In addition, motor skills promote exploration and learning, sparking further development not only in motor skills but in multiple developmental domains [2]. The impact abnormalities or delays in developing these early foundational motor skills can have on socialization, communication [5, 6], cognition, and perceptual necessary for function, ADLs, career, and recreation over a lifespan cannot be overstated [4, 7]. In the early twentieth century, Bayley began documenting and establishing a typical development framework, allowing for a method to monitor and identify delays [8]. Ultimately, identifying irregularities and delays in a child's development allows for intervention to eliminate or reduce the impact of motor delays.

IntechOpen

2. Normal motor development

Although variability exists among individuals, movement and clusters of motor skills emerge in young children and infants, typically within similar age ranges. In early infancy, spontaneous elicited, and reflexive movements dominate [9, 10], fostering movement exploration [1, 9, 10]. Gradually, intentional movements begin to develop, replaced with controlled movements [9, 11]. These controlled movements lead to the acquisition of motor skills and milestones, each new skill built upon previously acquired skills [4]. When referring to motor skills, there are two main categories: gross motor, involving large movements such as sitting, crawling, and walking, and fine motor, more precise movements such as manipulative skills, grasping, and handling objects [1, 12]. Internal factors promoting learning through exploration of movement and environment guide trajectories and patterns.

Motor skill development tends to occur directionally in a cephalocaudal and proximal to distal manner. Typically, the cephalocaudal maturation and progression of motor skills occur by gaining control, first in the areas closest to the brain or CNS, then extending downward into the legs. The neck develops control, followed by the trunk and eventual extremities [1, 13]. The initial development of neck control allows the child to interact with the environment, particularly visual engagement, promoting further motor, sensory-perceptual, and cognitive growth. This engagement facilitates further development of milestones, including reaching, propulsion, crawling, and walking. Control of the body progresses proximally to distally, with earlier skills acting as building blocks for more complex skills [4, 13]. In alignment with this proximal-distal growth, the gross motor tends to proceed with multifaceted fine motor developmental tasks [13]. For example, mastery of large proximal *muscles* for gross motor independent sitting proceeds the ability to perform upright distal muscles for the fine motor task of manipulating a toy [14].

Reflexes and synergistic patterns dominate early in development, and through experience, movements become more flexible and adaptable [1–3, 9]. Spontaneous and primitive reflexes are internally driven and sometimes triggered by external stimuli leading to learning through engagement of the body with the environment. Example: The primitive reflex of an ATNR promotes eye-hand engagement, which leads to the development of eye-hand coordination by proprioceptors responding to the position of the neck. When turning to the right, the right arm extends, placing the eyes in the direction of the hand, fostering an early connection between visual and motor systems [1]. Initially, in synergistic patterns, a group of muscles activate as a unit and dominate the movement; however, through practice, one gains flexibility and variability in controlling and isolating movements and muscle group activation [3]. In sitting and standing, postural reactions activate groups of muscles to keep the body within the center of gravity, maintaining an upright posture [15]. As people develop, they advance, becoming flexible and able to adapt when encountering changing terrains. Early movement is innate and becomes increasingly controlled, allowing for variability, and flexibility to adapt to the environment [2, 3].

Action required for motor skill development is not only influenced by the individual; however, environmental factors, task exposure and practice, socioeconomic factors, and cultural factors also play a role [3, 11]. Movement is embodied and dependent on the individual's current status, which constitutes physical and physiological factors such as musculoskeletal, sensory, cardiopulmonary. As well as motor control with sensory-perceptual and cognition [2, 3]. Perception action coupling plays a crucial role in the motor process [16]. The environmental influences include factors such as space to engage in practice, availability of toys or stairs, nutrition, and social interactions [2, 3, 17]. Through experience and engagement in different environments and levels of practice, children learn to adapt and refine their actions [17]. Greater practice walking improved onset of independent and overall walking skills Hospodan, [18]. The availability of these opportunities influences the progression and mastery of motor skills. Social and cultural influences such as customs and interactions with siblings, peers, and parents. Caregivers may or may not promote social engagement [2]. Thus, development is multifaceted and dependent on the individual, environment, and experiences during the process, which is particularly important during early life.

3. Abnormal motor development

Motor developmental delay can manifest as a delay or deviation in the age of typical acquisition of movement and motor skills. Often, minor or transitory delays in attaining motor skills fall within a normal range of variation [19]. However, when a child presents with a continual or substantial delay, it may reflect abnormalities in their environment, movement experiences, and/or social and cultural factors. The individual infant or child may have an underlying condition or deficit during critical periods of early development. For example, genetic abnormalities such as Down Syndrome [19–21] often present with hypotonia and congenital heart defect and cognitive deficits [22], which can negatively influence motor development. Similarly, children with Developmental Coordination Disorder (DCD) impairments in motor processing and control, which impact their ability to acquire motor skills [23].

Musculoskeletal and neuromuscular changes also can result in abnormal or delayed motor development. Condition like cerebral palsy, which result from central nervous system (CNS) damage, frequently leads to neuromuscular and musculoskeletal changes. These individuals often present with muscle spasticity, resulting in decreased range of motion, abnormal bony alignment, and interfere with motor function [24]. Preterm infants with underdeveloped systems often experience delays in overall motor skill acquisition. The risk for motor developmental delay increases exponentially with decreased gestational age [25]. Additionally, physical changes such as Diastrophic Dysplasia which includes short stature is associated with a motor developmental delay [26].

Environmental and external factors also play significant roles in motor development. Infants exposed to alcohol (Fetal Alcohol Syndrome), toxins, infection and malnourishment prenatally are at risk for motor deficits [12, 19, 20, 27]. Engagement and practice of motor skills are critical for development and progression. One study found that daycares with larger areas for the child to explore after 6 months facilitated motor development more effectively than in environments with a higher caregiver-to-infant ratio [17]. Increased daily tummy time has been associated with earlier onset of prone skills [28]. A greater amount of time practicing walking led to an earlier age and improved walking skills [14, 18].

Socioeconomic status, cultural practices, and the mother's education level can also influence motor development [2]. The cultural practice of binding girls' feet in China [29] impaired walking, and cradling in Tajik delayed the achievement of crawling, standing, and walking later [30]. The amount of time spent watching television below the age of two showed an inverse relationship with motor development [31].

Motor development delays are typically multifactorial rather than resulting from a single alteration in the individual or environment. For example, children with cystic fibrosis (CF), a genetic disorder with an 8% greater prevalence of developmental delay, experience malabsorption in the gastrointestinal system, leading to malnourishment and chronic obstructive pulmonary disease (COPD), causing respiratory problems. Frequent and lengthy hospitalizations particularly with those exceeding 60 days are associated with developmental delays [32]. As previously noted, the ability to explore and move were at risk for developmental delay [17, 29]. Conditions in individual and environmental factors impacting motor development are often interconnected and do not occur in isolation.

4. Identification of a motor developmental delay

Children with considerable variation in the child's age of motor skill acquisition on milestone checklists, screens, and norm-referenced testing establish suspicion or identification or classification of a developmental delay [33]. Most are administered by observing the infant or child's movement and skill, performing a physical examination, and/or completing questionnaires. Untrained individuals play a crucial role in identifying abnormal development, such as parents being the first to identify whether a child achieves typical motor milestones such as sitting, standing, and walking [12]. Delays and the absence of meeting milestones can be a red flag for a potential developmental delay [1, 19, 20].

Routine developmental screenings administered by physicians and healthcare providers through parent surveys, physical examinations, and checklists often identify infants and young children with a potential gross motor delay [19, 34]. When a developmental delay or abnormality is suspected based on history, screens, or parental concerns, a referral to specialists, including physical therapists, early interventionalists, developmental pediatricians, or other specialists where a more specific norm-referenced developmental test may assist the physician or psychologist to establish a "diagnosis" or classification of a developmental delay. Age equivalents, z scores [20] and percentiles signify the degree of delays where the child falls in relation to their peer [35]. The delay may result from a cluster or a scattering of missed or abnormal skills. The identification of the type and extent of delay informs the intervention strategies.

The motor domain in developmental tests is typically divided into gross and fine motor skills, often each further broken down into components. For example, the Peabody Developmental Motor Scales, Second Edition (PDMS-2) categorizes the gross motor quotient into reflexes, locomotion, and object manipulation and the fine motor quotient into grasping and visual-motor integration [35, 36]. The Bayley III breaks motor down based on posture, dynamic movement and balance [36, 37]. Generally, observing movement and/or motor skills provides scores, with assessments including unfacilitated movement found on the Bayley and/or facilitated movement with verbal instruction on the PDMS-2. Tools will also use elicited examination and/or questionnaires like the Ages and Stages Questionnaire [36]. Most developmental tests use a quantitative approach, scoring whether a child performs or does not perform a particular skill. However, some assessments, like the Alberta Infant Motor Scale (AIMS), also assess the quality of the skill performance, providing a more nuanced view of the child's motor development and providing additional information to direct intervention [38, 39].

4.1 Selection of developmental tools based and purpose and other characteristics

The selection of developmental assessment tools depends on the purpose and characteristics of the infant or child being evaluated. Short-duration tools and parent questionnaires are particularly valuable for individualized identification and large-group screening due to quick administration. Such as the Ages and Stages Questionnaire (ASQ) and the Parents' Evaluation of Developmental Status (PEDS) which require less expertise. These tests are also designed to identify potential deficits or delays in motor skills that require further investigation and referrals [22, 40].

Comprehensive developmental assessments are used to pinpoint specific areas of deficit. For example, the Peabody Developmental Motor Scales, Second Edition (PDMS-2), includes detailed sections with 225–241 questions on Motor Quotient's, offering precise insights [35]. In contrast, the Ages and Stages Developmental Inventory Screening Tool relies on only 30 questions which includes all domains [41]. The comprehensive tools assist in developing tailored intervention plans. They also often assist in diagnosing DD and establishing the need for further evaluation of underlying conditions [20].

Other tests focus on early motor development used to facilitate early identification and predict potential delays or underlying conditions. Tools like the Test of Infant Motor Performance (TIMP) and Gross Motor Assessment (GMA) have the potential for identifying infants at risk for conditions such as respectively Cerebral Palsy (CP) [42] and motor delays [43] enabling timely interventions and serving as outcome measures in research. Recent tests administered in early infancy emphasize the observation of the quality and presence of spontaneous movements occurring prior to the development of controlled motor skills such as the GMA and TIMP. These observations help to identify early motor patterns [44, 45].

Unlike norm-referenced tests, which determine where a child falls relative to the general population, criterion-based developmental tests assess a child's performance of specific motor skills. Results assist in the development of interventions. The Hawaii Early Learning Profile (HELP) Checklist tests for defined skills and provides possible curriculum for you to use to assist in the growth of the skills the child has not mastered.

Selecting the appropriate tool also is dependent on factors, such as the child's age range, cognitive level, attention span, and developmental delays in other domains. Example: the PDMS-2 has detailed instructions and requires the child to follow specific directions [25], thus the test may not be suitable for children with attention deficits. A more observational or less instructional tool like the Ages and Stages may be more appropriate in such cases [41].

The population based on the condition of the child influences the selection of the tool. Some tests have been validated in one population but not the other, so results may not be as reliable or valid for that group. Such as PDMS-2 is norm-referenced test to the general population and Cerebral Palsy, but not for Muscle Dystrophy [35].

The child's age significantly impacts the selection of developmental tests, as each test design assesses motor development within a specific age range. For example, the Alberta Infant Motor Scale (AIMS) focuses on motor skills in infants [39], while the Bruininks-Oseretsky Test of Motor Proficiency, Second Edition (BOT-2) assesses older children [36].

5. Interventions

Generally, if a child's delay is more than −2 standard deviations from the norm, they are considered to have a significant delay [20, 46], qualifying them for intervention [47]. Intervention for developmental delays is provided through outpatient services and state or locally run programs. Early Intervention services are available for children from birth to 3 years old and children over 4 years old typically transition to School-Based Services [48]. However, school-based interventions have a limitation: the impairment must interfere with the educational process to qualify [34]. Therefore, many families also rely on outpatient services.

Early identification of developmental delays is essential, as early intervention can alter a child's development trajectory across multiple domains, not just motor skills. Early movement and motor skills are measurable and observable earlier in development than other domains. Consequently, investigating early infant observational tools like the TIMP (Test of Infant Motor Performance) and GMA (General Movements Assessment) is on the front as tools for early indicators of developmental conditions. Movement assessment results have been found to be associated with future diagnoses of Cerebral Palsy and Autism Spectrum Disorder (ASD) [45, 49]. Early motor skill delays identified through the DAYC (Developmental Assessment of Young Children) and BSID (Bayley Scales of Infant Development) indicate a higher risk for cerebral palsy [50].

Additionally, early intervention for motor delays can impact multiple developmental domains due to their interdependency with motor skills. For example, motor skill development has been predictive of expressive language deficits [51]. An association was found between Motor skill development and the development of social cognition [52], cognitive abilities [53], language [54], problem-solving skills [55], and communication [56]. Locomotion is associated with perception, spatial cognition, and emotional development [5] while crawling has been linked to anger-emotion regulation [57], and receptive language development [5, 58]. Example: It has been speculated that this relationship is the motor skill, locomotion, promotes exploration and social interaction [14], exploration of objects [6], and greater caregiver interaction allowing for development of these other domains.

Author details

Daphne Golden
University of St. Augustine St. San Marcos Campus, San Marcos, CA, United States

*Address all correspondence to: dkgolden@udel.edu

References

[1] Gerber RJ, Wilks T, Erdie-Lalena C. Developmental milestones: motor development. Pediatrics in Review. 2010;**31**(7):267-277

[2] Adolph KE, Hoch JE. Motor development: Embodied, embedded, enculturated, and enabling. Annual Review of Psychology. 2019;**70**(1):141-164

[3] Shumway-Cook A. Motor Control: Translating Research into Clinical Practice. Philadelphia, Pennsylvania: Lippincott Williams and Wilkins; 2007

[4] Haywood KM, Getchell N. Life Span Motor Development. Chaplain, Illinois: Human Kinetics; 2018

[5] Campos JJ, Anderson DI, Barbu-Roth MA, Hubbard EM, Hertenstein MJ, Witherington D. Travel broadens the mind. Infancy. 2000;**1**(2):149-219

[6] Dumuids-Vernet MV, Provasi J, Anderson DI, Barbu-Roth M. Effects of early motor interventions on gross motor and locomotor development for infants at-risk of motor delay: A systematic review. Frontiers in Pediatrics. 2022;**10**:877345

[7] Golden D, Getchell N. Developmental delay, developmental coordination disorder, and motor behavior. In: Disability and Motor Behavior: A Handbook of Research, Rowman-Littlefield. Blue Ridge Summit, PA; 2023

[8] Bayley N. Bayley Scales of Infant Development. New York, New York: The Psychological Corporation; 1969

[9] Thelen E. Dynamic mechanisms of change in early perceptual-motor development. In: Mechanisms of Cognitive Development. New York, New York: Psychology Press; 2001. pp. 173-196

[10] Kloze A, Brzuszkiewicz-Kuzmicka G, Czyzewski P. Use of the TIMP in assessment of motor development of infants with down syndrome. Pediatric Physical Therapy (Philadelphia, Pennsylvania). 2016;**28**(1):40-45

[11] Adolph K, Robinson SR. Motor development. In: Liben L, Muller U, editors. Cognitive Processes. Hoboken, New Jersey: Wiley; 2015. pp. 114-157. (Handbook of child psychology and developmental science)

[12] Centers for Disease Control (CDC). Developmental Disability Basics; 2024. Available from: https://www.cdc.gov/child-development/about/developmental-disability-basics.html [Accessed: 07 January 2025]

[13] Emre O, Keskinkılıç AU. Child and Child Education in the 21st Century

[14] Franchak JM, Adolph KE. An Update of the Development of Motor Behavior. Malden, Massachusetts: Wiley Interdisciplinary Reviews: Cognitive Science; 2024. p. e1682

[15] Krishnamoorthy V, Goodman S, Zatsiorsky V, Latash ML. Muscle synergies during shifts of the center of pressure by standing persons: Identification of muscle modes. Biological Cybernetics. 2003;**89**:152-161

[16] Schmebreuckler MA. Perception-action coupling in infancy. Advances in Psychology. 1993;**97**:137-173

[17] Mulligan L, Specker BL, Buckley DD, O'Connor LS, Ho M. Physical and environmental factors affecting motor

development, activity level, and body composition of infants in child care centers. Pediatric Physical Therapy. 1998;**10**(4):156-161

[18] Hospodar CM, Hoch JE, Lee DK, Shrout PE, Adolph KE. Practice and proficiency: Factors that facilitate infant walking skill. Developmental Psychobiology. Nov 2021;**63**(7):e22187. DOI: 10.1002/dev.22187. PMID: 34674233; PMCID: PMC8550266

[19] Choo YY, Agarwal P, How CH, Yeleswarapu SP. Developmental delay: Identification and management at primary care level. Singapore Medical Journal. 2019;**60**(3):119

[20] Khan I, Leventhal BL. Developmental Delay. Treasure Island, Florida: StatPearls Publishing; 2021

[21] Malak R, Kostiukow A, Krawczyk-Wasielewska A, Mojs E, Samborski W. Delays in motor development in children with down syndrome. Medical Science Monitor: International Medical Journal of Experimental and Clinical Research. 2015;**21**:1904

[22] Centers for Disease Control (CDC). Birth Defects: Down's Syndrome; 2024. Available from: https://www.cdc.gov/child-development/about/developmental-disability-basics.html [Accessed: 07 January 2025]

[23] Castellucci G, Singla R. Developmental coordination disorder (dyspraxia). In: StatPearls [Internet]. Treasure Island, Florida: StatPearls Publishing; 2024

[24] Jr ME. Treatment of neuromuscular and musculoskeletal problems in cerebral palsy. Pediatric Rehabilitation. 2001;**4**(1):5-16

[25] Kerstjens JM, De Winter AF, Bocca-Tjeertes IF, Bos AF, Reijneveld SA. Risk of developmental delay increases exponentially as gestational age of preterm infants decreases: A cohort study at age 4 years. Developmental Medicine and Child Neurology. 2012;**54**(12):1096-1101

[26] Crockett MM, Carten MF, Hurko O, Sponseller PD. Motor milestones in children with diastrophic dysplasia. Journal of Pediatric Orthopaedics. 2000;**20**(4):437-441

[27] Chattopadhyay N, Saumitra M. Developmental outcome in children with malnutrition. Journal of Nepal Paediatric Society. 2016;**36**(2):170-177

[28] Dudek-Shriber L, Zelazny S. The effects of prone positioning on the quality and acquisition of developmental milestones in four-month-old infants. Pediatric Physical Therapy. 2007;**19**(1):48-55

[29] Ebrey PB. Gender and sinology: Shifting western interpretations of footbinding, 1300-1890. Late Imperial China. 1999;**20**(2):1-34

[30] Karasik LB, Adolph KE, Fernandes SN, Robinson SR, Tamis-LeMonda CS. Gahvora cradling in Tajikistan: Cultural practices and associations with motor development. Child Development. 2023;**94**(4):1049-1067

[31] Lin LY, Cherng RJ, Chen YJ, Chen YJ, Yang HM. Effects of television exposure on developmental skills among young children. Infant Behavior and Development. 2015;**38**:20-26

[32] de Almeida TP, de Miranda Chaves CR, Pássaro CP, Meio MD. Motor delay in cystic fibrosis infants: An observational study. Early Human Development. 2011;**87**(12):769-773

[33] Piek JP, Dawson L, Smith LM, Gasson N. The role of early fine and

gross motor development on later motor and cognitive ability. Human Movement Science. 2008;**27**(5):668-681

[34] Lipkin PH, Okamoto J, Council on Children with Disabilities and Council on School Health, Norwood KW Jr, Adams RC, Brei TJ, et al. The individuals with disabilities education act (IDEA) for children with special educational needs. Pediatrics. 2015;**136**(6):e1650-e1662

[35] Ryan S. Peabody Developmental Motor Scales-Second Edition. Chicago, Illinois: AbilityLab; 2025. Available from: https://www.sralab.org/rehabilitation-measures/peabody-developmental-motor-scales-second-edition [Accessed: 07 January 2025]

[36] Griffiths A, Toovey R, Morgan PE, Spittle AJ. Psychometric properties of gross motor assessment tools for children: A systematic review. BMJ Open. 2018;**8**(10):e021734

[37] Ryan S. Bayley Scales of Infant and Toddler Development. 4th ed. Chicago, Illinois: AbilityLab; 2025. Available from: https://www.sralab.org/rehabilitation-measures/bayley-scales-infant-and-toddler-development-fourth-edition [Accessed: 07 January 2025]

[38] Piper MC, Darrah J. Motor Assessment of the Developing Infant. (No Title); 1994

[39] Eliks M, Gajewska E. The Alberta infant motor scale: A tool for the assessment of motor aspects of neurodevelopment in infancy and early childhood. Frontiers in Neurology. 2022;**13**:927502

[40] Vitrikas K, Savard D, Bucaj M. Developmental delay: When and how to screen. American Family Physician. 2017;**96**(1):36-43

[41] Ryan S. Ages and Stages Questionnaires. Chicago, Illinois: AbilityLab; 2025. Available from: https://www.sralab.org/rehabilitation-measures/ages-and-stages [Accessed: 07 January 2025]

[42] Bosanquet M, Copeland L, Ware R, Boyd R. A systematic review of tests to predict cerebral palsy in young children. Developmental Medicine and Child Neurology. 2013;**55**(5):418-426

[43] Caesar R, Colditz PB, Cioni G, Boyd RN. Clinical tools used in young infants born very preterm to predict motor and cognitive delay (not cerebral palsy): A systematic review. Developmental Medicine and Child Neurology. 2021;**63**(4):387-395

[44] Aizawa CY, Einspieler C, Genovesi FF, Ibidi SM, Hasue RH. The general movement checklist: A guide to the assessment of general movements during preterm and term age. Jornal de Pediatria. 2021;**97**:445-452

[45] Einspieler C, Peharz R, Marschik PB. Fidgety movements–tiny in appearance, but huge in impact. Jornal de Pediatria. 2016;**92**(3 Suppl 1):64-70

[46] Bellman M, Byrne O, Sege R. Developmental assessment of children. BMJ. 2013;**346**:e8687

[47] Delgado CE, Vagi SJ, Scott KG. Identification of early risk factors for developmental delay. Exceptionality. 2007;**15**(2):119-136

[48] Clarke CD. IDEA part C proposed rules released: ASHA submits comments on personnel qualifications, early intervention, other issues. The ASHA Leader. 2007;**12**(9):1-6

[49] Herrero D, Einspieler C, Aizawa CY, Mutlu A, Yang H, Nogolová A, et al.

The motor repertoire in 3-to 5-month old infants with down syndrome. Research in Developmental Disabilities. 2017;**67**:1-8

[50] Maitre NL, Slaughter JC, Aschner JL. Early prediction of cerebral palsy after neonatal intensive care using motor development trajectories in infancy. Early Human Development. 2013;**89**(10):781-786

[51] Bedford R, Pickles A, Lord C. Early gross motor skills predict the subsequent development of language in children with autism spectrum disorder. Autism Research. 2016;**9**(9):993-1001

[52] Leonard HC, Bedford R, Pickles A, Hill EL, Basis Team. Predicting the rate of language development from early motor skills in at-risk infants who develop autism spectrum disorder. Research in Autism Spectrum Disorders. 2015;**13**:15-24

[53] Veldman SL, Santos R, Jones RA, Sousa-Sá E, Okely AD. Associations between gross motor skills and cognitive development in toddlers. Early Human Development. 2019;**132**:39-44

[54] Holloway JM, Long TM. The interdependence of motor and social skill development: Influence on participation. Physical Therapy. 2019;**99**(6):761-770

[55] Molinini RM, Koziol NA, Marcinowski EC, Hsu LY, Tripathi T, Harbourne RT, et al. Early motor skills predict the developmental trajectory of problem solving in young children with motor delays. Developmental Psychobiology. 2021;**63**(6):e22123

[56] Valla L, Slinning K, Kalleson R, Wentzel-Larsen T, Riiser K. Motor skills and later communication development in early childhood: Results from a population-based study. Child: Care, Health and Development. 2020;**46**(4):407-413

[57] Pemberton Roben CK, Bass AJ, Moore GA, Murray-Kolb L, Tan PZ, Gilmore RO, et al. Let me go: The influences of crawling experience and temperament on the development of anger expression. Infancy. 2012;**17**(5):558-577

[58] Walle EA, Campos JJ. Infant language development is related to the acquisition of walking. Developmental Psychology. 2014;**50**(2):336

Chapter 7

Heterogeneity in the Neurocognitive Characteristics of Developmental Dyslexia: Theoretical Approaches and Research Findings

Maria Chalmpe and Filippos Vlachos

Abstract

The aim of this chapter is to reveal the heterogeneity in the neurocognitive profiles of children with developmental dyslexia. Over several decades of research on developmental dyslexia, various hypotheses, both cognitive and biological, have been proposed regarding the causes of the disorder. Most of these hypotheses suggest the presence of a single deficit as the primary cause of the disorder. However, recent studies have indicated that children with dyslexia often exhibit combinations of deficits across different cognitive domains. Furthermore, recent findings have suggested that the single deficit hypotheses are insufficient to explain the full spectrum of symptoms associated with developmental dyslexia. The observed diversity in cognitive profiles aligns with modern theoretical models that highlight the importance of multiple neurocognitive deficits in developmental dyslexia. At the same time, recent studies have confirmed the existence of distinct cognitive subtypes among individuals with dyslexia, emphasizing the heterogeneity of the disorder. A deeper understanding of this heterogeneity can lead to more sophisticated diagnoses with the use additional tests that assess a broader range of abilities that would help describe a more complete individual neurocognitive profile for each child diagnosed with dyslexia. This would result in the design and implementation of more targeted interventions that would meet the individual needs of each student with dyslexia, allowing them to develop their full potential.

Keywords: developmental dyslexia, neurocognitive deficits, single deficit hypotheses, multiple-deficit models, children

1. Introduction

Developmental dyslexia (DD) is classified as a neurodevelopmental disorder [1, 2] with a genetic and neurobiological basis, affecting an individual's ability to develop and acquire adequate reading skills. Despite having a normal intellectual level and receiving appropriate education, individuals with dyslexia face difficulties in word recognition, decoding, and phonological processing. This disorder is considered the most common learning disability among the school population [3], with prevalence rates ranging from 5% to 15% [4].

Frith [5] attempts to describe DD by identifying three distinct but interconnected levels. The first level is biological (genetic and neurobiological), where the causes of dyslexia can be investigated. The second level is cognitive, providing information on how biological causes are linked to individual behavior. The third level is behavioral, where one can directly observe the difficulties exhibited by individuals with dyslexia. Thus, Frith proposes an etiological model within which theoretical approaches to DD should be framed [5]. According to this model, in addition to the cognitive and biological hypotheses that have been proposed, the symptoms of the disorder, as well as environmental factors (social and cultural), that influence individuals with dyslexia should also be considered.

Modern perspectives on DD and its causes, based on Frith's etiological model and its three levels of analysis, aim to describe the disorder by uncovering the relationships between these levels [6]. However, various cognitive and biological approaches have been proposed, often differing in terms of etiology and the interpretation of the diverse linguistic, sensory, and motor symptoms observed in individuals with dyslexia.

The inability of these single deficit theories to fully account for the etiology of dyslexia, along with ongoing disagreements among scientists regarding the establishment of a universally accepted definition of the disorder, has led the scientific community in recent years to develop multifactorial approaches. These theories attempt to explain the causes of dyslexia and its symptoms by considering multiple factors [7–11].

The aim of this chapter is to reveal the heterogeneity in the neurocognitive profiles of children with developmental dyslexia. The following sections will explore the main cognitive and biological approaches regarding the causes of DD. Additionally, the multiple deficit models will be presented, highlighting the heterogeneity of the disorder and suggesting that most children with DD exhibit a combination of neurocognitive deficits while also acknowledging cases of individuals with isolated deficits. These contemporary models support the heterogeneity of the disorder and the existence of distinct subtypes among children with dyslexia, characterized by their performance in different tasks. We expect that through the documented presentation of these approaches and models, the reader will be able to understand the complex nature of DD, as well as the heterogeneity of its neurocognitive characteristics. A deeper understanding of this heterogeneity can lead to more sophisticated diagnoses with the use additional tests that assess a broader range of abilities which would help describe a more complete individual neurocognitive profile for each child diagnosed with dyslexia. This would result in the design and implementation of more targeted interventions that would meet the individual needs of each student with dyslexia, allowing them to develop their full potential.

2. Cognitive approaches of DD

Researchers who have investigated the causes of DD from the perspective of cognitive processes seek to explain the difficulties faced by people with DD by focusing on differences in their cognitive functioning. The aim of these approaches was to identify the central deficit responsible for these difficulties. In this context, several theoretical approaches have been proposed that highlight the multidimensional challenges exhibited by children with DD. In this chapter, the most significant cognitive hypotheses on DD will be presented, as derived from the study of the existing literature.

2.1 Phonological deficit hypothesis

The most dominant and widely recognized cognitive hypothesis for DD is the phonological deficit hypothesis [12, 13]. This hypothesis argues that the core deficit in DD is a phonological deficit that is present in most individuals with DD. A possible dysfunction in phonological processing is considered responsible for the difficulties in written language, particularly in reading, experienced by students with dyslexia [14, 15]. According to the phonological deficit hypothesis, individuals with dyslexia struggle with tasks requiring phonological awareness [16], phonological memory [17], and rapid automatized naming [18, 19].

Experimental studies suggest that the phonological deficits in individuals with dyslexia cannot be explained by dysfunctions in auditory mechanisms but are instead linked to deeper linguistic deficits [20]. A recent longitudinal study [21] has highlighted that children at high risk of developing a phonological deficit are five times more likely to develop dyslexia as they grow. In the same direction, a study [22] involving 56 children with dyslexia from Hong Kong showed significant differences in phonological performance between subgroups of children with dyslexia and control groups, confirming the presence of a phonological deficit. Moreover, research indicates that for a large percentage of children with dyslexia, difficulties in phonological processing are directly related to their reading difficulties [23]. Deficits in phonological skills and processing have been associated with deficits in verbal short-term memory [24–26].

Research [27] demonstrated that individuals with dyslexia exhibit lower levels of phonological awareness compared to proficient readers, regardless of age or reading level. Similar findings suggest that children with dyslexia experience deficits in short-term memory, reinforcing the connection between memory and reading ability [28].

At the same time, researchers studying the neurobiological basis of dyslexia confirm that the phonological deficit is associated with brain dysfunctions, particularly in the left angular gyrus and Wernicke's area, which are crucial for phonological processing and reading [16, 29].

Although the phonological deficit hypothesis has gained wide recognition, in recent years, it has come under examination and does not have general acceptance [18]. While the hypothesis of a single phonological deficit dominated the dyslexia literature from the 1980s to 2000 [6], more recent research has identified additional deficits, in visual or auditory processing as well as motor impairments in students with dyslexia [8, 30]. Such studies have led some researchers to argue that the co-occurrence of these additional difficulties, along with the phonological deficit in individuals with dyslexia, cannot be fully explained by the phonological deficit hypothesis as the sole cause of dyslexia [31, 32].

2.2 Temporal processing deficit hypothesis

The temporal processing deficit hypothesis suggests that individuals with dyslexia struggle to efficiently process visual and/or auditory stimuli, especially when these stimuli alternate rapidly [33–35]. This generalized difficulty in temporal processing may explain the phonological, visual, and motor difficulties that children with dyslexia exhibit [36].

In 1985, Tallal and his colleagues [35], using six variables related to rapid sensory processing and reproduction, classified their sample into two groups: individuals with language disorders and those without. A decade later, Farmer and Klein [33], in a review of studies evaluating visual and auditory discrimination, confirmed that individuals with dyslexia show significant differences compared to typically developing individuals. Furthermore, other research on stimulus sequence discrimination showed lower performance in individuals with dyslexia compared to control groups in 9 out of 15 conditions studied [35]. These findings support the idea that dyslexia could be due to a deficit in brain circuits that process auditory information at a fast rate [36].

However, this hypothesis has faced criticism, mainly due to confusion between temporal and sequential processing [37]. Mody and colleagues [37] demonstrated that individuals with dyslexia exhibit deficits in temporal sequence perception that are more related to phonemic distance than to temporal sequencing. Nevertheless, in clinical practice, cases of children with dyslexia who experience difficulties in various aspects of temporal processing are observed, such as difficulty in naming sequences of temporal concepts, perceiving temporal duration, and organizing memory events in a temporal sequence [38].

A study that investigated the nature of DD in the Spanish language revealed lower performance in children with dyslexia in all tasks assessing temporal processing. This finding was observed in comparison to two control groups: the first comprised children matched by chronological age, while the second included children matched by reading age [39]. Additionally, a study using eye-tracking technology with university students with dyslexia [40] revealed that dyslexic students took longer to process information and respond, indicating problems with temporal processing. Difficulties in auditory system temporal processing at early stages were also shown in a study using electroencephalography (EEG) [41]. The difficulty in temporal processing of visual information may result from dysfunction in visual-auditory coordination, which affects grapheme recognition and their connection with abstract concepts in verbal memory [42].

The temporal processing deficit hypothesis may be linked to the phonological deficit hypothesis and the magnocellular deficit hypothesis (a biological hypothesis for DD, which is presented at Section 3.2.2), as all seem to be related to difficulties in sensory processing of stimuli that change rapidly and sequentially [36].

2.3 Automatization deficit hypothesis

Automaticity is defined as the process that allows individuals to perform skills without conscious control, making them automatic [43]. Individuals with DD often struggle with fluency in skills that typically become automatic through repeated practice [43, 44]. Consequently, they face notable challenges in areas like reading, needing additional time and effort to develop automaticity [36].

Additionally, some behavioral symptoms of dyslexia have been attributed to deficits in automatization [43]. More specifically, besides phonological deficits, individuals with dyslexia may exhibit deficits in balance and motor skills [43, 45], in the speed of processing visual and auditory stimuli [46], as well as in skills that require closed eyes [47]. In a study evaluating children with dyslexia, through cerebellar tests and phonological assessments, researchers found that all children exhibited phonological deficits, while 50% of them also displayed motor difficulties [48]. Another study [49] found that children with dyslexia demonstrated deficits in motor skills. Similarly, more recent research [50] revealed reduced automatized functioning in dyslexic readers, with delays in naming and visual-orthographic processing. In another study [51] involving children with dyslexia, it was found that these children exhibited deficits in automatization during reading, leading them to develop specific strategies for text comprehension.

These deficits of dyslexics in automatization have been linked to dysfunction of the cerebellum, a structure of nervous system that is responsible for motor control and adaptive learning [36]. Cerebellar dysfunction may sufficiently explain motor, visual, auditory, and cognitive difficulties that dyslexic people often experience [52].

2.4 Attention deficit hypothesis

Another hypothesis that attempts to explain the deficits associated with DD is the attention deficit hypothesis [53–55]. According to this hypothesis, attention deficits interfere with the process of encoding letter sequences, leading individuals with dyslexia to confuse letters and the forms of visual words [55]. Such a visual attention deficit may reduce perceptual capacity and coexist with the phonological deficit in DD [53].

In their study, Zoubrinetzky and colleagues assessed 142 children with dyslexia and classified them into four cognitive subgroups: children with a phonological disorder, children with a visual attention disorder, children with a combination of both, and children with no disorder [56]. Although the research did not identify clear subtypes of dyslexia based on cognitive profiles, it showed that cognitive deficits may be associated with different behaviors in reading and spelling. Another study [53] assessed phonological skills and visual attention in a large sample from France and United Kingdom indicated that visual attention skills, like phonological skills, are critical for reading and that dyslexia may be due either to a phonological deficit or to a visual attention deficit.

An additional study evaluating children from France highlighted that 92.1% of children with dyslexia exhibited a phonological deficit, while 28.1% also displayed visual attention deficits [57]. Similarly, recent research [58] has found that visual attention deficits are directly related to reading fluency and may be influenced by the reading strategies children use.

Furthermore, studies have shown that visual attention deficits often coexist with auditory attention deficits [59]. Facoetti and his colleagues found that children with dyslexia display both visual and auditory attention deficits, which may hinder the development of phonological skills [54]. Finally, Vidyasagar and Pammer [60] proposed that phonological deficits in individuals with dyslexia result from a visuo-spatial attention deficit, while Ruffino and colleagues [61] demonstrated that there is a correlation between spatiotemporal attention and phonology.

Overall, several studies the last two decades indicate that children with dyslexia exhibit attention deficits, which often coexist with phonological deficits.

2.5 Memory deficit hypothesis

Memory is a fundamental brain function involved in the continuous processing of incoming information [62]. It is defined as the ability of an individual to encode, process, and recall information received in the past [63], and it is categorized into three levels: short-term, long-term, and working memory [64].

Working memory, as a higher cognitive skill, is involved in many activities, from simple linguistic tasks to complex verbal comprehension tasks [65]. It is defined as the system responsible for retaining and processing new information. Research has shown that deficits in working memory play a significant role in dyslexia [66]. In children with dyslexia, working memory deficits affect phonological and visuospatial skills, and these deficits often persist in adulthood [24, 67].

Difficulties in written language, particularly reading, are also associated with problems in verbal memory [24, 25, 67, 68]. These difficulties appear both in childhood and in young adults [68]. Research found that the performance of children with dyslexia on phonological memory tasks, such as nonword repetition, depends on their capacity for phonological storage, making these tasks reliable indicators for predicting dyslexia deficits [69].

A recent study by Gray et al. [70], which evaluated many children with and without language disorders, has demonstrated that children with dyslexia exhibit significant deficits in working memory. The authors emphasized that evaluating working memory provides critical information about children's broader cognitive function. In another study, Schuchardt and colleagues assessing children with dyslexia, dyscalculia, or both disorders found that children with dyslexia primarily exhibited deficits in phonological and working memory [68]. Deficits in both phonological and visuospatial memory in children with dyslexia have been confirmed in a recent study in Greece [71]. Additionally, a study [41] involving students with dyslexia or dyscalculia showed that children with dyslexia had deficits in verbal memory and processing speed.

Finally, neuroimaging studies using functional magnetic resonance imaging (fMRI) suggest that brain structures related to working memory, such as the frontal lobes and the cerebellum, show reduced activation in individuals with dyslexia, indicating the neurobiological basis of the obtained deficit and supporting the neurological origin of the disorder [72].

2.6 Anchoring deficit hypothesis

The anchoring deficit hypothesis [73] attempts to explain the difficulties faced by individuals with dyslexia. According to this hypothesis, the problems exhibited by dyslexic individuals are attributed to the inability to form specialized anchors during stimulus perception, which disrupts the dynamic relationship between perception and perceptual memory. These anchors function as reference points that facilitate the sensory processing of future stimuli and enhance the ability to retain and recall them [73].

This hypothesis is supported by research data indicating that difficulties in the dynamics of perception, which also affect short-term memory, may explain a wide range of challenges experienced by individuals with dyslexia [73]. These difficulties are related to phonology, working memory, auditory and visual perception, as well as sensitivity to environmental stimuli [73].

In typically developing individuals, the ability to create "anchors" around stimuli is observed, allowing for faster and more accurate processing of stimuli upon subsequent appearances [73, 74]. In contrast, individuals with dyslexia seem to be unable to sufficiently utilize stimulus repetitions, which contributes to their difficulties in processing information.

2.7 Double deficit hypothesis

The double deficit hypothesis offers an alternative approach to understanding DD, positioned between hypotheses that attribute the disorder to a single deficit and those that propose multiple deficits. According to this hypothesis, individuals with dyslexia exhibit deficits in both phonological processing and naming speed, which refers to the ability to quickly name words or objects [75]. These two deficits are not considered independent but complementary, with individuals who exhibit both being more likely to experience severe reading difficulties [76].

This hypothesis identifies four subtypes of DD, based on the presence or absence of phonological deficits and deficits in naming speed [77]. Specifically, it includes individuals with phonological deficits, individuals with naming speed deficits, individuals with both deficits, and those with neither deficit. Supporters of the hypothesis emphasize that children exhibiting both phonological and naming speed deficits face more severe reading difficulties compared to those presenting only one of these deficits.

Research supports the double deficit hypothesis and confirms the existence of different subtypes of dyslexia. A study that evaluated a large number (671) of children with reading difficulties confirmed the heterogeneity of DD, identifying subtypes with and without phonological deficits [78]. Additionally, a longitudinal study showed that those with a double deficit had significantly lower reading and spelling performance compared to children with only a phonological deficit or only a deficit in naming speed [79].

Further research [80] also confirms that children with written language difficulties simultaneously exhibit deficits in phonological awareness and naming speed, reinforcing the close relationship between these two deficits. Moreover, studies [49, 81] support that children with low performance in both phonological awareness tasks and naming speed tasks are at a higher risk of developing reading difficulties later.

However, supporters of the phonological deficit hypothesis view the double-deficit hypothesis as a variation of the phonological theory, arguing that deficits in naming speed and working memory are part of a broader phonological disorder [76].

In sum, many studies have tried to reveal the cognitive basis of DD and several relevant hypotheses have been formulated. This body of research is continued in our days, and hypotheses are still evaluated to enrich the understanding of DD, recognizing the complexity of the disorder and the heterogeneity of its manifestations.

3. Biological approaches

In recent years, significant advances in the field of biology, particularly in the branches of genetics and neurobiology, have expanded our ability to understand the causes of the deficits exhibited by individuals with dyslexia in these areas. Biological approaches suggest that the difficulties faced by individuals with dyslexia have a genetic and neurological basis [5, 36]. The differences observed in individuals with dyslexia may be related to abnormalities in brain structure [82] and/or variations in their brain activation patterns during cognitive activities [18].

3.1 Genetic basis of DD

Many studies have documented the complex genetic etiology of DD [83]. Genetic factors play an important role in the emergence of the disorder, with difficulties in written language exhibiting a considerable heritability [84].

The first studies in this examined families of dyslexics and an increased prevalence of dyslexia observed in such families [36, 85]. Additionally, twins' studies and molecular-genetic studies in families with members presenting specific reading difficulties further support the hereditary basis of dyslexia [86]. The research shows that children are more likely to develop dyslexia when there is a family history of the disorder.

The last decades, research have focused on identifying genetic markers on specific chromosomes associated with dyslexia [85]. Studies examine genetic regions that are inherited alongside genes linked to the reading disorder, with the aim of identifying genetic vulnerability loci [85]. The literature has reported 12 genetic loci and several genes that are potentially associated with the occurrence of dyslexia [85, 87]. A study that examined 165 families with members who had dyslexia [88] showed that the interactions between genes involved in brain development and environmental factors can explain dyslexia through a predisposition/stress model.

Overall, the research data demonstrate that the genetic predisposition to DD is strong, although the exact mechanism of inheritance remains unclear, as it does not follow Mendelian inheritance laws [36].

3.2 Neurobiological basis of DD

Studies aimed at examining the neurobiological basis of DD have for a history of more than five decades. In the early phases of research, in the late 1970s and mid-1980s, pioneers such as Galaburda and his colleagues [89, 90] studied the anatomy of the brains of individuals with dyslexia symptoms who had died [82]. Galaburda was the first to undertake such research, examining structural abnormalities in the brains of these individuals.

Over the past three decades, research in the field of dyslexia has advanced with the use of neuroimaging techniques, such as magnetic resonance imaging (MRI), functional magnetic resonance imaging (fMRI), magnetoencephalography (MEG), and other techniques that provide valuable information about the structure and the function of the brain in living individuals. From these studies, three main hypotheses have emerged regarding the neurobiological basis of DD.

3.2.1 Hypotheses of atypical structure and function in linguistics centers of brain

The research by Galaburda and his colleagues, which began in the late 1970s, revealed significant morphological differences and abnormalities in the cellular structure of the brains of individuals with dyslexia, particularly in the temporal region of the left hemisphere around the Sylvian fissure [90]. These areas are directly associated with language processing. Subsequent studies using positron emission tomography (PET) showed reduced activity in the left posterior parietal cortex during word recognition, suggesting structural and functional differences between the two hemispheres of the brain in individuals with dyslexia [29]. Additionally, dysfunction in the insula, which connects Wernicke's area to Broca's area, may contribute to reading difficulties, as these areas do not function collaboratively in dyslexic individuals [29].

The use of MRI has allowed for extensive study of the brains of living individuals with dyslexia. MRI studies have shown reduced gray and white matter volume, decreased brain gyrification, increased size of the corpus callosum, and asymmetries in the structures of the cerebellum and temporal lobe [91]. A recent study has also showed that the overall brain volume of individuals with dyslexia is smaller compared to that of typically developing individuals [82].

Studies using fMRI reveal reduced activation of cortical areas, such as the temporal gyrus and the area around the Sylvian fissure, in children with dyslexia [92]. Additionally, reduced activity has been recorded in the frontal cortex and the temporoparietal cortex, which are critical for language processing and reading [93].

Studies with magnetoencephalography (MEG) have also shown reduced activation in the temporoparietal region and the associative visual cortex, while simultaneously increased activation has been observed in the right temporoparietal region and the inferior frontal gyrus [94]. These findings support the existence of neurobiological differences related to DD.

Overall, the research data demonstrate significant differences in the structure and function of the brains of individuals with dyslexia, especially in the linguistic centers, compared to typically developing individuals. Such studies using various neuroimaging techniques highlight the contribution of neuroscience to understanding DD and explaining its symptoms through its neurobiological background.

3.2.2 Hypothesis of magnocellular deficit

According to the magnocellular deficit hypothesis, reading difficulties are attributed to the reduced development or dysfunction of magnocells, which are large neurons that play a significant role in temporal perception and motor processes [95]. Studies have shown that individuals with dyslexia may exhibit dysfunction in this system, which affects the processing of sensory information and, consequently, learning and language processing [36].

The magnocellular hypothesis was based on neuroanatomical studies [96] that revealed abnormalities in the visual and auditory magnocellular systems in individuals with dyslexia. These abnormalities may lead to difficulties in decoding rapidly changing sounds, which in turn create phonological deficits. Similar problems are observed in the visual magnocellular system, which is responsible for processing rapidly moving visual stimuli. Its dysfunction results in blurry visual representations, affecting the visual processing of letters and words [97].

Despite the evidence supporting the magnocellular hypothesis, some studies have questioned its broad application to all individuals with dyslexia [98]. The magnocellular hypothesis has faced criticism, primarily because it does not adequately explain all the symptoms of dyslexia in all individuals. Research does not always succeed in identifying the expected deficits in auditory and visual processing [36]. Furthermore, phonological deficits cannot be predicted solely based on difficulties in auditory processing [99], suggesting that the magnocellular hypothesis is insufficient for fully understanding the complexity of dyslexia.

3.2.3 Hypotheses of deficit in cerebellar function

The cerebellum is one of the main brain structures responsible for controlling motor functions and optimizing automatic motor skills [100]. Additionally, it actively participates in reading and cognitive skills in general [101]. Specifically, when processing information related to linguistic and magnocellular brain areas, this information passes through the cerebellum [36]. A dysfunction in the cerebellum could negatively impact reading and explain the various deficits exhibited by individuals with dyslexia [36, 52].

This notion is supported by neuroanatomical studies, neuropsychological data, and functional imaging research, indicating that cerebellar deficits may play a crucial role in the manifestation of DD. Based on this framework, the cerebellar dysfunction hypothesis was proposed, according to which mild motor difficulties and articulation problems in dyslexics may stem from cerebellar abnormalities [43, 52]. Articulation difficulties may lead to problems with the representation of phonological features of speech, which in turn affect the development of phonological awareness and, consequently, the reading ability [43, 52].

Cerebellar dysfunction may also explain the poor handwriting quality observed in individuals with dyslexia, as the cerebellum is critical for coordinating and automating the motor skills required during writing. Additionally, difficulties with articulation and spelling can be attributed to efforts to read correctly, which are accompanied by reduced phonological awareness and deficits in automatization [52].

According to the cerebellar dysfunction hypothesis, approximately 80% of children with dyslexia exhibit cerebellar deficits [52]. Studies over the past two decades have attempted to confirm this hypothesis. For example, a study involving elementary school students aged 8–12 demonstrated that children with dyslexia performed worse on cerebellar and cognitive tests compared to the control group and those with ADHD, as well as having slower articulation speed [102].

Similar studies have shown that children with dyslexia also exhibit motor difficulties, which may be due to cerebellar dysfunction [52]. Research assessing motor skills [103] confirmed that children with dyslexia performed worse on balance and motor coordination tests. Another study [104] found that children with dyslexia had reduced performance in static and dynamic balance tests, partially supporting the cerebellar deficit hypothesis.

However, the cerebellar deficit hypothesis faces two main limitations. First, not all individuals with dyslexia exhibit motor difficulties [97]. Second, this hypothesis does not account for the sensory processing difficulties observed in dyslexia. Nevertheless, proponents of this hypothesis acknowledge the existence of different dyslexia subtypes, which may stem from distinct dysfunctions of the cerebellum or the magnocellular system [52].

4. Contemporary models of multiple deficits

For several decades researchers considered DD as the result of a single deficit [7, 10]. However, advances in science and the complexity of the difficulties faced by individuals with dyslexia have led to a more multifaceted view of the disorder. Today, with the development of assessment methods and the study of dyslexia from various scientific disciplines, there is discussion of the heterogeneity of the disorder, and the prevailing view is that its causes are multiple [2]. The diverse and often conflicting hypotheses regarding the etiology of dyslexia lead some scientists to suggest that the disorder is likely the result of multiple deficits, with single or double deficit theories showing significant weaknesses to explain all the deficits of dyslexics [7].

The last decade, several researchers challenge the existence of a single deficit, emphasizing the heterogeneity of the disorder [105]. According to these studies, individuals with dyslexia face, in addition to phonological difficulties, other challenges such as visual, auditory, motor, and balance problems. While the phonological deficit may be the dominant cause of dyslexia, it can also occur independently of other sensory disorders [97]. Biological approaches support the idea that dyslexia may be due to brain differentiations, making its basis purely neurobiological.

At the same time, no single deficit has been identified that can explain the full range of dyslexia symptoms [11]. Moreover, the single deficit model cannot explain the comorbidity between various learning disorders, which often coexist without being independent [11, 106].

In conclusion, it is regarded necessary to transition from single deficit theories or dual-deficit theories to models of multiple deficits. These new models explore the relationships between different levels of analysis (genetic, biological, cognitive, behavioral, environmental, etc.) to further illuminate the causes of dyslexia [6, 11].

4.1 Multiple deficit model

Pennington [7] challenged the idea of a single cognitive deficit for the explanation of the causes of dyslexia, particularly due to its comorbidity with other developmental disorders, and introduced the Multiple Deficit Model (MDM) in the literature. This model is based on Frith's etiological approach [5], which asserts that understanding DD requires a combined study of biological and cognitive approaches, as well as the symptoms and environmental influences affecting individuals with dyslexia. MDM has since become one of the most contemporary and accepted theoretical approaches to the multifactorial etiology of dyslexia.

According to this model, DD can be understood through four levels of analysis: etiological, neurological, cognitive, and behavioral. At the etiological level, genetic and environmental risk and protective factors interact to lead to the onset of dyslexia. At the neurological level, differences in brain function are recorded, resulting from the influence of the etiological factors. At the cognitive level, the dominant cognitive deficits associated with structural and functional changes in the brain are highlighted. At the behavioral level, cognitive deficits manifest as symptoms and difficulties in individuals with DD [7].

Several recent studies have supported this model. Heim and colleagues [8] tested Pennington's model [7] by studying students with dyslexia in Germany. Their results identified three subcategories of dyslexia based on different cognitive deficits, such as phonological deficits, phonological and auditory deficits, as well as attention deficits. Similarly, Menghini and colleagues [9] studied children with dyslexia in Italy and confirmed the existence of multiple cognitive deficits, focusing on deficits in executive functions and phonological memory.

Other studies [12, 107] also support MDM, indicating that processing speed is a common risk factor for both dyslexia and ADHD, reinforcing the theory of comorbidity between the two disorders. Studies [30, 97] have also identify the existence of sensorimotor deficits in individuals with dyslexia, alongside phonological deficits. A study conducted on a sample of 78 children with dyslexia from Poland revealed the existence of three distinct subtypes of dyslexia, characterized by deficits in attention and visual search [108]. Additionally, a recent study in Greece [109] has also highlighted the existence of distinct neurocognitive subtypes of DD. In this study, 101 students diagnosed with dyslexia were classified into three different subtypes based on their performance across a wide range of tests that assessed the phonological domain, memory, attention, visual and auditory processing, visuomotor skills, and processing speed. In conclusion, recent research data have reinforced the view that dyslexia is the result of multiple deficits rather than a single deficit, supporting Pennington's model [7] and confirming the multifactorial nature of the disorder.

4.2 Hybrid model

A more recent theoretical approach that has emerged in the literature on the etiology of dyslexia is the hybrid model [10]. The hybrid model incorporates all previous hypotheses regarding the causes of dyslexia and allows for the formation of cognitive profiles in dyslexic individuals, which may include either a single deficit or a combination of multiple deficits. This model emphasizes the complexity of the disorder, and the heterogeneity observed among individuals with dyslexia.

This model was confirmed by a research conducted in Portugal, which included 36 children diagnosed with dyslexia [110]. The children were assessed in tasks of phonological awareness, rapid automatized naming, verbal short-term memory, and vocabulary. The results showed that the children could be divided into two subgroups: the first exhibited low performance in both phoneme deletion and rapid naming, while the second group had deficits only in phonological awareness, without problems in rapid naming. This confirms the existence of different cognitive profiles in dyslexia.

Similar findings were obtained in a study conducted with a sample of 285 students from Indonesia, 46 of whom were at risk of dyslexia [111]. The results indicated that some children at high risk for dyslexia exhibited either single or multiple deficits, while others showed no deficits in phonological tasks. These findings further support the hybrid model as an explanatory framework for DD, highlighting the heterogeneity of cognitive deficits that may present in individuals with dyslexia.

The hybrid model offers a comprehensive approach that reflects the complexity of dyslexia and emphasizes the need for flexible assessment and intervention methods, considering the unique cognitive profiles of everyone.

4.3 Intergenerational multiple deficit model

Just 2 years later, the Intergenerational Multiple Deficit Model (iMDM) appeared in the literature [11], building on the MDM [7] and adding a new level of analysis. The fifth level of analysis introduced focuses on parental characteristics and the family environment, highlighting the heritability and the intergenerational transmission of risk and protective factors. Heritability can provide insights into how these factors are passed from generation to generation through genes and the environment in which children are raised [11].

According to the iMDM, parents transmit genetic factors that influence their children's cognitive abilities, which interact with the environment to shape their cognitive profiles. The proportion of children with dyslexia who have at least one parent with the same disorder ranges between 34% and 66% [112]. A study of 182 children with a history of dyslexia confirmed that the reading abilities of parents are predictive factors for the development of dyslexia in children, especially through phonological awareness and processing speed, which are also linked to dyscalculia [11].

Thompson and his colleagues [113] continued in this direction, confirming the intergenerational nature of dyslexia and assessing phonological awareness, rapid automatized naming, and executive functions as predictive factors of the disorder. Additionally, research [114] confirmed that reading skills are 64% heritable, supporting the association across all family members.

In summary, contemporary multiple deficit models support the complexity and neurocognitive heterogeneity of DD. These models of DD emphasize the need for future research that considers both genetic and environmental influences in the study of the disorder.

5. Conclusion

The aim of the chapter was to reveal the heterogeneity in the neurocognitive profiles of children with developmental dyslexia. Through the presentation of various single deficit approaches that have been proposed in the literature regarding the causes of dyslexia, as well as more recent models suggesting the existence of multiple deficits, we sought to determine whether a stable and recurring set of cognitive characteristics can be systematically identified in a significant percentage of these children.

According to recent findings, DD is recognized as a complex and heterogeneous disorder [7–9, 11, 56, 109, 115], characterized by multifactorial deficits rather than single deficits, as earlier researchers had proposed [34, 35, 43]. Recent research data have confirmed that most individuals with DD exhibit a combination of neurocognitive deficits, although cases of individuals with single deficits are not excluded.

Contemporary scientific studies indicate that dyslexia is characterized by varied neurocognitive profiles, or "fingerprints," as Heim and Grande [18] describe. These profiles are related to differences in brain activation patterns in individuals with dyslexia, which supports the heterogeneous neurobiological nature of the disorder [18]. The heterogeneous and multifactorial neurobiological basis of dyslexia has been repeatedly confirmed in recent years. For example, differences have been identified in several brain regions (e.g., left inferior frontal gyrus, left superior temporal gyrus, fusiform gyrus) following neuropsychological and neuroimaging evaluations of a large sample of individuals with dyslexia [116]. These findings reinforce the multifactorial interpretation of the behavioral deficits that characterize dyslexia and its heterogeneity.

Recent findings have demonstrated differences in brain anatomy, particularly in the ratio of gray to white matter, between individuals with dyslexia and those with typical development. Individuals with dyslexia show reduced gray matter density in specific brain regions. Moreover, it has been observed that the gray-to-white matter ratio varies depending on the dominant cognitive deficit (phonological, magnocellular, auditory attention), confirming with neurobiological terms the heterogeneity of the disorder [115].

A meta-analysis of neuroimaging studies [117] revealed that the absence or reduced activation of the left temporo-occipital cortex during reading and visual-phonological tasks, as well as decreased function of the dorsal left parieto-frontal cortex, is linked to deficits in attention and motor skills. These findings support a multifactorial etiology of dyslexia, indicating that various neural networks may be involved in its manifestation.

The heterogeneity of this neurodevelopmental disorder and the observation that DD can affect abilities beyond language underscores the need for improving the diagnostic process. Currently, the diagnosis of this developmental disorder is primarily based on tests that assess children's intelligence and reading abilities, often overlooking other difficulties that these children may face, such as concentration, memory, visual and auditory perception, information processing, and motor coordination. However, a significant percentage of children with DD exhibit a combination of deficits rather than isolated difficulties.

As a result, a diagnostic system that does not consider variations across different neurocognitive domains fails to provide a comprehensive understanding of the causes of dyslexia for everyone. Although the results of reading tests provide useful information about reading progress, they do not adequately capture the cognitive deficits and disorders that contribute to its manifestation [56]. Administering additional tests that assess a broader range of abilities would help describe a more complete individual neurocognitive profile for each child diagnosed with dyslexia.

At the same time, the existence of neurocognitive subtypes of DD highlights the need for individualized educational programs that target the specific strengths and weaknesses of each student. To date, most educational interventions have focused on the phonological domain. However, research studies [8, 9, 30] indicate the presence of multiple deficits in individuals with dyslexia. Identifying the individual characteristics of each student can significantly contribute to the creation of more effective personalized educational interventions [110].

In summary, this chapter highlighted the heterogeneous and multifaceted nature of DD, emphasizing the need for a more comprehensive approach in both its diagnosis and treatment. The identification of distinct subtypes, with different neurocognitive deficits, among children with dyslexia leads to the conclusion that DD can no longer be viewed as the result of a single deficit but as a multifactorial disorder related to variations across several neurocognitive domains. Understanding these variations and documenting the individual neurocognitive profiles of each child with dyslexia could help to achieve for earlier and effective diagnosis using a variety of tests that assess a broader range of abilities that would help describe a more complete individual neurocognitive profile for each child. Such diagnosis would result in the development of personalized educational interventions, with more targeted strategies suited to the profiles of individual children.

Author details

Maria Chalmpe* and Filippos Vlachos
University of Thessaly/Hellenic Open University, Volos, Greece

*Address all correspondence to: mahalbe@uth.gr

References

[1] Brimo K, Dinkler L, Gillberg C, Lichtenstein P, Lundström S, Åsberg JJ. The co-occurrence of neurodevelopmental problems in dyslexia. Dyslexia. 2021;**27**:277-293. DOI: 10.1002/dys.1681

[2] Peterson RL, Pennington BF. Developmental dyslexia. Lancet. 2012;**379**(9830):1997-2007. DOI: 10.1016/S0140-6736(12)60198-6

[3] Vlachos F, Avramidis E. The difference between developmental dyslexia and dysgraphia: Recent neurobiological evidence. International Journal of Neuroscience and Behavioral Science. 2020;**8**:1-5

[4] Vlachos F, Avramidis E, Dedousis G, Chalmpe M, Ntalla I, Giannakopoulou M. Prevalence and gender ratio of dyslexia in Greek adolescents and its association with parental history and brain injury. American Journal of Educational Research. 2013;**1**(1):22-25. DOI: 10.12691/education-1-1-5

[5] Frith U. Paradoxes in the definition of dyslexia. Dyslexia. 1999;**5**(4):192-214. DOI: 10.1002/(SICI)1099-0909(199912)5:4<192::AID-DYS144>3.0.CO.2-N

[6] Ramus F. Neurobiology of dyslexia: A reinterpretation of the data. Trends in Neurosciences. 2004;**27**(12):720-726. DOI: 10.1016/j.tins.2004.10.004

[7] Pennington BF. From single to multiple deficit models of developmental disorders. Cognition. 2006;**101**(2):385-413. DOI: 10.1016/j.cognition.2006.04.008

[8] Heim S, Tschierse J, Amunts K, Vossel S, Wilms M, Willmes K, et al. Cognitive subtypes of dyslexia. Acta Neurobiologiae Experimentalis (Wars). 2008;**68**:73-82. DOI: 10.55782/ane-2008-1674

[9] Menghini D, Finzi A, Benassi M, Bolzani R, Facoetti A, Giovagnoli S, et al. Different underlying neurocognitive deficits in developmental dyslexia: A comparative study. Neuropsychologia. 2010;**48**(4):863-872. DOI: 10.1016/j.neuropsychologia.2009.11.003

[10] Pennington BF, Santerre-Lemmon L, Rosenberg J, MacDonald B, Boada R, Friend A, et al. Individual prediction of dyslexia by single versus multiple deficit models. Journal of Abnormal Psychology. 2012;**121**(1):212-224. DOI: 10.1037/a0025823

[11] van Bergen E, van der Leij A, de Jong PF. The intergenerational multiple deficit model and the case of dyslexia. Frontiers in Human Neuroscience. 2014;**8**:346. DOI: 10.3389/fnhum.2014.00346

[12] Vellutino FR, Fletcher JM, Snowling MJ, Scanlon DM. Specific reading disability (dyslexia): What have we learned in the past four decades? Journal of Child Psychology and Psychiatry. 2004;**45**(1):2-40. DOI: 10.1046/j.0021-9630.2003.00305.x

[13] Vellutino FR, Fletcher JM. The Science of Reading: A Handbook. Malden: Blackwell Publishing; 2005. pp. 362-378

[14] Pickering S. Working memory in dyslexia. In: Alloway TP, Gathercole SE, editors. Working Memory in Neurodevelopmental Conditions. Hove: Psychology Press; 2006. pp. 7-40

[15] Provazza S, Adams AM, Giofre D, Roberts DJ. Double trouble: Visual and phonological impairments in English dyslexic readers. Frontiers in Psychology. 2019;**10**. DOI: 10.3389/fpsyg.2019.02725

[16] Shaywitz SE, Shaywitz BA, Pugh KR, Fulbright RK, Constable RT, Mencl WE, et al. Functional disruption in the organization of the brain for reading in dyslexia. Proceedings of the National Academy of Sciences of the United States of America. 1998;**95**:2636-2641. DOI: 10.1073/pnas.95.5.2636

[17] Wagner RK, Torgesen JK. The nature of phonological processing and its causal role in the acquisition of reading skills. Psychological Bulletin. 1987;**101**(2):192-212. DOI: 10.1037/0033-2909.101.2.192

[18] Heim S, Grande M. Fingerprints of developmental dyslexia. Trends in Neuroscience and Education. 2012;**1**(1):10-14. DOI: 10.1016/j.tine.2012.09.001

[19] Sprenger-Charolles L, Siegel L, Béchennec D, Serniclaes W. Development of phonological and orthographic processing in reading aloud, in silent reading, and in spelling: A four-year longitudinal study. Journal of Experimental Child Psychology. 2003;**84**(3):194-217

[20] Snowling M. From language to reading and dyslexia. Dyslexia. 2001;**7**(1):37-46. DOI: 10.1002/dys.185

[21] Catts HW, McIlraith A, Bridges MS, Nielsen DC. Viewing a phonological deficit within a multifactorial model of dyslexia. Reading and Writing. 2017;**30**(3):613-629. DOI: 10.1007/s11145-016-9692-2

[22] Ho CSH, Law TPS, Ng PM. The phonological deficit hypothesis in Chinese developmental dyslexia. Reading and Writing. 2000;**13**(1):57-79. DOI: 10.1023/A:1008040922662

[23] Gillon GT. Phonological Awareness: From Research to Practice. New York: The Guilford Press; 2004

[24] Jeffries S, Everatt J. Working memory: Its role in dyslexia and other specific learning difficulties. Dyslexia. 2004;**10**(3):196-214. DOI: 10.1002/dys.278

[25] Kibby MY, Marks W, Morgan S, Long CJ. Specific impairment in developmental reading disabilities: A working memory approach. Journal of Learning Disabilities. 2004;**37**(4):349-363. DOI: 10.1177/00222194040370040601

[26] Perez TM, Majerus S, Mahot A, Poncelet M. Evidence for a specific impairment of serial order short-term memory in dyslexic children. Dyslexia. 2012;**18**(2):94-109. DOI: 10.1002/dys.1438

[27] Bruck M. Persistence of dyslexics' phonological awareness deficits. Developmental Psychology. 1992;**28**(5):874-886. DOI: 10.1037/0012-1649.28.5.874

[28] Rack JP. Dyslexia: The phonological deficit hypothesis. In: Fawcett A, Nicolson R, editors. Dyslexia in Children. London: Routledge; 2017. pp. 3-33. DOI: 10.4324/9781315504773

[29] Paulesu E, Frith U, Snowling M, Gallagher A, Morton J, Frackowiak R, et al. Is developmental dyslexia a disconnection syndrome? Evidence from PET scanning. Brain. 1996;**119**:143-157. DOI: 10.1093/brain/119.1.143

[30] White S, Milne E, Rosen S, Hansen P, Swettenham J, Frith U, et al. The role of sensorimotor impairments

in dyslexia: A multiple case study of dyslexic children. Developmental Science. 2006;**9**(3):237-255. DOI: 10.1111/j.1467-7687.2006.00483.x

[31] Fletcher JM. Dyslexia: The evolution of a scientific concept. Journal of the International Neuropsychological Society. 2009;**15**:501-508. DOI: 10.1017/S1355617709090900

[32] Pennington BF. Diagnosing Learning Disorders: A Neuropsychological Framework. 2nd ed. New York: Guilford Press; 2009

[33] Farmer M, Klein R. The evidence for a temporal processing deficit linked to dyslexia: A review. Psychonomic Bulletin & Review. 1995;**2**:460-493. DOI: 10.3758/BF03210983

[34] Tallal P. Language and reading: Some perceptual prerequisites. Bulletin of the Orton Society. 1980;**30**(1):170-178. DOI: 10.1007/BF02653716

[35] Tallal P, Stark R, Mellits E. Identification of language-impaired children on the basis of rapid perception and production skills. Brain and Language. 1985;**25**:314-322. DOI: 10.1016/0093-934X(85)90087-2

[36] Vlachos F. Dyslexia: A synthetic approach to causal theories. Hellenic Journal of Psychology. 2010;7:205-240. (In Greek)

[37] Mody M, Studdert-Kennedy M, Brady S. Speech perception deficits in poor readers: Auditory processing or phonological coding? Journal of Experimental Child Psychology. 1997;**64**:199-231. DOI: 10.1006/jecp.1996.2343

[38] Habib M. The neurological basis of developmental dyslexia: An overview and working hypothesis. Brain. 2000;**123**(12):2373-2399. DOI: 10.1093/brain/123.12.2373

[39] Serrano F, Defior S. Dyslexia speed problems in a transparent orthography. Annals of Dyslexia. 2008;**58**(1):81. DOI: 10.1007/s11881-008-0013-6

[40] Jones MW, Obregón M, Kelly ML, Branigan HP. Elucidating the component processes involved in dyslexic and non-dyslexic reading fluency: An eye-tracking study. Cognition. 2008;**109**(3):389-407. DOI: 10.1016/j.cognition.2008.10.005

[41] Moll K, Göbel SM, Gooch D, Landerl K, Snowling MJ. Cognitive risk factors for specific learning disorder: Processing speed, temporal processing, and working memory. Journal of Learning Disabilities. 2016;**49**(3):272-281. DOI: 10.1177/0022219414547221

[42] Le Jan G, Le Bouquin-Jeannès R, Costet N, Trolès N, Scalart P, Pichancourt D, et al. Multivariate predictive model for dyslexia diagnosis. Annals of Dyslexia. 2011;**61**(1):1-20. DOI: 10.1007/s11881-010-0038-5

[43] Nicolson RI, Fawcett AJ. Automaticity: A new framework for dyslexia research? Cognition. 1990;**35**(2):159-182. DOI: 10.1016/0010-0277(90)90013-A

[44] Fawcett AJ, Nicolson RI. Automatisation deficits in balance for dyslexic children. Perceptual and Motor Skills. 1992;**75**:507-529. DOI: 10.2466/pms.1992.75.2.507

[45] Nicolson RI, Fawcett AJ, Berry EL, Jenkins IH, Dean P, Brooks DJ. Association of abnormal cerebellar activation with motor learning difficulties in dyslexic adults. Lancet. 1999;**353**(9165):1662-1667. DOI: 10.1016/S0140-6736(98)09165-X

[46] Nicolson RI, Fawcett AJ. Comparison of deficits in cognitive and motor skills among children with dyslexia. Annals of Dyslexia. 1994;**44**(1):147-164. DOI: 10.1007/BF02648159

[47] Nicolson RI, Daum I, Schugens MM, Fawcett AJ, Schulz A. Eyeblink conditioning indicates cerebellar abnormality in dyslexia. Experimental Brain Research. 2002;**143**(1):42-50. DOI: 10.1007/s00221-001-0969-5

[48] Ramus F, Pidgeon E, Frith U. The relationship between motor control and phonology in dyslexic children. Journal of Child Psychology and Psychiatry. 2003;**44**:712-722. DOI: 10.1111/1469-7610.00157

[49] Kirby JR, Parrila RK, Pfeiffer SL. Naming speed and phonological awareness as predictors of reading development. Journal of Educational Psychology. 2003;**95**(3):453-464. DOI: 10.1037/0022-0663.95.3.453

[50] Jones MW, Snowling MJ, Moll K. What automaticity deficit? Activation of lexical information by readers with dyslexia in a rapid automatized naming Stroop-switch task. Journal of Experimental Psychology. Learning, Memory, and Cognition. 2016;**42**(3):465-474. DOI: 10.1037/xlm0000186

[51] van Daal V, van der Leij A. Developmental dyslexia: Related to specific or general deficits? Annals of Dyslexia. 1999;**49**(1):71-104. DOI: 10.1007/s11881-999-0020-2

[52] Nicolson RI, Fawcett AJ, Dean P. Developmental dyslexia: The cerebellar deficit hypothesis. Trends in Neurosciences. 2001;**24**(9):508-511. DOI: 10.1016/S0166-2236(00)01896-8

[53] Bosse ML, Tainturier MJ, Valdois S. Developmental dyslexia: The visual attention span deficit hypothesis. Cognition. 2007;**104**(2):198-230. DOI: 10.1016/j.cognition.2006.05.009

[54] Facoetti A, Lorusso ML, Paganoni P, Cattaneo C, Galli R, Umiltà C, et al. Auditory and visual automatic attention deficits in developmental dyslexia. Cognitive Brain Research. 2003;**16**(2):185-191. DOI: 10.1016/S0926-6410(02)00270-7

[55] Valdois S, Bosse ML, Ans B, Carbonnel S, Zorman M, David D, et al. Phonological and visual processing deficits can dissociate in developmental dyslexia: Evidence from two case studies. Reading and Writing. 2003;**16**(6):541-572. DOI: 10.1023/A:1025501406971

[56] Zoubrinetzky R, Bielle F, Valdois S. New insights on developmental dyslexia subtypes: Heterogeneity of mixed reading profiles. PLoS ONE. 2014;**9**(6):e99337. DOI: 10.1371/journal.pone.0099337

[57] Saksida A, Iannuzzi S, Bogliotti C, Chaix Y, Démonet JF, Bricout L, et al. Phonological skills, visual attention span, and visual stress in developmental dyslexia. Developmental Psychology. 2016;**52**(10):1503-1516. DOI: 10.1037/dev0000184

[58] Zhao J, Liu M, Liu H, Huang C. The visual attention span deficit in Chinese children with reading fluency difficulty. Research in Developmental Disabilities. 2018;**73**:76-86. DOI: 10.1016/j.ridd.2017.12.017

[59] Sperling AJ, Lu ZL, Manis FR, Seidenberg MS. Deficits in perceptual noise exclusion in developmental dyslexia. Nature Neuroscience. 2005;**8**(7):862-863. DOI: 10.1038/nn1474

[60] Vidyasagar TR, Pammer K. Dyslexia: A deficit in visuo-spatial attention, not

in phonological processing. Trends in Cognitive Sciences. 2010;**14**(2):57-63. DOI: 10.1016/j.tics.2009.12.003

[61] Ruffino M, Trussardi AN, Gori S, Finzi A, Giovagnoli S, Menghini D, et al. Attentional engagement deficits in dyslexic children. Neuropsychologia. 2010;**48**(13):3793-3801. DOI: 10.1016/j.neuropsychologia.2010.09.002

[62] Eichenbaum H, Cohen NJ. From Conditioning to Conscious Recollection. Oxford, UK: Oxford University Press; 2001

[63] Swanson HL. Working memory and reading disabilities: Both phonological and executive processing deficits are important. In: Alloway TP, Gathercole SE, editors. Working Memory and Neurodevelopmental Disorders. Hove and New York: Psychology Press; 2006. pp. 59-88

[64] Baddeley A. The episodic buffer: A new component of working memory? Trends in Cognitive Sciences. 2000;**4**(11):417-423. DOI: 10.1016/S1364-6613(00)01538-2

[65] Cowan N, Alloway TP. The development of working memory in childhood. In: Courag M, Cowan N, editors. Development of Memory in Infancy and Childhood. 2nd ed. Hove: Psychology Press; 2008. pp. 303-342

[66] McLoughlin D, Leather C, Stringer P. The Adult Dyslexic. Interventions and Outcomes. London: Whurr; 2002

[67] Smith-Spark J, Fisk J, Fawcett A, Nicolson R. Investigating the central executive in adult dyslexics: Evidence from phonological and visuospatial working memory performance. European Journal of Cognitive Psychology. 2003;**15**(4):567-587. DOI: 10.1080/09541440340000024

[68] Schuchardt K, Maehler C, Hasselhorn M. Working memory deficits in children with specific learning disorders. Journal of Learning Disabilities. 2008;**41**(6):514-523. DOI: 10.1177/0022219408317856

[69] van der Leij A, van Daal VHP. Automatization aspects of dyslexia: Speed limitations in word identification, sensitivity to increasing task demands, and orthographic compensation. Journal of Learning Disabilities. 1999;**32**(5):417-428. DOI: 10.1177/002221949903200507

[70] Gray S, Fox AB, Green S, Alt M, Hogan TP, Petscher Y, et al. Working memory profiles of children with dyslexia, developmental language disorder, or both. Journal of Speech, Language, and Hearing Research. 2019;**62**(6):1839-1858. DOI: 10.1044/2019_JSLHR-L-18-0148

[71] Chalmpe M, Vlachos F, Avramidis H, Andreou G. Investigation of phonological and visual-spatial memory in children with dyslexia. Hellenic Review of Special Education. 2017;**5**:37-58. DOI: 10.12681/edusc.3185 (In Greek)

[72] Beneventi H, Tønnessen FE, Ersland L, Hugdahl K. Working memory deficit in dyslexia: Behavioral and fMRI evidence. The International Journal of Neuroscience. 2010;**120**(1):51-59. DOI: 10.3109/00207450903275129

[73] Ahissar M. Dyslexia and the anchoring-deficit hypothesis. Trends in Cognitive Sciences. 2007;**11**:458-465. DOI: 10.1016/j.tics.2007.08.015

[74] Menghini D, Hagberg G, Caltagirone C, Petrosini L, Vicari S. Implicit learning deficits in dyslexic adults: An fMRI study. NeuroImage. 2006;**33**:1218-1226. DOI: 10.1016/j.neuroimage.2006.08.024

[75] Wolf M, Bowers PG. The double-deficit hypothesis for the developmental dyslexias. Journal of Education & Psychology. 1999;**91**(3):415-438. DOI: 10.1037/0022-0663.91.3.415

[76] Nicolson RI, Fawcett AJ. Development of dyslexia: The delayed neural commitment framework. Front. Behavioral Neuroscience. 2019;**13**(112). DOI: 10.3389/fnbeh.2019.00112

[77] Wolf M, Bowers PG, Biddle K. Naming-speed processes, timing, and reading: A conceptual review. Journal of Learning Disabilities. 2000;**33**(4):387-407. DOI: 10.1177/002221940003300409

[78] O'Brien BA, Wolf M, Lovett MW. A taxometric investigation of developmental dyslexia subtypes. Dyslexia. 2012;**18**(1):16-39. DOI: 10.1002/dys.1431

[79] Papadopoulos TC, Georgiou GK, Kendeou P. Investigating the double-deficit hypothesis in Greek: Findings from a longitudinal study. Journal of Learning Disabilities. 2009;**42**(6):528-547. DOI: 10.1177/0022219409338745

[80] Constantinidou M, Stainthorp R. Phonological awareness and reading speed deficits in reading disabled Greek-speaking children. Educational Psychologist. 2009;**29**(2):171-186. DOI: 10.1080/01443410802613483

[81] Catts HW, Fey ME, Tomblin JB, Zhang X. A longitudinal investigation of reading outcomes in children with language impairments. Journal of Speech, Language, and Hearing Research. 2002;**45**(6):1142-1157. DOI: 10.1044/1092-4388(2002/093)

[82] Ramus F, Altarelli I, Jednoróg K, Zhao J, Scotto di Covella L. Neuroanatomy of developmental dyslexia: Pitfalls and promise. Neuroscience and Biobehavioral Reviews. 2018;**84**:434-452. DOI: 10.1016/j.neubiorev.2017.08.001

[83] Francks C, MacPhie IL, Monaco AP. The genetic basis of dyslexia. Lancet Neurology. 2002;**1**(8):483-490. DOI: 10.1016/S1474-4422(02)00221-1

[84] Fisher SE, DeFries JC. Developmental dyslexia: Genetic dissection of a complex cognitive trait. Nature Reviews. Neuroscience. 2002;**3**(10):767-780. DOI: 10.1038/nrn936

[85] Vlachos F, Nisiotou-Mantelou I. Genes of dyslexia. Pediatriki. 2013;**76**:20-25. (In Greek)

[86] Harlaar N, Dale PS, Plomin R. From learning to read to reading to learn: Substantial and stable genetic influence. Child Development. 2007;**78**(1):116-131. DOI: 10.1111/j.1467-8624.2007.00988.x

[87] Papadopoulou AK, Vlachos F, Papadatou-Pastou M. Cerebral lateralization of language in children at risk for dyslexia: A review of neuroscientific evidence. Dialogues in Clinical Neuroscience & Mental Health. 2022;**5**(2):89-97. DOI: 10.26386/obrela.v5i2.228

[88] Mascheretti S, Bureau A, Battaglia M, Simone D, Quadrelli E, Croteau J, et al. An assessment of gene-by-environment interactions in developmental dyslexia-related phenotypes. Genes, Brain, and Behavior. 2013;**12**(1):47-55. DOI: 10.1111/gbb.12000

[89] Galaburda AM, Kemper TL. Cytoarchitectonic abnormalities in developmental dyslexia: A case study. Annals of Neurology. 1979;**6**(2):94-100. DOI: 10.1002/ana.410060203

[90] Galaburda AM, Sherman GF, Rosen GD, Aboitiz F, Geschwind N. Developmental dyslexia: Four consecutive

patients with cortical anomalies. Annals of Neurology. 1985;**18**(2):222-233. DOI: 10.1002/ana.410180210

[91] Vanderauwera J, Wouters J, Vandermosten M, Ghesquière P. Early dynamics of white matter deficits in children developing dyslexia. Developmental Cognitive Neuroscience. 2017;**27**:69-77. DOI: 10.1016/j.dcn.2017.08.003

[92] Cao F, Bitan T, Chou T, Burman D, Booth J. Deficient orthographic and phonological representations in children with dyslexia revealed by brain activation patterns. Journal of Child Psychology and Psychiatry. 2006;**47**:1041-1050. DOI: 10.1111/j.1469-7610.2006.01684.x

[93] Gabrieli JDE. Dyslexia: A new synergy between education and cognitive neuroscience. Science. 2009;**325**(5938):280-283. DOI: 10.1126/science.1171999

[94] Papanicolaou AC, Simos PG, Breier JI, Fletcher JM, Foorman BR, Francis D, et al. Brain mechanisms for reading in children with and without dyslexia: A review of studies of normal development and plasticity. Developmental Neuropsychology. 2003;**24**(2-3):593-612. DOI: 10.1080/87565641.2003.9651912

[95] Stein J. The magnocellular theory of developmental dyslexia. Dyslexia. 2001;**7**(1):12-36. DOI: 10.1002/dys.186

[96] Galaburda AM, Menard MT, Rosen GD. Evidence for aberrant auditory anatomy in developmental dyslexia. Proceedings of the National Academy of Sciences of the United States of America. 1994;**91**(17):8010-8013. DOI: 10.1073/pnas.91.17.8010

[97] Ramus F, Rosen S, Dakin SC, Day BL, Castellote JM, White S, et al. Theories of developmental dyslexia: Insights from a multiple case study of dyslexic adults. Brain. 2003;**126**(4):841-865. DOI: 10.1093/brain/awg076

[98] Kronbichler M, Hutzler F, Wimmer H. Dyslexia: Verbal impairments in the absence of magnocellular impairments. Neuroreport. 2002;**13**(5):617-620. DOI: 10.1097/00001756-200204160-00016

[99] Bishop DVM, Bishop SJ, Bright P, James C, Delaney T, Tallal P. Different origin of auditory and phonological processing problems in children with language impairment. Journal of Speech, Language, and Hearing Research. 1999;**42**(1):155-168. DOI: 10.1044/jslhr.4201.155

[100] Ito M. A new physiological concept of cerebellum. Revue Neurologique (Paris). 1990;**146**:564-569

[101] Vlachos F, Papathanasiou I, Andreou G. Cerebellum and reading. Folia Phoniatrica et Logopaedica. 2007;**59**:177-183. DOI: 10.1159/000102929

[102] Kasselimis DS, Margarity M, Vlachos F. Cerebellar function, dyslexia and articulation speed. Child Neuropsychology. 2008;**14**(4):303-313. DOI: 10.1080/09297040701550138

[103] Getchell N, Padreja P, Needle K, Carrio V. Comparing children with and without dyslexia on the movement assessment battery for children and the test of gross motor development. Perceptual and Motor Skills. 2007;**105**:207-214. DOI: 10.2466/PMS.105.5.207-214

[104] Petropoulou P, Vlachos F, Avramidis H. Investigating balance skills in children with dyslexia. In: Proceedings

of the 3rd Panhellenic Conference on Special Education. Athens: Grigori Publications; 2013. pp. 1-8. ISBN: 978-960-333-781-220

[105] Ramus F, Ahissar M. Developmental dyslexia: The difficulties of interpreting poor performance, and the importance of normal performance. Cognitive Neuropsychology. 2012;**29**(1-2):104-122. DOI: 10.1080/02643294.2012.677420

[106] Pavlidou M, Teliou E, Vlachos F. Heterogeneity in the cognitive profile of dyslexics. Hellenic Review of Special Education. 2017;**5**:17-36. (In Greek)

[107] McGrath LM, Pennington BF, Shanahan MA, Santerre-Lemmon LE, Barnard HD, Willcutt EG, et al. A multiple deficit model of reading disability and attention-deficit/hyperactivity disorder: Searching for shared cognitive deficits. Journal of Child Psychology and Psychiatry. 2011;**52**(5):547-557. DOI: 10.1111/j.1469-7610.2010.02346.x

[108] Lewandowska M, Milner R, Ganc M, Włodarczyk E, Skarżyński H. Attention dysfunction subtypes of developmental dyslexia. Medical Science Monitor. 2014;**20**:2256-2268. DOI: 10.12659/MSM.890969

[109] Chalmpe M, Vlachos F. Are there distinct subtypes of developmental dyslexia?. Frontiers in Behavioral Neuroscience. 2025;**18**:1512892. DOI: 10.3389/fnbeh.2024.1512892

[110] Pacheco A, Reis A, Araújo S, Inácio F, Petersson KM, Faísca L. Dyslexia heterogeneity: Cognitive profiling of Portuguese children with dyslexia. Reading and Writing. 2014;**27**(9):1529-1545. DOI: 10.1007/s11145-014-9504-5

[111] Borleffs E, Jap BAJ, Nasution IK, Zwarts F, Maassen BAM. Do single or multiple deficit models predict the risk of dyslexia in Standard Indonesian? Applied PsychoLinguistics. 2018;**39**(3):675-702. DOI: 10.1017/S0142716417000625

[112] Snowling MJ, Gallagher A, Frith U. Family risk of dyslexia is continuous: Individual differences in the precursors of reading skill. Child Development. 2003;**74**(2):358-373. DOI: 10.1111/1467-8624.7402003

[113] Thomson JB, Chenault B, Abbott RD, Raskind WH, Richards T, Aylward E, et al. Converging evidence for attentional influences on the orthographic word form in child dyslexics. Journal of Neurolinguistics. 2005;**18**(2):93-126. DOI: 10.1016/j.jneuroling.2004.11.005

[114] Swagerman SC, van Bergen E, Dolan C, de Geus EJC, Koenis MMG, Hulshoff Pol HE, et al. Genetic transmission of reading ability. Brain and Language. 2017;**172**:3-8. DOI: 10.1016/j.bandl.2015.07.008

[115] Jednoróg K, Gawron N, Marchewka A, Heim S, Grabowska A. Cognitive subtypes of dyslexia are characterized by distinct patterns of grey matter volume. Brain Structure & Function. 2014;**219**(5):1697-1707. DOI: 10.1007/s00429-013-0595-6

[116] Pernet C, Andersson J, Paulesu E, Demonet JF. When all hypotheses are right: A multifocal account of dyslexia. Human Brain Mapping. 2009;**30**:2278-2292. DOI: 10.1002/hbm.20670

[117] Paulesu E, Danelli L, Berlingen M. Reading the dyslexic brain: Multiple dysfunctional routes revealed by a new meta-analysis of PET and fMRI activation studies. Frontiers in Human Neuroscience. 2014;**8**:830. DOI: 10.3389/fnhum.2014.00830

Chapter 8

Autism: Its Foundation and Practical Implications

Wenn B. Lawson

Abstract

The following chapter explores and explains what 'lies beneath' the diagnosis of autism. The foundation for this chapter is based on original knowledge grounded in the theory of monotropism, heralded in the 2005 paper by Murray, Lesser and Lawson. The work on monotropism began in the 90's and has been followed through until present times. Current research is supportive of the monotropism theory of autism which posits autism as 'a matter of attention', specifically 'monotropic attention'. When attention is captured by interest (for whatever reason) it occupies the whole of one's attention. This impacts concepts such as being literal (not reading between the lines), missing the subtle cues of social interaction and highlighting or underwhelming our sensory systems, challenges with object permanence and being misunderstood. But it also leads to incredible strengths and allows for one's passion to be a source of joy, stability and an aid to mental fitness. When an individual's autism is understood and accommodated, self-compassion can flourish and we can live life to the best of our ability. This chapter offers original knowledge to aid the understanding of autism that has not previously been accommodated.

Keywords: autism, monotropism, object permanence, interoception, attention

1. Introduction

The DSM-5 [1] lays out the criteria for an autism assessment (challenges with communication, social interaction and the experiences of human senses) but it does not explain why these exist or what lies 'beneath' the criteria for autism. This chapter explains what the very foundation of autism is, neurologically, and the impact our Autistic monotropic cognitive style has upon how we understand and process daily life. It is this unique understanding that adds knowledge to our overall understanding of autism and how best to support Autistic individuals. Like other developmental differences autism appears to change over time but can be hard to understand and accommodate. This chapter seeks to explain what autism is and where its challenges stem from. It is written by an Autistic researcher and British Psychologist who is a theorist on the concept of 'monotropism'.

The Autism Spectrum includes developmental differences from regular development that impact how an individual communicates, how they relate socially and how they experience the information from their external and internal sensing systems [1]. Currently between 1 in 100/1 in 40 individuals being born will be somewhere on the Autism spectrum; which is more than 1% of the world's population [2, 3]. Autism is only one spectrum area of developmental differences, but the recognised numbers have increased dramatically over the past two decades [4]. Maybe the world is ready for us!

Traditionally, autism was recognised as occurring mainly in children and males; females did not occur in the statistics. Autism was largely viewed as a catastrophe that cost society financially and emotionally [5–9]. Also, autism was only viewed as a tragic 'deficit disorder' and millions of dollars were spent on finding a cure [10, 11]. However, questioning these long-held beliefs has led to a broader understanding of autism as part of neurodiversity [12] and the further term within neurodiversity, that of neurodivergence (See: Ref. [13]): Legault et al. [14], due to diverging from the typical. No longer, however, do we view Autism as a tragedy and increasingly, we are listening to the experiences and voices of autistic people. This does not mean that being in a world that does not accommodate autism is without its challenges; there are many. But the more understanding we have of autism and monotropism, and how it impacts on us as Autistic people, the better it will be for everyone (http://monotropism.org).

Possibly a big part of the shift away from the 'medical model' and towards the biopsychosocial model [15] (all minds are of equal value in their diversity) adding to the richness of humanity, has led to being open to listening to the Autistic Voice. As such, Autistic people are adding to the discourse and to autism research as Autistic researchers [16]. Once it was believed that Autistic people lacked empathy and we did not have 'a theory of mind' [17, 18] but this has radically changed in the last decade or so [19, 20]. Now, as we move into the age of neurodiversity and the understanding that 'all minds' contribute to the wonderfully colourful world of being human, we recognise neurodivergence as simply diverging from the majority but not from being human [21].

Another development that has occurred, building on from the work of Murray et al. [22, 23] and Lawson [24, 25] is the notion of monotropism. The authors of the 2005 paper suggest that monotropism is responsible for all the criteria used to assess for autism [1] and all the social and communication differences experienced by autistic people [24–28].

Monotropism is explained as 'single attention' focussed and complete in that, as a scarce resource, being 'mono' means having all of one's attention captured and not having any free attention for other things. It is illustrated by the image of a torch beam illuminating a narrow field and only highlighting those 'things' captured by the narrow light. Whereas non-autistic people operate on the 'polytropic' channel of attention, which is like the wider, broader and less intense torch beam.

Behaviourally we see in autism a tendency to notice only that which is within the attention tunnel and not to notice other aspects outside of the focussed attention. This is different in non-autistic people. The non-autistic or polytropic cognitive style allows non-autistic individuals to change attentional focus quite quickly, moving them between various interests and even allowing them to show interest when they are not interested [22, 23, 25]. For social connectivity, rapid shifting of attention and general societal connection is important. So, the polytropic cognitive style is more suited than the monotropic cognitive style to social interaction, unless the interaction is based upon shared interest. Monotropic individuals thrive when they can use passionate interests that lead to deeper connections, possible new inventions, flow states and productivity [28]. The downside of the monotropic cognitive style are times of inertia [29], rumination [30] and awkwardness in social situations outside of mutual interest [31].

As we come to understand the autistic monotropic cognitive style in autistic individuals we will notice other challenges that impact autistic lives. These are connected to areas of poor object permanence and a lack of noticing the information from the internal sensing system (interoception) as well as a heightened or underwhelming experience of the external sensory world [1, 27].

1.1 Object permanence (OP)

Object permanence is the understanding that things continue to exist even when we can not see or sense them. It is like knowing your pet, (family, bedroom, clothes, iPad and so on), are at home even when you are away and cannot see them [27]. The flip side to the 'coin' of 'OP' is that moving on from comprehending the 'permanence' of an object, person, place, season, time and so on, is the generalisation of that meaning. This means something can be permanent, but also temporary. For example, a person could be choking on food eaten but then move on from choking to being able to swallow and not be choking anymore. Typically, individuals appreciate and accommodate both sides of the OP coin. We understand something can be both permanent and temporary, as well as only permanent or only temporary. This generalisation of knowledge allows us to move past and beyond an understanding that may be 'black and white' to various shades of grey, but without losing context. OP understanding in autism, however, can be challenging.

For most people, understanding OP develops before the age of 12–18 months [27]. However, for many of us as Autistic individuals, we might experience OP differently. Experiencing OP differently is a flow on state from being monotropic and having all our attention taken over by the one thing currently before us [22–24]. This 'occupied attention' can affectively 'knock out' any connection to aspects of our usual daily lives, including people, seasons, expectations and objects around us, if we ca not see them.

1.2 How being 'mono' might impact our sense of OP

As an autistic individual, object permanence differences might show up in our life in several ways:

1. Emotional reactions:

   - We might feel worried or upset when familiar objects are moved or are out of sight.
   - We may feel confused or unsure when loved ones leave the room.
   - We might find it challenging to manage our emotions during changes or transitions due to not knowing what comes next or what to expect.

2. Daily life impact:

   - We may find it difficult to handle changes in our routines because it is difficult to forward think. Forward thinking requires a split in our attention. We attend to 'now' but also to 'after'. Being monotropic and having all our attention only on 'now' makes it very difficult to appreciate consequences or attend to the 'after'.

- We might become very attached to specific objects or places because they keep us grounded, are familiar and 'protect' against 'change'.

- We may find it hard to adapt when things in our surroundings change because we can not imagine or picture what it means when things change. For example, is it really the same room, the same person? This occurs because the person may belong to that setting and is understood only in that context. For example, a child encounters a teacher from their school in the Supermarket and says to them; 'What are you doing here, you should be at school'!

3. Relationships and attachment:

- We might find it challenging to form or maintain relationships because people seem so changeable and unpredictable, so how can we trust or be sure? The flip side of this can be that we 'over attach' and become possessive.

- We may feel anxious when separated from caregivers or loved ones as they are part of 'us' and it feels wrong without them. It is hard to imagine them still in our world if they are out of sight.

- We might find it difficult to understand people still care about us even when they are not physically present because we may lose connection with the feeling that we usually have when we are with them in person.

4. How we process information as Autistic people:

- We may have unique ways of understanding and interacting with our environment that often depend upon familiarity.

- We might find it challenging to think about things we can not see or touch.

1.3 Helpful strategies

Here are some strategies that might help manage object permanence challenges [24]:

1. Plans:

- We can use picture schedules or calendars to show our daily activities and any expected changes. For unexpected or unanticipated changes put a comment into our calendar, diary or schedule that says: 'sometimes changes occur that we were not expecting, this is uncomfortable but is OK. We can prepare/think of what to do instead'. This might mean checking in with our list of 'alternative ideas', with a family member or a friend for support.

- We may like to create photo albums or digital galleries of important people and places. I have these on my mobile phone and can look at them (helping to keep them present) whenever I want to.

- We may prefer to have picture cards to represent objects or people that are temporarily away. I keep mine in my wallet (e.g., a family photo).

2. Consistent routines:

  - We can try to keep our daily routines as regular as possible. If this leads to more anxiety though, it is OK to make plans as we think about things, allow for changes, and have important contact information on our phones.

  - We can ask family and friends to give us clear explanations and visual cues (if we think these might help) before changes happen. For example, an idea of colour changes before someone redecorates.

  - We can create a predictable environment that helps us feel comfortable and safe. For example, use a headset to reduce noise levels, wear shades (sunglasses) and have an item of clothing/or fiddle object (cap, umbrella, bracelet, etc.) that we can interact with and help us feel calm.

3. Comfort objects:

  - We can have a special item that helps us feel good (in our pocket or on our person). I have a particular T-shirt I wear, a soft bear keyring I can hold, and pictures I like to look at on my phone.

  - We can use these during transitions/times of change or when separated from others, to help us feel OK.

4. Using technology:

  - We can use video calls to see and talk to someone when they are away, this helps reassure us they are still 'here'.

  - We can use apps with picture schedules, reminders or location tracking for reassurance.

  - We can use countdown timers or apps to help us know when to expect changes or when to expect someone to return.

5. Calming techniques:

  - Practicing mindfulness (focussing on the present moment) or on our breathing can help us manage if we are worried.

  - We can develop personalised ways to calm ourselves when feeling stressed. For example, I like to hum or look at pictures on my phone.

  - We can write a social story (short description of a particular situation, event or activity) to help us understand and prepare for changes. For example, The bus usually leaves at 9.00 am. But sometimes the bus is delayed. I can wait longer for the bus or/and I can phone family or a friend to let them know and check in on what to do next.

6. Adapting our environment:

- We can try to keep our home or workspace consistent and familiar. I try to put the linen in my linen cupboard in a space labelled for it, such as single sheets, double sheets, Queen sized sheets, hand towels, bath towels and so on.
- I try to keep any room changes (furniture, etc.) to a minimum. I avoid unnecessary changes to how my room is arranged.
- I make the spaces in my home sensory friendly. This helps to reduce the overall stress in my environment. I also have lots of soft animals, fidget things and dim lights. These help me, but we are all different, so we need to explore what works for us.

7. Gradual practice:
    - If we want to, we could slowly increase the time we are separated from important objects or people... knowing we can connect with them again.
    - We can practice games or activities related to object permanence in a safe, supportive setting (like hide and seek with family).
    - We can celebrate our successes in managing separations, no matter how small, but it is also OK if we still feel uncomfortable.

1.4 Remember

- Our autistic experience with object permanence is unique to us, so it might be different for different people.
- It is okay to feel challenged or frustrated sometimes – our feelings are valid. Having a feeling does not make something 'true', it is a feeling that could change with our circumstances.
- These strategies are suggestions – feel free to adjust them to what works best for you.

1.5 Professional support

Working with a psychologist or therapist can provide additional support in managing object permanence challenges:

1. Supportive strategies:
    - Develop personalised ways to build an understanding of object permanence, (e.g., read about the concept, explore what others have found helpful, practice using photos, taking an object with you, wearing an item of clothing that connects you to past and present, use text or messaging as reminders to self and others).
    - Use techniques, *as outlined above*, and even gradual exposure to being separated, but with support, to reduce anxiety related to separation.

2. Thought strategies:

    - Learn techniques to challenge worried thoughts: look up concepts associated with Mindfulness: https://www.wisebrain.org/wellspring-institute.

    - Develop different ways of thinking about our understanding of object permanence (e.g., nothing really leaves our world (unless in a spaceship) because our planet has gravity; We carry 'love' and those close to us in our 'emotions heart'; I can always ask and check in with trusted friends and/or family).

3. Managing emotions:

    - We can learn and practice techniques to handle distress and anxiety (e.g., our emotions are all OK to experience, no emotion is bad. But, they are feeling states that change and will go away; it is OK to miss someone or/and something, it's also OK to connect differently with other good things that help us feel good again, like speaking with a friend, listening to our music, reading a favourite book or watching our programmes on TV or on our streaming media, spending time with our community where we feel safe and belong) See: https://langleygroup.com.au/10-strategies-for-managing-emotions/.

    - We can develop personalised coping strategies that support us in challenging situations (sometimes we need help to do this, and we may find spending time with friends who help us or seeing a counsellor/psychologist can be useful). But we need to be sure whatever we do it needs to involve people who GET autism and GET us!

1.6 External sensing system

Our external senses, such as: seeing, hearing, tasting, touching, smelling, Proprioception (knowing which part of our body is in touch with another body part) and vestibular (knowing where we are in time and space) all contribute towards feeding our brain information to help keep us upright, safe from harm, connected to our external world and aware of things outside of our body [32, 33]. They usually operate by co-operating with each other and helping us build an appropriate picture of our world. For example, we can see flowers, birds, water, sky and so on, as well as hear the buzz of insects, smell the flowers, know if it is day or night and avoid walking places that are not safe. But these senses do not alert us to being hungry or needing the toilet [33, 34].

Usually, our external senses work in synchrony but, being monotropic can mean that our sensing system is easily overwhelmed by one sense over another, meaning we notice information from one sense but not the other. So, being in a situation where sound is experienced as being too loud might mean we do not notice we are walking into danger, or we need to stop to avoid danger (e.g., crossing a road) [32]. This is a processing issue and happens due to our monotropic cognitive style as Autistic people [24].

Adapting our environment so it is 'sensory friendly' is OK at home because hopefully, we are in control of what's going on inside our own home. We can wear clothes that are not scratchy, we can have soft furnishings, avoid bright lights, use colour and décor that suit us and enable us to be comfortable. We can choose the level of sound we need, whether to eat amongst/with other people or on our own, and choose to eat food we are happy with that does not feel uncomfortable due to texture, colour or taste. But, outside of home life can be very different! The sounds can be too loud, the lights too bright, it is difficult to avoid being amongst too many people and becoming overwhelmed and overloaded! I have my shades (sunglasses) with me, my headset or noise cancelling headphones, my cap that I can pull down over my eyes if the light is too bright, and I can eat Take Out or away from others. It is easier for me to take what I need into the outside world, often not designed for monotropic people, so I can cope better.

Exploring what we each need to enable us to function well in a sensory world that might not cater to us is vital. There are a number of 'online' checklists for sensory functions such as https://www.sensorysmarts.com/sensory-checklist.pdf building a profile of what works for you is so important and this is your 'Right' to enable you to be safe and comfortable in the world we all share.

1.7 Internal sensing system (interoception)

Interoception is our eighth sense [33]. It refers to our perceptions of what is going on inside our bodies. Interoception helps develop our connection to self because when we understand how we feel, we learn to connect to ourselves and connect to others. In autism, because we are monotropic our internal sensing system can be 'offline' or not noticed due to our attention being occupied by whatever has captured us (passionate interest, our emotive state such as anxiety, feeling unwell, an expectation and so on). Interoception comes from our Neuroception which is the autonomic, unconscious sense that warns the body of danger [34]. But interoception is a whole system of sensing that includes messages from inside our body being sent to our brain so we can act on this if needed. It lets us know when we are hungry, thirsty, tired, unwell, in need of the bathroom, the temperature we feel so we can wear the appropriate clothing, sexual desire, heart rate and related breathing and much more [33]. Interoception connections appropriately allow us to know our mood and how to respond to it [35].

Overarching theme: Interoception contributes to bodily autonomy which is crucial for a sense of self and quality of life. As Autistic people, we may need to be supported in developing adaptive interoceptive skills that support our wellbeing.

Currently not a whole heap of research exists in connection to interoception in autism which means there are aspects of theory and knowledge we are missing.

Some questions to ask ourselves as Autistic individuals or for others to be aware of as they live, love and/or work with us. What are the interoceptive differences seen and experienced by autistic monotropic individuals?

1. Both benefits and challenges

    - What are the implications for differentiation between sensations? Is this more about processing and if so, what are the implications for meaning-making and emotion, as well as self-care, autonomy and relating to others?

    - In monotropism there are fluctuations in interoception perception according to available attention, our environment, our age and current demand on us [24].

    - As such they will not be static but changeable. Being context-dependent means we might notice at some times but not at other times.

- Stress and arousal impact interoception connection in a big way, so lowering stress and, at times, heightening arousal can be useful [33, 34].
- The interventions that work best for us as autistic people must be individually planned with us and suit our personality, socioeconomic status and general culture.

2. Inter-individual variability will mean:

- There will be differences between hypo- and hyper-awareness according to those things named above.

The implications for wellbeing are manifold

- As we learn how to 'notice' our interoceptive senses our ability to self-manage and build a sense of autonomy is increased.
- Once our interoception connection flows more positively we will be better able to regulate our responses to our own feelings and to what we notice about others.
- We can build awareness of pain and mood changes which will lead to better emotional and physical health.

This all comes together as we build a better sense of body ownership and mental fitness.

Research has found that a great way to build interoceptive awareness is by pairing physical activity with mental focus [33]. So, as we practice particular exercises and attend/focus on specifics of these our brain works to link them together. As I notice my breathing, for example, I can help reduce my heart rate which lowers 'panic' mode and reduces anxiety.

A great helpful site is: https://neurodivergentinsights.com/blog/autism-interoception.

Also see: https://studentwellbeinghub.edu.au/media/erkfigg4/swh_getreadytolearn_selfregulationresource-2023.pdf

And: https://reframingautism.org.au/interoception-knowing-yourself-inside-and-out/

2. Conclusion

The original contribution in this chapter increases knowledge of autism and why we are who we are. This chapter has uncovered and explored the detail beneath the criteria for an assessment for autism. Just telling us that, as Autistic people, we have challenges with communication and social interaction, as well as we experience our senses differently from non-autistic people, does not tell us why or what's causing this or how to help us be better equipped to live in this world we all share, which is not set up for us. By looking at what's 'beneath our autism' we can better understand ourselves, better equip ourselves to live differently, better arm ourselves to have an answer for who we are, and be better able to live a life that leads to autonomy and mental fitness. Every Autistic person is different. As well as being monotropic we each have our own personality, our own likes and dislikes, our own culture and so on. These aspects of who we are also need consideration and will contribute to the experience of our daily lives. Focussing upon our strengths and finding support for our challenges is every human's right. This chapter helps to put the above into focus and enable the reader to understand autism and themselves in a positive light. A great free resource for Autistic individuals to help us build mental fitness as we work to understand our autism can be found here: https://www.edx.org/learn/mental-health/curtin-university-autism-and-mental-health

Author details

Wenn B. Lawson
Curtin University, Australia

*Address all correspondence to: wenbe2@outlook.com

References

[1] American Psychiatric Association. Diagnostic & Statistical Manual of Mental Disorders. 5th ed. Arlington, VA: American Psychiatric Association; 2013

[2] Kogan MD, Vladutiu JC, Schieve LA, Ghandour RM, Blumberg SJ, Zablotsky B, et al. The prevalence of parent-reported autism spectrum disorder among US children. Paediatrics. 2018;**142**(6):e20174161

[3] Zeidan J, Fombonne E, Scorah J, Ibrahim A, Durkin MS, Saxena S, et al. Global prevalence of autism: A systematic review update. Autism Research. 2022;**15**(5):778-790. DOI: 10.1002/aur.2696

[4] Shenouda J, Barrett E, Davidow AL, Sidwell K, Lescott C, Halperin W, et al. Prevalence and disparities in the detection of autism without intellectual disability. Pediatrics. 2023;**151**(2):e2022056594

[5] Cruz S, Zubizarreta SCP, Costa AD, et al. Is there a bias towards males in the diagnosis of autism? A systematic review and meta-analysis. Neuropsychology Review. 2024. DOI: 10.1007/s11065-023-09630-2

[6] Hurley-Hanson AE, Giannantonio CM, Griffiths AJ. The costs of autism. In: Autism in the Workplace. Palgrave Explorations in Workplace Stigma. Cham: Palgrave Macmillan; 2020. DOI: 10.1007/978-3-030-29049-8_3

[7] Mussey JL, Ginn NC, Klinger LG. Are males and females with autism spectrum disorder more similar than we thought? Autism. 2017;**21**(6):733-737. DOI: 10.1177/1362361316682621

[8] Pisula E, Pudło M, Słowińska M, Kawa R, Strząska M, Banasiak A, et al. Behavioral and emotional problems in high-functioning girls and boys with autism spectrum disorders: Parents' reports and adolescents' self-reports. Autism. 2017;**21**(6):738-748. DOI: 10.1177/1362361316675119

[9] Rogge N, Janssen J. The economic costs of autism spectrum disorder: A literature review. Journal of Autism and Developmental Disorders. 2019;**49**:2873-2900. DOI: 10.1007/s10803-019-04014-z

[10] Ebben H. The desire to recognize the undesirable: De/constructing the autism epidemic metaphor and contagion in autism as a discourse. Feminist Formations. 2018;**30**(1):141-163. DOI: 10.1353/ff.2018.0007

[11] Gombosi PG. Parents of autistic children: Some thoughts about trauma, dislocation, and tragedy. The Psychoanalytic Study of the Child. 1998;**53**(1):254-275

[12] Dwyer P. The neurodiversity approach(es): What are they and what do they mean for researchers? Human Development. 2021;**66**(2):73-92. DOI: 10.1159/000523723

[13] Why Everything You Know about Autism is Wrong. Jac Den Houting: AiraBreeze AU V89 B17 16x9 VO1 ND. Available from: https://www.youtube.com/watch?v=A1AUdaH-EPM

[14] Legault M, Bourdon JN, Poirier P. From neurodiversity to neurodivergence: The role of epistemic and cognitive marginalization. Synthese. 2021;**199**(5):12843-12868

[15] Bölte S, Lawson WB, Marschik PB, Girdler S. Reconciling the seemingly

irreconcilable: The WHO's ICF system integrates biological and psychosocial environmental determinants of autism and ADHD. BioEssays. 2021;**43**:e2000254. DOI: 10.1002/bies.202000254

[16] Lebenhagen C. Including speaking and nonspeaking autistic voice in research. Autism in Adulthood. 2020;**2**(2):128-131

[17] Frith U. Autism and "theory of mind". In: Diagnosis and Treatment of Autism. Boston, MA: Springer US; 1989. pp. 33-52

[18] Mathersul D, McDonald S, Rushby JA. Understanding advanced theory of mind and empathy in high-functioning adults with autism spectrum disorder. Journal of Clinical and Experimental Neuropsychology. 2013;**35**(6):655-668

[19] Hume R, Burgess H. "I'm human after all": Autism, trauma, and affective empathy. Autism in Adulthood. 2021;**3**(3):221-229

[20] Nicolaidis C, Milton D, Sasson NJ, Sheppard E, Yergeau M. An expert discussion on autism and empathy. Autism in adulthood. 2018;**1**(1):4-11

[21] Holt A, Bounekhla K, Welch C, Polatajko H. "Unheard minds, again and again": Autistic insider perspectives and theory of mind. Disability and Rehabilitation. 2022;**44**(20):5887-5897

[22] Murray D, Lesser M, Lawson W. Attention, monotropism and the diagnostic criteria for autism. Autism. 2005;**9**(2):139-156

[23] Murray D. Monotropism: An interest-based account of autism. In: Encyclopedia of Autism Spectrum Disorders. Cham: Springer International Publishing; 2021. pp. 2954-2956

[24] Lawson W. The passionate mind: How people with autism learn. In: Lawson W, editor. 'Autism Taking Over': Lambert Pubs. Germany: Jessica Kingsley Publishers; 2011

[25] Lawson W. Sensory connection, interest/attention and gamma synchrony in autism or autism, brain connections and preoccupation. Medical Hypothesis. 2012;**80**(3):284-288

[26] Lawson W. Autism spectrum conditions: The pathophysiological basis for inattention and the new diagnostic and statistical manual of mental disorders (DSM-V). OA Autism. 2013;**1**(1):1

[27] Lawson W, Dombroski B. Problems with object permanence: Rethinking traditional beliefs associated with poor theory of mind in autism. Journal of Intellectual Disability-Diagnosis and Treatment. 2017;**5**(1):1-6

[28] Pellicano E, Fatima U, Hall G, Heyworth M, Lawson W, Lilley R, et al. A capabilities approach to understanding and supporting autistic adulthood. Nature Reviews Psychology. 2022;**1**(11):624-639

[29] Rapaport H, Clapham H, Adams J, Lawson W, Porayska-Pomsta K, Pellicano E. "In a state of flow": A qualitative examination of autistic adults' phenomenological experiences of task immersion. Autism in Adulthood. 2024;**6**(3):362-373

[30] Dwyer P, Williams ZJ, Lawson WB, Rivera SM. A trans-diagnostic investigation of attention, hyper-focus, and monotropism in autism, attention dysregulation hyperactivity development, and the general population. Neurodiversity. 2024;**2**:27546330241237883

[31] Browne K, Lawson W, McGarry S, Scott M, Girdler S, Milbourn B. "Consistent support is good for my mental health"—Exploring the lived experience of autistic mental health. Autism in Adulthood. 2024

[32] Boyd L. Sensory processing in autism. In: The Sensory Accommodation Framework for Technology: Bridging Sensory Processing to Social Cognition. Switzerland AG: Springer Nature; 2024. pp. 27-40

[33] Goodall E. Thriving at School: How Interoception Is Helping Children and Young People Engage in Learning Everyday. Toowoomba, Australia: University of Southern Queensland; 2020

[34] Porges SW. Neuroception: A Subconscious System for Detecting Threats and Safety. Vol. 24. USA: Zero to Three; 2004. pp. 19-24

[35] Palser ER, Fotopoulou A, Pellicano E, Kilner JM. The link between interoceptive processing and anxiety in children diagnosed with autism spectrum disorder: Extending adult findings into a developmental sample. Biological Psychology. 2018;**136**:13-21

Chapter 9

Autism Spectrum Condition: An Update on its Understanding and Clinical Perspective

Sambhu Prasad, Soni Kisku, Rituparna Sahana and Sweta Gupta

Abstract

Autism spectrum condition (ASC) is a multifaceted neurobiological entity characterized by challenges in communication, social interaction, and a propensity for repetitive behaviors. The conceptualization of ASC has evolved significantly since Paul Eugen Bleuler first introduced the term "autism" in 1912. This chapter traces the historical development of ASC, emphasizing its trajectory from a focus on deficits for a recognition of individual strengths and diversity within the spectrum. Current estimates suggest a rising prevalence of ASC, attributed to both expanded diagnostic criteria and increased awareness. The clinical perspective on ASC underscores a range of symptoms affecting various domains, from social communication to emotional regulation, informing a comprehensive diagnostic and intervention framework. As research continues to illuminate the genetic, neurobiological, and environmental underpinnings of the condition, effective management strategies—ranging from psychological to pharmacological interventions—are being refined. Despite advancements, challenges remain in understanding ASC's complexities and improving support systems for affected individuals and their families.

Keywords: autism, spectrum, neurodevelopmental, etiological diversity, management principles

1. Introduction

Autism spectrum condition (ASC) is a complex neurobiological entity which holds challenges in communication and social interaction, and has some repetitive behavior. The term "*spectrum*" contains a wide range of symptoms, which varies across individuals affecting their daily usual activities [1]. The affected individual has an inherent focus on its own internal world which very much fits the term autism meaning autos in Greek literature. This idea was first introduced in 1912 by Swiss psychiatrist Paul

Eugen Bleuler, who used it to describe a form of self-centeredness in individuals with schizophrenia, highlighting difficulties in social engagement [2, 3]. Over time, the concept evolved, with Hans Asperger and Leo Kanner expanding its meaning in the 1930s to include specific behavioral patterns observed in children, leading to today's classification of ASC. In the modern context, autism encompasses a broad range of behaviors and developmental challenges, particularly in social communication. The term reflects both strengths and difficulties experienced by individuals on the spectrum. Its etymological roots underscore the unique internal experiences of those with ASC, emphasizing the need for empathy and supportive interventions to help them navigate the external social world. Additionally, broadening diagnostic criteria might explain the increasing prevalence, though other factors cannot be ruled out [4]. The outlook for individuals with ASC has improved over the past 50 years with more people able to speak, read, and live in the community. However, many still face challenges in working full time or living independently [5].

2. Historical perspective of autism spectrum condition

In 1908, Eugen Bluerler used the word autism to describe a subset of schizophrenic patients who were especially withdrawn and self-absorbed. In 1943, Leo Kanner, an American Psychologist, published a paper describing 11 highly intelligent

Specific description of ASD	DSM-4 classification	DSM-5 classification	ICD-10 classification	ICD-11 classification	Relevance
General classification	Utilized a multiaxial system for diagnosis, categorizing disorders into five axes.	ASD is a single diagnosis encompassing several previously separate disorders.	ASD is classified under the Pervasive Developmental Disorders umbrella, with specific codes.	ASD closely aligns with the DSM-5, using a single "Autism Spectrum Disorder" diagnosis and specifying associated features such as intellectual and language impairments.	Critical for diagnosis and treatment planning.
Autism	Included multiple specific categories: Autistic Disorder, Asperger Syndrome, PDD-NOS, Childhood Disintegrative Disorder.	Classified as part of ASD; requires deficits in social communication and restricted behaviors.	F84.0 - Autism Spectrum Disorder.	6A02: Autism Spectrum Disorder	Facilitates understanding of social interaction difficulties.

Specific description of ASD	DSM-4 classification	DSM-5 classification	ICD-10 classification	ICD-11 classification	Relevance
Asperger Syndrome	Defined as a distinct diagnosis with criteria focusing on social interaction difficulties and restricted behaviors.	Now included under ASD; lacks significant language delay.	F84.5 - Asperger's Syndrome, distinctly recognized.	No differential classification merged with ASD.	Facilitates understanding of social interaction difficulties.
Rett Syndrome	Classified as one of the characteristics of ASD with specific diagnostic criteria.	Considered a separate diagnosis; not included under ASD criteria.	F84.2 - Rett Syndrome, classified separately due to genetic origins and distinct features.	Merged with ASD.	Distinguishes genetic-based conditions; impacts treatment approaches and research focus on genetic factors in autism.
Childhood Disintegrative Disorder	Classified as a separate disorder, characterized by regression of acquired skills after a period of normal development.	Recognized as one of the conditions previously classified under ASD but now part of the broader ASD diagnosis.	F84.3 - Childhood Disintegrative Disorder; characterized by a significant regression in skills.	Merged with ASD.	Highlights the need for specific diagnostic recognition; indicates significant regression of skills over time, guiding different intervention strategies.
Pervasive Developmental Disorder Not Other Specified (PDD-NOS)	A catch-all diagnosis for individuals exhibiting some but not all criteria for other PDDs.	Incorporated as part of ASD; previously used for cases not fitting specific categories.	F84.9 - PDD-NOS; used for children who demonstrate ASD symptoms but do not fully meet criteria for any specific ASD diagnosis.	Merged with ASD.	Important for capturing cases that don't fit neatly into the other categories; emphasizes the need for individualized diagnostic and treatment approaches.

It is classified as ASD in a single diagnosis encompassing several previously separate disorders as per DSM 5 and even in ICD11 ASC closely aligns with the DSM-5, using a single "Autism Spectrum Disorder" diagnosis and specifying associated features such as intellectual and language impairments.

Table 1.
Nosological variation in the description of autism spectrum condition across classificatory system.

children who displayed "*a powerful desire for aloneness*". Later their condition was named "*early infantile autism.*" Hans Asperger a German scientist in 1944 described a "*milder*" form of autism now known as *Asperger's syndrome.* "Refrigerator mothers" was the term popularized by Bruno Bettelheim in 1967 suggesting that lack of warmth and affection was the cause of autism. In 1980, "*Infantile autism*" was listed in the DSM for the first time. In 1988, a popular movie "*Rain Man*" was released to create public awareness of autism. In 2007, the United Nations adopted the slogan "*Light it Up Blue*". In 2013, DSM-5 folds all subcategories of the condition into one umbrella diagnosis of ASC.

ASC encompasses five specific conditions: "*Autism, Asperger's Syndrome, Rett Syndrome, Childhood Disintegrative Disorder, and Pervasive Developmental Disorder Not Otherwise Specified (PDD-NOS),*" which are characterized across different nosological classifications (**Table 1**). [Since DSM-5 and ICD-11, ASC has been unified into a single diagnosis, which replaces previously separate disorders such as Asperger's, Childhood Disintegrative Disorder, and PDD-NOS. This shift toward a single "autism spectrum condition" classification with specific criteria for intellectual and language impairments aligns these systems and enhances clarity for diagnosis and treatment planning. This unified approach acknowledges the spectrum nature of autism and helps clinicians focus on individual symptoms and support needs, rather than categorizing patients into rigid subtypes.]

It gives the description of ASC across various classificatory nosology [6]. It is classified as ASD in a single diagnosis encompassing several previously separate disorders as per DSM-5 and even in ICD-11, and ASC closely aligns with the DSM-5, using a single "autism spectrum disorder" diagnosis and specifying associated features such as intellectual and language impairments.

3. Epidemiology of autism spectrum condition

The prevalence of ASC varies across several studies. In one study, around 1% of children aged 9–10 years exhibit some form of ASC. This estimate aligns with earlier studies but higher than several other studies with narrower definitions of autism. The male-female ratio was 3.3:1, increasing to 8.3:1 for consensus autism. Additionally, lower identification rates are observed among children of less educated parents, highlighting the necessity of standardized screening and diagnosis methods to reduce bias [6]. Globally, the prevalence of ASC has been steadily increasing. In the United States, current estimates suggest that approximately 1 in 36 children are diagnosed with this condition, a significant rise in the condition from 1 in 150 in 2000 and 1 in 44 in 2018 [7, 8]. The increase can be attributed to expanded diagnostic criteria and heightened awareness rather than a true rise in incidence. This condition is notably more common in boys than girls, with boys nearly four times more likely to receive a diagnosis. Current estimates show that 1 in 34 boys and 1 in 154 girls are identified with ASC [6], emphasizing the need for improved understanding of how autism may present differently in males and females. The prevalence varies across racial and ethnic groups. According to data from the "*Centers for Disease Control and Prevention (CDC),*" the highest prevalence rates are found among Hispanic and Asian/Pacific Islander children in the United States, followed by Black and White children. These differences may reflect the variations in healthcare access, awareness, and diagnostic practices [8].

4. Etiopathogenesis of autism spectrum condition

4.1 Neurobiological factors involved in etiopathogenesis of autism spectrum condition

Brain growth patterns: ASC is associated with abnormal brain growth, with reduced head size at birth followed by rapid growth in early infancy, particularly in the frontal lobe, cerebellum, and limbic structures. This growth slows later in childhood and is linked to deficits in social, communication, and motor abilities [9, 10]. Studies show overall brain enlargement, increased subcortical white matter, and disruptions in white matter tracts involved in social functioning. The functional MRI *(fMRI)* reveals reduced functional connectivity in areas related to language, memory, and social cognition [11]. ASC is associated with abnormal neuronal organization, such as smaller and more numerous cortical mini-columns, and a loss of Purkinje cells in the cerebellum [12]. The abnormalities suggest that key events in ASC development occur during early gestation, although the specific timing remains uncertain [13]. The *HGF/MET* pathway, crucial for neuronal development, shows genetic variations in ASC, affecting immune regulation and brain structure. Reelin is crucial for neuronal migration and cortical layering. Genetic studies have found associations between *RELN* and ASC, with some evidence showing altered levels of Reelin in autistic brains. However, results have been inconsistent, and further research is needed [14]. Neurotrophins like *Brain-Derived Neurotrophic Factor (BDNF)* play significant roles in the neuronal development and plasticity. Abnormal levels of *BDNF* might be involved in autism pathogenesis. Genetic changes in *CADPS2*, a gene related to *BDNF* regulation, have also been linked to autism. The "*FMR protein (FMRP)*" contributes to neuronal plasticity and regulation of "*group I (mGluR).*" Loss of *FMRP* leads to increased "*mGluR5*" signaling activity and adversely affects synaptic plasticity [15].

Postmortem neuroimaging: The social, linguistic, and behavioral challenges indicate that the disorder impacts a variety of neural systems with different functions. The initial damage was localized but later spread, leading to more extensive impairments. Individuals who struggle with processing complex information show the broad cortical abnormalities. Those with emotional and social difficulties exhibit issues within the limbic system. In the cerebellum, there is a reduction in the number of Purkinje and granule cells. These irregularities, along with an absence of gliosis, suggest a prenatal origin. Within the limbic system, there are decreases in neuronal size, less branching of dendrites, and a higher density of neurons. The enlargement of the amygdala in autism is accompanied by a reduction in the total number of neurons. One theory is that autism primarily arises from abnormalities in the amygdala-cortical loop system, which helps regulate social and cognitive processes related to social perception [16].

In reaction to socially important stimuli, individuals with ASC experience increased amygdala activity. During "theory of mind" tasks, which involve recognizing and attributing emotional states to others, fMRI studies show activation of the right temporal lobe and other regions in typically developing individuals. This difference is thought to stem from a dysfunction in the "mirror neuron system (MNS)." Furthermore, atypical patterns of frontal lobe activation have been observed during tasks related to face processing [17].

In ASC, there are several biomarkers that result from interactions of genes and environmental factors. These biomarkers result from abnormal signaling in the *5-HT* system, the *mTOR-linked synaptic plasticity* mechanisms, and alterations of the GABA inhibitory system. Changes in *5-HT* cause alterations in neuronal migration and growth in the brain may be associated with autism. Several studies found increased total brain volume in children <4 years of age, whose neonatal head circumferences were normal. By about age 5 years, however, 15 to 20% develop macrocephaly in autistic children with alteration of the size of amygdala. The size of the striatum has also been found in several studies to be enlarged, with a positive correlation of striatal size with the frequency of repetitive behaviors [18, 19].

4.2 Neurotransmitters involved in etiopathogenesis of autism spectrum condition

There are multiple biological neurochemicals found to alter in the patient of ASC as highlighted in **Table 2** [20].

4.3 Genetical factors associated with autism spectrum condition

There are multiple genes and their interaction with the environment plays a vital role in the pathogenesis of ASC (**Table 3**) [21].

4.4 Suspected immunological factors in genesis of autism spectrum condition

Various studies have suggested that immunological incompatibility, where maternal antibodies target the fetus, could contribute to the development of autistic traits. In children with autism, their lymphocytes interact with maternal antibodies, which raises the possibility that the fetal neural tissue might be damaged during pregnancy. This theory is still under investigation. Additionally, there have been instances of autism linked to viral infections. A major debate exists regarding whether the MMR (measles, mumps, rubella) vaccine could be a potential cause. However, the majority of research does not support any causal connection between vaccination and autism [22, 23].

Aspect	Points
Serotonin	Altered serotonin levels and receptor binding in ASD; both elevated and reduced serotonin levels observed. Genetic variations in serotonin-related genes and pharmacological responses suggest its involvement in ASD.
Glutamate and GABA	Abnormalities in glutamatergic and GABAergic signaling in ASD. Changes in glutamate receptor genes and GABA receptor levels may affect cortical development and plasticity.
Synaptic and dendritic changes	Disruptions in synaptic proteins like Neuroligins, Neurexins, and SHANK3, which are crucial for synaptic formation and function. Mutations in these proteins impact neurodevelopment.
Abnormalities in brain growth	Macrocephaly (enlarged head size) is common in some autistic individuals, linked to genetic factors like mutations in the PTEN gene. Tuberous sclerosis, with high autism comorbidity, also affects similar pathways.
Role of non-genetic factors	Genetic factors alone do not account for all ASD phenotypes. Non-genetic factors such as environmental influences, epigenetic changes, and maternal factors play a significant role.

Disturbance of functional connectivity together with alteration of neurochemicals are the consistent findings in the patient of autism. The abnormal binding of serotonin, GABA, glutamate, etc., at dendritic and synaptic level may explain the poor development of communicative, language, and social aspect in autism [20].

Table 2.
Neurotransmitters involved in autism spectrum condition.

Aspect	Details
Heritability	Autism is highly heritable, with estimates ranging from 50 to 90%.
Twin studies	Higher concordance rates in monozygotic (identical) twins (up to 90%) compared to dizygotic (fraternal) twins (up to 30%).
Family studies	Siblings of individuals with autism have a 10–20% increased risk of developing autism. First-degree relatives often show milder autistic traits.
Chromosomal abnormalities	Associated with conditions like *Fragile X Syndrome* and *Rett Syndrome*. *Chromosome 15q11-13* duplications and deletions have been linked to autism.
Gene mutations and variants	Single-gene mutations (e.g., *SHANK3, NRXN1, PTEN*) associated with autism. Copy number variations (CNVs), deletions, or duplications in specific genes increase risk.
Common gene pathways	Genes involved in *synapse formation and function*, *neuronal communication*, and *brain development* are often implicated (e.g., *CNTNAP2, NLGN3, NRXN1*).
Polygenic risk	Autism is polygenic, meaning multiple genes contribute to the risk, each with a small effect size.
Epigenetics	Environmental factors can influence gene expression through *DNA methylation* and *histone modification*, potentially affecting autism risk.
Gene-environment interaction	Genetic predisposition may interact with environmental factors (e.g., prenatal exposure to toxins, maternal infections) to increase the likelihood of developing autism.
De novo mutations	Some cases of autism are associated with *de novo (new) mutations* not inherited from parents, often affecting critical genes for brain function.
Mitochondrial dysfunction	Evidence suggests that mitochondrial dysfunction may be linked to autism, with maternal inheritance patterns sometimes observed.
Syndromic autism	Autism associated with specific genetic syndromes, such as: *Fragile X Syndrome* *Rett Syndrome* *Tuberous Sclerosis Complex* *Down Syndrome*
Non-syndromic autism	Cases without known syndromic causes but influenced by multiple genetic and environmental factors.
Gender differences	Autism is 4–5 times more common in males. *X-linked genes* and *hormonal factors* (e.g., fetal testosterone) may play a role.
Gene editing and future research	Advancements in *CRISPR* and other gene-editing technologies offer potential for understanding and potentially addressing genetic mutations linked to autism.

Autism has no genetic variability and has complex interaction with the environment. The salient features are polygenic pattern, gene-environmental interaction, syndromic association, epigenetic changes, some degree of mutation, and heritability [21].

Table 3.
Genetical association of autism spectrum condition.

4.5 Fetal environmental factors in genesis of autism spectrum condition

The fetal environment, including maternal conditions such as obesity, diabetes, hypertension, infections, and prenatal exposure to drugs "(e.g., *Valproate, SSRIs*)" and hormones, may contribute to ASC by affecting fetal brain development through neuroinflammation, oxidative stress, and neurotransmitter disruptions [24–26]. Lifestyle factors such as smoking, alcohol use, and poor nutrition also increase the risk. Additionally, toxic exposures, including air pollution, heavy metals, and pesticides, are linked to a higher risk of ASC.

Infants who are later diagnosed with ASC appear to have a higher occurrence of prenatal and perinatal complications. These complications include advanced maternal and paternal age at the time of birth, maternal bleeding during pregnancy, gestational diabetes, birth trauma, fetal distress, low birth weight, low Apgar scores, congenital malformations, ABO or Rh factor incompatibility, and hyperbilirubinemia. Many obstetric complications that increase the risk for ASC also contribute to hypoxia, which could serve as a potential underlying risk factor [27, 28].

Parental age: Advanced parental age, especially paternal, increases the risk of ASC due to genetic mutations, DNA methylation changes, and possible intergenerational effects. Meta-analysis shows that each 10-year increase in maternal age raises the risk by 18%, while paternal age increases it by 21% [29].

Sex steroids: Elevated fetal exposure to sex steroids, particularly testosterone, is linked to ASC. The "*male brain theory*" suggests that ASC reflects an extreme form of male cognition, with higher fetal testosterone levels associated with traits like reduced eye contact, vocabulary, and empathy. Genes involved in sex steroid synthesis are also related to ASC traits, and studies of amniotic fluid show increased sex steroids in ASC cases, supporting this connection [19].

Polycystic ovarian syndrome in mother: Mothers with PCOS, especially with comorbid obesity, have a higher risk of having children with ASC. Women with PCOS also show a higher prevalence of ASC [30].

Obesity: Mixed evidence exists, but extreme maternal weight conditions, such as obesity or underweight, are linked to a 36% increased ASC risk, especially with additional pregnancy weight gain [31].

Maternal diabetes: Maternal diabetes raises ASC risk by 48–62%, with early gestational diabetes (before 26 weeks) increasing the risk by 42% [32].

Maternal hypertension: Pregnancy-related hypertensive disorders, like "*preeclampsia*", increase ASC risk by 35% [33].

Maternal infections: Maternal infections during pregnancy, especially with fever, double the ASC risk, potentially through immune system activation and inflammation [34].

Perinatal factors: Prematurity, cesarean delivery, low birth weight, and hypoxia are linked to ASC, though they are not primary causes [35].

Medications during pregnancy: Drugs like valproic acid and SSRIs during pregnancy may elevate ASC risk, with valproate strongly linked to malformations and developmental delays [36].

Maternal smoking and alcohol consumption: Maternal smoking is possibly linked to ASC, particularly with intellectual disabilities. Alcohol shows no strong connection to ASC [37].

Maternal nutrition: Deficiencies in vitamins like D and iron, short inter-pregnancy intervals, and mineral imbalances *(e.g., zinc and copper)* may increase ASC risk [38].

Vaccination: The MMR vaccine has been scientifically disproven as a cause of ASC [39].

Toxic exposures: Air pollutants, heavy metals (mercury, lead), and pesticides are associated with higher ASC risk [24].

Psychosocial factors: While not a cause, maternal stress, migration, and adverse conditions can affect ASC severity and developmental challenges [40].

Protective factors: Prenatal supplementation with *folate, omega-3 s,* and *probiotics* may offer some protection, though more research is needed [41].

5. Clinical characteristics of autism spectrum condition across various domain of classification

ASC has a variety of symptoms and behaviors [42–46] that vary from person to person as highlighted in **Table 4**. [The core symptoms can generally be grouped into: lack of social communication, difficulty interpreting social cues and engaging effectively, poor language development, delays in speech and conversational difficulties, and repetitive and eccentric behaviors, including sensory sensitivities and preferences for routines. Additionally, emotional regulation challenges, struggles with managing

Characteristic	Description	Relevance
Issues with social interaction	• Difficulty interpreting and responding to social cues. • Challenges in forming and maintaining friendships. • Preference for being alone or engaging in solitary activities. • Limited eye contact or facial expressions.	• This can lead to misunderstandings and conflict in social settings, affecting relationships and social integration. • Struggles in building social connections can result in feelings of isolation or loneliness, impacting emotional well-being. • Indicates potential avoidance of social situations, which can further hinder social skills development. • May signal disinterest or discomfort, making social interactions less engaging and effective.
Issues with communication	• Speech or language development delays. • Difficulty initiating or maintaining conversations. • Unusual speech patterns, such as echolalia (repetition of words). • Less frequent use of gestures and nonverbal communication.	• Early delays can affect children's ability to communicate effectively, limiting their social interactions and relationships. • Impairs the ability to connect with others, which is essential for building relationships. • Can be viewed as unusual in typical settings, making meaningful communication difficult. • Nonverbal cues are crucial for effective communication; absence can create misunderstandings.
Repetitive actions and narrow interests	• Repetitive movements like hand flapping or rocking. • Strong preference for routines and distress over changes. • Intense interest in specific topics or hobbies. • Attachment to unusual objects or parts of items.	• These behaviors can serve as self-soothing mechanisms, helping individuals manage anxiety or sensory overload. • A need for structure can lead to anxiety during transitions, complicating daily functioning. • These interests can provide individuals with a sense of identity and opportunities for social connection with like-minded peers. • Such attachments can be comforting and serve a purpose in emotional regulation.
Sensitivity to sensory inputs	• Heightened or diminished reactions to sensory stimuli, such as lights and sounds. • Unique interest in sensory experiences, like specific smells or bright lights, etc.	• -Sensory sensitivities can lead to discomfort or overwhelm in various environments, impacting daily activities. • May indicate a unique perspective and can be harnessed for engagement in recreational or therapeutic activities.

Characteristic	Description	Relevance
Regulating emotions and behavior	• Difficulty managing emotions and behavior. • Struggles with anxiety, depression, or other mental health issues. • Meltdowns or shutdowns during stress or sensory overload.	• Can lead to miscommunication and conflict with others, further complicating social interactions. • These challenges can exacerbate social interaction issues and hinder effective communication. • Such responses can disrupt social situations, leading to isolation and difficulties in social integration.

The gross category of the symptoms ASC may be grouped into lack of social communication, poor language developmental, repetitive eccentric behavior, emotional numbness, poor sensitivity to sensory inputs.

Table 4.
Clinical descriptive of various domains characterized the autism spectrum condition.

emotions, may complicate social relationships.] [This structured table can assist in understanding the multifaceted challenges individuals with ASC may face, informing diagnostic and intervention approaches.]

The gross category of the symptoms may be grouped into lack of social communication, poor language development, repetitive eccentric behavior, emotional numbness, and poor sensitivity to sensory inputs. They have poor communication or deficit in communication creating conflict with others, further complicating social interactions, leading to isolation and difficulties in social integration.

6. Assessment of autism spectrum condition

Diagnosing ASC involves a comprehensive evaluation that includes clinical observations, standardized tools, and input from parents, caregivers, and sometimes teachers. The process typically includes multiple steps and tools to ensure a reliable and valid diagnosis.

6.1 Screening tools for autism spectrum condition

Autism detection in early childhood (ADEC): This manual was developed by Young in 2007. It was created to incorporate various domains necessary as screening tools for detecting autism in children aged 12 to 36 months. It consists of 16 specific behaviors that are believed to reflect the core deficits of autism in very young children. These behaviors were identified through retrospective parental reports and video analysis and have been clearly defined to allow for reliable measurement [47]. The ADEC manual demonstrates strong reliability, as evidenced by Cronbach's alpha values ranging from .85 to .93 (indicating robust internal consistency), a test-retest reliability coefficient of r = .83, and an interrater reliability intraclass correlation coefficient (ICC) of .83 [48].

Modified checklist for autism in toddlers, revised (M-CHAT R/F) is a screening tool of two stages based on parent reports developed to evaluate the risk in children aged 16 to 30 months, which consists of 20 yes-or-no questions that focus on key developmental areas related to ASC, enabling quick identification of children who may need further evaluation. The reliability and validity of the M-CHAT-R/F have been confirmed, with optimal scoring identified through receiver operating characteristic curves. Children with an initial total score of ≥3 and a follow-up score of ≥2 have a 47.5% risk of being diagnosed with ASC and a 94.6% risk of any developmental delay or concern. An algorithm using three risk levels is recommended to enhance clinical utility, reduce the age of diagnosis, and facilitate early intervention [49].

Scoring: Except for 2, 5, and 12, in all other responses, "NO" indicates ASC risk; and for items 2, 5, and 12, "YES" indicates ASC risk. The M-CHAT R algorithm maximizes psychometric properties: LOW RISK: Total Score is 0–2; if the child is under 24 months, rescreen to be done after 2 years of age. No further action is required unless surveillance indicates risk. MEDIUM RISK: Total score is 3–7; follow-up to be administered (second stage of M-CHAT-R/F) to get additional information about at-risk responses. If the M-CHAT R/F score is 2 or more, it indicates that the child has screened positively. In this case, the necessary action is to refer the child for a diagnostic assessment as well as an eligibility evaluation for early intervention services. Conversely, if the follow-up score ranges from 0 to 1, the child has screened negatively, and no further action is needed unless monitoring suggests a potential risk. The child should undergo rescreening at upcoming well-child visits. For those classified as HIGH RISK with a total score between 8 and 20, it is permissible to skip the follow-up and refer the child directly for diagnostic assessment and eligibility evaluation for early intervention [50, 51].

The Autism Spectrum Screening Questionnaire (ASSQ) is an initial screening tool with 27 question assessments completed by parents or teachers for children and adolescents aged 6 to 17, particularly for those with high or normal IQs or mild intellectual disabilities. A total score between 0 and 54 with higher scores indicates more characteristics. A score of 13 or above suggests a probable diagnosis, with a 90% true positive rate and a 22% false positive rate [52]. The total scale has a high internal consistency with an alpha reliability coefficient of 0.90 and good convergent validity, as evidenced by a strong *Pearson correlation of* $r = .75$ between parent ratings on the *ASSQ* and the *Rutter scale* [53, 54].

The First Year Inventory (FYI): It is a 63-item parent-report screening tool for 12-month-old infants at risk. It focuses on two developmental domains: social communication and sensory regulatory functions. The FYI uses a scoring algorithm with risk scores (0, 1, or 2 points) based on item response frequencies in a normative sample. Each of the eight constructs and the two domains generates a quasi-logarithmic risk score ranging from 0 to 50. The domain scores are averaged to produce a total FYI risk score, with higher scores indicating more atypical behaviors. The FYI risk score is then converted to a percentile score for easier interpretation [54, 55]. In a large community sample study by Turner Brown et al. [55], the First Year Inventory (FYI) 2.0 demonstrated the following diagnostic accuracy for predicting ASC at age 3 when using a two-domain cutoff criterion (Social Communication domain score ⩾22.5 and Sensory Regulatory domain score ⩾14.75) at 12 months. It has a sensitivity of 44.4% and a specificity of 98.9% [56].

6.2 Diagnostic tools for autism spectrum condition

International Clinical Epidemiology Network (INCLEN) Diagnostic Tool for ASC (INDT-ASC) [57] consists of two sections: Section A with 29 symptoms/items, and Section B with 12 questions aligned with DSM-IV-TR criteria, including details about time of onset, symptom duration, scoring, and a diagnostic algorithm. The tool takes 45–60 minutes to administer and uses a trichotomous response option ("yes," "no," "unsure/not applicable"). Clinicians or psychologists must observe and score the child's behavior, and in case of discrepancies between parental reports and interviewer observations, the tool specifies which should take precedence. A diagnosis of ASC requires ≥ six symptoms/items, with two from impaired communication and restricted repetitive behavior. The tool demonstrated high diagnostic accuracy, with a 0.97 AUC, 98% sensitivity, 95% specificity, a 91% positive predictive value, and a 99% negative predictive value when compared to expert diagnoses based on DSM-IV-TR criteria.

Autism Diagnostic Observation Schedule, Second Edition (ADOS2) is a semi-structured assessment designed to evaluate communication, social interaction, and play in individuals with ASC. Behavioral and language observations are coded across five areas: language and communication, social interaction, play and imagination, stereotyped behaviors, and other behaviors with codes ranging from 0 (no abnormal behavior) to 3 (markedly abnormal behavior), with additional codes for specific language abilities or unscored items. It has a sensitivity of 60–95% and a specificity of 75–100% [58–60].

Autism Diagnostic Interview-Revised (ADIR) is a revised edition of the original Autism Diagnostic Interview (ADI). It is a standardized, semi-structured interview designed for caregivers of individuals. It provides a diagnostic algorithm based on the "*ICD-10 and DSM-IV*" criteria. Scoring is based on the interviewer's judgment of the behaviors described by the caregiver, using a coding system similar to the original ADI. Most items are scored as 0 (no definite behavior), 1 (probably present but not fully meeting criteria), or 2 (definite abnormal behavior), with a score of 3 indicating extreme severity. The scoring typically reflects current behavior, with specific age-related items having age restrictions [61]. Internal consistency of the domain scores ranged from .54 to .84. While there were some similarities with other measures of adaptive behavior, psychopathology, and autism, the ADIR was shown to uniquely measure autism [62].

Social Responsiveness Scale, Second Edition (SRS2): The Social Responsiveness Scale, Second Edition (SRS2) is a 65-item rating scale designed to assess social behavior deficits related to ASC, as defined by the *DSM-IV-TR*. It can be completed by multiple raters who know the individual well, takes 15–20 minutes, and can be scored by hand or computer. The results are presented as T-Scores across five subscales: Social Awareness, Social Communication, Social Cognition, Restricted Interests, and Repetitive Behaviors, and Social Motivation in addition to an overall score. Norms for the School-Age Form vary by the examinee's gender and the rater's relationship (parent or teacher). The SRS2 has strong reliability, with internal consistency ranging from .94 to .96 and interrater reliability from .61 to .92. It also demonstrated strong content validity, effectively distinguishing individuals with ASC, with high sensitivity and specificity (both .92) for the School-Age Form, though the Adult Form had lower specificity at .60. Construct validity aligns with the *DSM-5*'s two-factor model of ASC [63].

The Indian Scale for Assessment of Autism (ISAA): It is an objective tool designed to diagnose autism. It evaluates individuals through observation, clinical behavior assessments, interaction-based testing, and input from parents or caretakers. It consists of 40 items categorized into six distinct domains: Emotional Responsiveness, Social Relationship and Reciprocity, Speech Language and Communication, Behavior Patterns, Sensory Aspects, and Cognitive Component. Each, rated on a five-point scale from 1(never) to 5(always), demonstrated a sensitivity of 93.3% and specificity of 97.4%, with positive and negative likelihood ratios of 85.7 and 98.7, respectively. The positive predictive value was 35.5%, and the negative predictive value was 0.08. The reliability of the ISAA was good, but its validity was suboptimal in four out of six domains. The optimal threshold for distinguishing autism from non-autism was an ISAA score of 70, according to the Receiver Operating Characteristic curve. However, the agreement with the "*Childhood Autism Rating Scale (CARS)*" was low, with a *Kappa coefficient of 0.14* [64].

6.3 Assessments of behavioral and adaptive functioning of autism spectrum condition

Vineland Adaptive Behavior Scales, Third Edition (Vineland3): The Vineland Social Maturity Scale (VSMS), developed by "*American psychologist Edgar Arnold Doll in 1935,*" is a widely used tool for assessing social and adaptive functions in individuals from birth to about 25 years. The test consists of 117 items across eight domains and is typically administered by a caregiver. It provides valuable insights into a child's day-to-day functioning and has a strong correlation with intelligence (approximately 0.80). The VSMS has been adapted for various cultures, with differences in the number of items, age range, and other aspects. The version standardized in India, for example, has 89 items and assesses children from 0 to 15 years [65].

6.4 Electrophysiological assessment of autism spectrum condition

Some objective findings of autism include "Electroencephalographic *(EEG)*" abnormalities, which may include diffuse and focal spikes, paroxysmal spike-and-wave patterns, multifocal spike activity, and a mixed discharge. Abnormal EEGs are significantly higher in mentally retarded autistic individuals. The high incidence of EEG abnormalities and seizure disorders in autism was one of the first compelling evidence of a biological basis [66]. A study found that individuals with ASC exhibit abnormalities in P300 components, which may reflect deficits in cognition, attention, orientation and working memory processing, particularly in decision making conditions [67].

7. Diagnosis of autism spectrum condition

The diagnosis has evolved with different versions of DSM and ICD to reflect the update in understanding.

In *DSM-IV (1994) and ICD-10 (1992)*, ASC was categorized under "*Pervasive Developmental Disorders (PDD),*" which included *Autistic Disorder, Asperger's Disorder, PDD NOS, Rett's Disorder, and Childhood Disintegrative Disorder*. The diagnostic criteria focused on social interaction, communication, and repetitive behaviors. The major issues were overlapping diagnoses, subjectivity in interpretation, and high comorbidity with other disorders. In *DSM-5 (2013) and ICD-11 (2018)*, ASC has criteria of deficits in social communication, restricted behaviors, and early childhood symptoms with issues of loss of specific labels like "*Asperger's,*" subjectivity in severity levels, and the risk of missing subtle ASC presentations. Thus, we can draw the following conclusion: overlap with other conditions like ADHD complicates diagnosis, evolving definitions hinder research comparisons, and cultural differences impact the applicability of criteria [68–71].

7.1 Differential diagnosis of autism spectrum condition

The ASC has several differential diagnoses, some are described below [70]:

Rett syndrome: Social interaction may be disrupted during a regressive phase (1–4 years), resembling ASC. However, social communication improves after this period, unlike ASC.

Selective mutism: Unlike ASC, children with selective mutism can communicate effectively in certain environments, and they do not exhibit the restricted behaviors typically associated with ASC.

Schizophrenia: Childhood-onset schizophrenia (COS) may resemble ASC early on, but hallucinations and delusions distinguish it (as given in **Table 5**). [Although some clinical features of ASC and COS can appear similar, key distinctions help differentiate these conditions: Age of onset: ASC typically appears in the early developmental years, whereas COS is very rare in children under 5. Behavioral patterns: ASC is characterized by social and communication difficulties with repetitive behaviors, while COS includes hallucinations, delusions, and thought disorders. Level of intelligence and IQ patterns: Individuals with ASC often show a performance-verbal IQ discrepancy, while COS typically presents with more evenly distributed IQ levels. Seizure incidence: Higher in ASC than in COS. These criteria aid in distinguishing between ASC and COS, particularly focusing on unique aspects of behavior, intelligence, communication, and emotional expression.]

Intellectual disability without ASC: Differentiating ASC from intellectual disability can be challenging, but ASC is diagnosed when social communication is more impaired than nonverbal skills.

Stereotypic movement disorder: Motor stereotypies seen in ASC may overlap, but both can be diagnosed if self-injurious behavior is present.

ADHD: Attention issues and hyperactivity may coexist with ASC but can be diagnosed separately if symptoms are more severe.

Criteria	Autism spectrum disorder (ASC)	Childhood-onset Schizophrenia
Age of onset	Early developmental period	Rarely under the age of 5
Incidence	1%	<1 in 10,000
Sex ratio (M)	4:1	1.67:1 (slight preponderance of males)
Family history of schizophrenia	Not increased	Likely increased
Prenatal and perinatal complications	Increased	Not increased
Behavioral characteristics	Poor social relatedness; aberrant language, speech, or echolalia; stereotyped phrases; repetitive behaviors	Hallucinations, delusions, thought disorder
Adaptive functioning	Impaired	Deterioration in functioning
Level of intelligence	Wide range, maybe intellectually disabled (30%)	Usually within normal range, maybe low average
Pattern of IQ	Typically higher performance than verbal	More even
Grand mal seizures	4–32%	Low incidence

The clinical feature of ASC and Schizophrenia closely resemble, however salient feature such as age of onset, behavioral pattern, level of intelligence, communication skill, emotional expression help to differentiate such to entities in details.

Table 5.
Autism spectrum condition and childhood-onset Schizophrenia.

Criteria	Autism spectrum condition (ASC)	Language disorder (LD)
Incidence	1%	5 of 10,000
Sex ratio (M)	4:1	Equal or almost equal
Family history of speech delay or language problems	<25% of cases	<25% of cases
Associated deafness	Very infrequent	Not infrequent
Nonverbal communication (e.g., gestures)	Impaired	Actively utilized
Language abnormalities (e.g., echolalia)	Present in a subset	Uncommon
Articulation problems	Infrequent	Frequent
Intellectual level	Impaired in a subset (about 30%)	Uncommon, less frequently severe
Patterns of intelligence quotient (IQ) tests	Typically lower on verbal than performance	Often verbal scores lower than performance
Impaired social communication, restricted behaviors	Present	Absent or mild if present
Imaginative play	Often impaired	Usually intact

It describes the salient features which help to understand ASC and learning disorders such as level of intelligence, communication pattern, language abnormality, and associated comorbidities.

Table 6.
Autism spectrum condition in comparison with language disorder.

Language disorders/social (pragmatic) communication disorder: Language disorders impact a child's ability to understand and use language but do not necessarily involve the social interaction deficits and repetitive behaviors characteristic of ASC (as given in **Table 6**).

8. Management strategies

8.1 Psychosocial interventions

8.1.1 Early intensive behavioral and developmental interventions

The UCLA (*University of California Los Angeles*)/*Lovaas-based Model*: It is an intensive and manualized intervention primarily utilizing techniques derived from *Applied Behavior Analysis (ABA)*. This model is administered on a one-to-one basis for many hours per week. In this setting, a therapist works with a child to practice specific social skills, language usage, and other target play skills, with reinforcement and rewards provided for accomplishments and mastery of skills [72].

Early Start Denver Model (ESDM): These interventions are administered in naturalistic settings such as daycare, at home, and during play with other children. Parents are typically trained to be co-therapists, providing training at home to develop basic play and relationship skills. This model integrates applied behavior analysis techniques and is focused on aiding very young children within their daily routines [73].

Parent training approaches: It includes Pivotal Response Training, which teaches parents to facilitate social and communication development within the home. This method targets pivotal social behaviors for mastery by the child, which promotes the natural generalization of social skills. Additional training focuses on language acquisition, where interventions occur throughout the day with the child. The Hanen More Than Words Program is another example of a parent training approach [74, 75].

8.2 Social skills approaches

Social skills training: Therapists typically provide social skills training to children of various ages in a group setting. During these sessions, children receive guided practice initiating social conversations, greetings, games, and joint attention. The program often includes emotion identification and regulation instruction, teaching children to label emotions and attribute emotional reactions in social situations. The overall goal is for children to apply these techniques in everyday settings [76].

8.3 Behavioral interventions and cognitive behavioral therapy (CBT)

Behavioral therapy: Applied behavior analysis has proven somewhat effective in reducing certain repetitive behaviors associated with autism. Early intervention is particularly crucial for self-injurious repetitive behaviors. It may be necessary to combine behavioral interventions with pharmacological treatments to adequately manage symptoms [77].

Cognitive-behavioral therapy: This therapy has a significant evidence base from randomized controlled trials demonstrating its efficacy in treating anxiety, depression, and obsessive-compulsive disorders in children. Although there are fewer controlled trials specific to children with ASC, at least two published studies have discussed using CBT to treat repetitive behaviors in this population [78].

8.4 Interventions for comorbid symptoms

Neurofeedback: This is administered to influence symptoms of ADHD and anxiety and to promote increased social interaction. This modality uses computer games that reinforce desired behaviors while the child wears electrodes monitoring brain activity. The objective is to prolong the electrical activity present during desired behaviors [79].

Management of insomnia in ASC: This may involve both behavioral and pharmacological interventions. The most common behavioral intervention focuses on altering the parent's behavior toward the child at bedtime and throughout the night. Reinforcement and attention to being awake are gradually reduced, leading to a decrease in "staying awake" behaviors. Studies have indicated that massage therapy before bedtime can improve sleep and provide relaxation [80].

8.5 Educational interventions

Treatment and Education of Autistic and Communication-Related Handicapped Children (TEACCH) was developed in the 1970s at the University of North Carolina at Chapel Hill. It employs structured teaching to assist children with ASC who struggle with perception. This approach incorporates visual supports and picture schedules to aid in teaching academic subjects and socially appropriate responses. The physical environment is organized to support visual learning, promoting autonomy and social interactions [81].

Computer-based approaches and virtual reality utilize programs and games designed to teach language acquisition and reading skills. For instance, *let us face it!* The program teaches children to recognize faces through interactive computer games targeting emotional expressions. Research demonstrates that children using this program have improved focus on the eye region of a face and enhanced face-processing skills. Various studies support the effectiveness of virtual reality environments in facilitating social interactions and skills [82].

8.6 Pharmacological management of autism spectrum condition

Among the medications, "*Risperidone*" stands out as the most extensively studied and effective option, particularly for children aged 5 years and older. It significantly reduces symptoms such as tantrums and self-injury but is associated with common side effects including weight gain and drowsiness. "*Aripiprazole*" has also shown efficacy in treating irritability in slightly older children, though it shares similar adverse effects. In contrast, "*Clozapine and Haloperidol*" are less favored due to significant side effects, and sertraline has limited evidence for use in this domain. For hyperactivity and inattention, methylphenidate and venlafaxine show promise, but their effectiveness varies and must be weighed against potential side effects. Ongoing research is critical to refine dosages better and identify effective treatment protocols for these aspects of ASC [83–85].

Addressing repetitive behaviors, both "*fluoxetine*" and "*fluvoxamine*" have demonstrated effectiveness in reducing symptoms in children and adults, respectively, with minor side effects noted. These pharmacological treatments offer additional avenues for managing specific symptoms associated with ASC [86].

9. Challenges encountered by autism spectrum condition

Familiar issues: Families, with children diagnosed, face difficulties associated with caregiving, service access, and managing behavior. These underscore the need for effective coping strategies and support systems.

Social: Children with distinct behavioral and communication styles are at higher risk of bullying and social exclusion, primarily due to their challenges in social interactions and understanding social cues. This vulnerability can lead to negative consequences, both psychosocial and emotional.

Academic: Face significant challenges in school settings due to rigid thinking patterns, sensory sensitivities, and communication and executive functioning difficulties. These challenges lead to increased stress and decreased participation in educational activities, negatively affecting their learning experiences and outcomes.

Employment: Face significant difficulties that can extend into adulthood, particularly in finding and maintaining employment, achieving independent living, and navigating adult responsibilities. These challenges lead to inherent social and cognitive difficulties associated with ASC, which can impact their ability to interact effectively in social settings and manage the complexities of daily life.

10. Conclusion

Our understanding of autism has changed over time, initially being viewed as a form of developmental delay or mental retardation. Today, however, it is recognized as an independent neurological disorder of considerable significance, representing a major public health issue and an area of extensive research. Researchers have faced challenges in identifying precise causes for the disorder with limited success. Autism has undergone various diagnostic changes and encompasses several areas, including difficulties with social interaction and communication, repetitive behaviors, restricted interests, heightened sensitivity to sensory stimuli, and struggles with emotional regulation and behavior. The proposed causes of ASC involve a combination of genetic, neurobiological, and environmental factors, along with their complex interactions. Various strategies are being developed to assist these children in reaching their full potential and improving their social skills. Despite progress in genetics and neuroscience, practical applications remain limited, and further research is essential to better understand the disorder's causes and how to manage it. Consequently, significant efforts are necessary to provide personalized support, help families find appropriate resources, and prepare for life transitions.

Acknowledgements

The authors acknowledge the usage of Grammarly and Gemini for language polishing of the manuscript.

Author details

Sambhu Prasad[1*], Soni Kisku[1], Rituparna Sahana[1] and Sweta Gupta[2]

1 All India Institute of Medical Sciences, Patna, Bihar, India

2 Patna Dental College and Hospital, Patna, Bihar, India

*Address all correspondence to: sambhu3011@gmail.com

References

[1] National Autistic Society. Varying Support Needs. National Autistic Society; 2024. Available from: https://www.autism.org.uk/advice-and-guidance/what-is-autism/varying-support-needs [Accessed: September 13, 2024]

[2] Kuhn R, Cahn CH. Eugen Bleuler's concepts of psychopathology. History of Psychiatry. 2004;**15**(3):361-366

[3] Bleuler E. Zur Theorie des schizophrenen Negativismus. Psychiatrisch-Neurologische Wochenschrift. 1910;**12**:171-198

[4] Baird G, Simonoff E, Pickles A, Chandler S, Loucas T, Meldrum D, et al. Prevalence of disorders of the autism spectrum in a population cohort of children in South Thames: The special needs and autism project (SNAP). The Lancet. 2006;**368**(9531):210-215

[5] Lord C, Elsabbagh M, Baird G, Veenstra Vanderweele J. Autism spectrum disorder. The Lancet. 2018;**392**(10146):508-520

[6] Loomes R, Hull L, Mandy WPL. What is the male-to-female ratio in autism spectrum disorder? A systematic review and meta-analysis. Journal of the American Academy of Child & Adolescent Psychiatry. 2017;**56**(6):466-474

[7] Maenner MJ. Prevalence and characteristics of autism spectrum disorder among children aged 8 years—Autism and developmental disabilities monitoring network, 11 sites, United States, 2020. MMWR Surveillance Summaries. 2023;**72**:1-14

[8] Centers for Disease Control and Prevention. Data & Statistics on Autism Spectrum Disorder. Centers for Disease Control and Prevention; 2022

[9] Ha S, Sohn IJ, Kim N, Sim HJ, Cheon KA. Characteristics of brains in autism spectrum disorder: Structure, function and connectivity across the lifespan. Experimental Neurobiology. 2015;**24**(4):273

[10] Courchesne E. Brain development in autism: Early overgrowth followed by premature arrest of growth. Mental Retardation and Developmental Disabilities Research Reviews. 2004;**10**(2):106-111

[11] Minshew NJ, Keller TA. The nature of brain dysfunction in autism: Functional brain imaging studies. Current Opinion in Neurology. 2010;**23**(2):124-130

[12] Peng Y, Lu Z, Li G, Piechowicz M, Anderson M, Uddin Y, et al. The autism-associated MET receptor tyrosine kinase engages early neuronal growth mechanism and controls glutamatergic circuits development in the forebrain. Molecular Psychiatry. 2016;**21**(7):925-935

[13] Peng Y, Huentelman M, Smith C, Qiu S. MET receptor tyrosine kinase as an autism genetic risk factor. International Review of Neurobiology. 2013;**113**:135-165

[14] Campbell DB, Li C, Sutcliffe JS, Persico AM, Levitt P. Genetic evidence implicating multiple genes in the MET receptor tyrosine kinase pathway in autism spectrum disorder. Autism Research. 2008;**1**(3):159-168

[15] Lammert DB, Howell BW. RELN mutations in autism spectrum disorder. Frontiers in Cellular Neuroscience. 2016;**10**:84

[16] Fetit R, Hillary RF, Price DJ, Lawrie SM. The neuropathology of autism: A systematic review of post-mortem studies of autism and related disorders. Neuroscience & Biobehavioral Reviews. 2021;**129**:35-62

[17] Dichter GS. Functional magnetic resonance imaging of autism spectrum disorders. Dialogues in Clinical Neuroscience. 2012;**14**(3):319-351

[18] Muller CL, Anacker AM, Veenstra-Vander Weele J. The serotonin system in autism spectrum disorder: From biomarker to animal models. Neuroscience. 2016;**321**:24-41

[19] Baron-Cohen S, Auyeung B, Nørgaard-Pedersen B, Hougaard DM, Abdallah MW, Melgaard L, et al. Elevated fetal steroidogenic activity in autism. Molecular Psychiatry. 2015;**20**(3):369-376

[20] Almandil NB, Alkuroud DN, Abdul Azeez S, AlSulaiman A, Elaissari A, Borgio JF. Environmental and genetic factors in autism spectrum disorders: Special emphasis on data from Arabian studies. International Journal of Environmental Research and Public Health. 2019;**16**(4):658

[21] Choi L, An JY. Genetic architecture of autism spectrum disorder: Lessons from large-scale genomic studies. Neuroscience & Biobehavioral Reviews. 2021;**128**:244-257

[22] Robinson-Agramonte MDLA, Noris García E, Fraga Guerra J, Vega Hurtado Y, Antonucci N, Semprún-Hernández N, et al. Immune dysregulation in autism spectrum disorder: What do we know about it? International Journal of Molecular Sciences. 2022;**23**(6):3033

[23] Rao TS, Andrade C. The MMR vaccine and autism: Sensation, refutation, retraction, and fraud. Indian Journal of Psychiatry. 2011;**53**(2):95-96

[24] Rossignol DA, Genuis SJ, Frye RE. Environmental toxicants and autism spectrum disorders: A systematic review. Translational Psychiatry. 2014;**4**(2):e360-e360

[25] Chun H, Leung C, Wen SW, McDonald J, Shin HH. Maternal exposure to air pollution and risk of autism in children: A systematic review and meta-analysis. Environmental Pollution. 2020;**256**:113307

[26] Kalkbrenner AE, Schmidt RJ, Penlesky AC. Environmental chemical exposures and autism spectrum disorders: A review of the epidemiological evidence. Current Problems in Pediatric and Adolescent Health Care. 2014;**44**(10):277-318

[27] Yong Z, Dou Y, Gao Y, Xu X, Xiao Y, Zhu H, et al. Prenatal, perinatal, and postnatal factors associated with autism spectrum disorder cases in Xuzhou, China. Translational Pediatrics. 2021;**10**(3):635

[28] Gardener H, Spiegelman D, Buka SL. Prenatal risk factors for autism: Comprehensive meta-analysis. The British Journal of Psychiatry. 2009;**195**(1):7-14

[29] Wu S, Wu F, Ding Y, Hou J, Bi J, Zhang Z. Advanced parental age and autism risk in children: A systematic review and meta-analysis. Acta Psychiatrica Scandinavica. 2017;**135**(1):29-41

[30] Jiang L, Tian L, Yuan J, Xu X, Qu F, Zhang R, et al. Associations between sex hormone levels and autistic traits in infertile patients with polycystic ovary syndrome and their offspring. Frontiers in Endocrinology. 2022;**12**:789395

[31] Surén P, Gunnes N, Roth C, Bresnahan M, Hornig M, Hirtz D, et al. Parental obesity and risk of autism spectrum disorder. Pediatrics. 2014;**133**(5):e1128-e1138

[32] Xu G, Jing J, Bowers K, Liu B, Bao W. Maternal diabetes and the risk of autism spectrum disorders in the offspring: A systematic review and meta-analysis. Journal of Autism and Developmental Disorders. 2014;**44**:766-775

[33] Xu RT, Chang QX, Wang QQ, Zhang J, Xia LX, Zhong N, et al. Association between hypertensive disorders of pregnancy and risk of autism in offspring: A systematic review and meta-analysis of observational studies. Oncotarget. 2018;**9**(1):1291

[34] Croen LA, Qian Y, Ashwood P, Zerbo O, Schendel D, Pinto-Martin J, et al. Infection and fever in pregnancy and autism spectrum disorders: Findings from the study to explore early development. Autism Research. 2019;**12**(10):1551-1561

[35] Fezer GF, Matos MBD, Nau AL, Zeigelboim BS, Marques JM, Liberalesso PBN. Características perinatais de crianças com transtorno do espectro autista. Revista Paulista de Pediatria. 2017;**35**:130-135

[36] Christensen J, Grønborg TK, Sørensen MJ, Schendel D, Parner ET, Pedersen LH, et al. Prenatal valproate exposure and risk of autism spectrum disorders and childhood autism. JAMA. 2013;**309**(16):1696-1703

[37] Tran PL, Lehti V, Lampi KM, Helenius H, Suominen A, Gissler M, et al. Smoking during pregnancy and risk of autism spectrum disorder in a Finnish National Birth Cohort. Paediatric and Perinatal Epidemiology. 2013;**27**(3):266-274

[38] Bener A, Khattab AO, Bhugra D, Hoffmann GF. Iron and vitamin D levels among autism spectrum disorders children. Annals of African Medicine. 2017;**16**(4):186-191

[39] DeStefano F, Shimabukuro TT. The MMR vaccine and autism. Annual Review of Virology. 2019;**6**(1):585-600

[40] Beversdorf DQ, Stevens HE, Margolis KG, Van de Water J. Prenatal stress and maternal immune dysregulation in autism spectrum disorders: Potential points for intervention. Current Pharmaceutical Design. 2019;**25**(41):4331-4343

[41] Rees G, Brough L, Orsatti GM, Lodge A, Walker S. Do micronutrient and omega-3 fatty acid supplements affect human maternal immunity during pregnancy? A scoping review. Nutrients. 2022;**14**(2):367

[42] American Psychiatric Association. Diagnostic and Statistical Manual of Mental Disorders. 4th ed. Washington, DC: American Psychiatric Association; 2000

[43] Kesherim R. Total Care Therapy. Autism Nursing Care Plan: Strategies for Transformative Care. 2024. Available from: https://www.totalcareaba.com/autism/autismnursingcareplan [Accessed: September 13, 2024]

[44] Gonyon A, ADHD. 2024. Available from: https://lighthouseautismcenter.com/blog/autismspectrumdisorderandadhd/ [Accessed: July 29, 2024]

[45] Yellowbusaba. Shedding Light on Autism: Unveiling the Spectrum Disorder. 2024. Available from: https://www.yellowbusaba.com/post/whatistheautismspectrumdisor der [Accessed: July 29, 2024]

[46] Patra S, Arun P. Use of Indian scale for assessment of autism in child guidance clinic: An experience. Indian Journal of Psychological Medicine. 2011;**33**(2):217

[47] Young R. Autism Detection in Early Childhood (ADEC) Manual. Camberwell, Australia: ACER Press; 2007

[48] Nah Y-H, Young RL, Brewer N, Berlingeri G. Autism detection in early childhood (ADEC): Reliability and validity data for a level 2 screening tool for autistic disorder. Psychological Assessment. 2014;**26**(1):215-226

[49] Robins DL, Casagrande K, Barton M, Chen CMA, Dumont Mathieu T, Fein D. Validation of the modified checklist for autism in toddlers, revised with follow up (MCHATR/F). Pediatrics. 2013;**133**(1):37-45

[50] Singh A, Squires J, Yeh CJ, Heo KH, Bian H. Validity and reliability of the developmental assessment screening scale. Journal of Family Medicine and Primary Care. 2016;**5**(1):1248

[51] Robins, Fein, & Barton. Modified Checklist for Autism in Toddlers, Revised, with FollowUp (MCHATR/F). 2009. Available from: https://www.mchatscreen.com/ [Accessed: September 26, 2024]

[52] NovoPsych. Autism Spectrum Screening Questionnaire (ASSQ). NovoPsych; 2025. Available from: https://novopsych.com.au/assessments/diagnosis/autism-spectrum-screening-questionnaire-assq/ [Accessed: August 22, 2024]

[53] Ehlers S, Gillberg C, Wing L. A screening questionnaire for Asperger syndrome and other high-functioning autism spectrum disorders in school age children. Journal of Autism and Developmental Disorders. 1999;**29**(2):129-141

[54] Posserud MB, Lundervold AJ, Gillberg C. Validation of the autism spectrum screening questionnaire in a total population sample. Journal of Autism and Developmental Disorders. 2009;**39**(1):126-134

[55] Turner-Brown LM, Baranek GT, Reznick JS, Watson LR, Crais ER. The First Year Inventory: A longitudinal follow-up of 12-month-old to 3-year-old children. Autism. 2012;**17**(5):527-540. DOI: 10.1177/1362361312439633 (Original work published 2013)

[56] Lee HY, Vigen C, Zwaigenbaum L, Smith IM, Brian J, Watson LR, et al. Construct validity of the first-year inventory (FYI version 2.0) in 12-month-olds at high-risk for autism spectrum disorder. Autism. 2020;**25**:33-43

[57] Juneja M, Mishra D, Russell PSS, et al. INCLEN diagnostic tool for autism spectrum disorder (INDT-ASD): Development and validation. Indian Pediatrics. 2014;**51**:359-365

[58] McCrimmon A, Rostad K. Test review: Autism diagnostic observation schedule, second edition (ADOS2) manual (part II): Toddler module. Journal of Psychoeducational Assessment. 2013;**32**(1):88-92

[59] Lord C, Luyster RJ, Gotham K, Guthrie W. Autism Diagnostic Observation Schedule, Second Edition (ADOS2) Manual (Part II): Toddler Module. Torrance, CA: Western Psychological Services; 2012

[60] Lord C, Rutter M, Di LavoreP C, Risi S, Gotham K, Bishop S. Autism Diagnostic Observation Schedule. 2nd ed. Torrance, CA: Western Psychological Services; 2012

[61] Lord C, Rutter M, Le Couteur A. Autism diagnostic interview-revised: A revised version of a diagnostic interview for caregivers of individuals with possible pervasive developmental disorders. Journal of Autism and Developmental Disorders. 1994;**24**(5):659-685

[62] Lecavalier L, Aman MG, Scahill L, McDougle CJ, McCracken JT, Vitiello B, et al. Validity of the autism diagnostic interview-revised. American Journal on Mental Retardation. 2006;**111**(3):199

[63] Bruni TP. Test review: Social responsiveness scale–second edition (SRS-2). Journal of Psychoeducational Assessment. 2014;**32**(4):365-369

[64] New Delhi: Ministry of Social Justice & Empowerment: Government of India. Report on Assessment Tool for Autism: Indian Scale for Assessment of Autism. ISAA; 2009. Available from: https://www.thenationaltrust.gov.in/upload/uploadfiles/files/ISAA%20TEST%20MANNUAL(2).pdf [Accessed: August 27, 2024]

[65] Roopesh BN. Advanced scoring and interpretation of vineland social maturity scale: Procedure to obtain 'impairment adjusted social quotient'. Indian Journal of Mental Health. 2022;**9**(1):1-6

[66] Wang J, Barstein J, Ethridge LE, Mosconi MW, Takarae Y, Sweeney JA. Resting state EEG abnormalities in autism spectrum disorders. Journal of Neurodevelopmental Disorders. 2013;**5**(1):24

[67] Cui T, Wang PP, Liu S, Zhang X. P300 amplitude and latency in autism spectrum disorder: A meta-analysis. European Child & Adolescent Psychiatry. 2017;**26**:177-190

[68] Lordan R, Storni C, De Benedictis CA. Autism Spectrum disorders: Diagnosis and treatment. In: Autism Spectrum Disorders. Brisbane (AU): Exon Publications; 2021

[69] World Health Organization. International Classification of Diseases (ICD). 10th ed. 1993

[70] American Psychiatric Association. Diagnostic and Statistical Manual of Mental Disorders. 5th ed. 2013

[71] World Health Organization. International Classification of Diseases. 11th ed. 2019

[72] Adams JB, Kirby JK, Sorensen JC, Pollard EL, Audhya T. Evidence based recommendations for an optimal prenatal supplement for women in the US: Vitamins and related nutrients. Maternal Health, Neonatology and Perinatology. 2022;**8**:4

[73] Food and Drug Administration FDA Approves the First Drug to Treat Irritability Associated with Autism, Risperdal. 2006. Available from: http://www.fda.gov/NewsEvents/Newsroom/PressAnnouncements/2006/ucm108759.htm [Accessed: September 1, 2024]

[74] Hardan AY, Gengoux GW, Berquist KL, Libove RA, Ardel CM, Phillips J, et al. A randomized controlled trial of pivotal response treatment group for parents of children with autism. Journal of Child Psychology and Psychiatry. 2014;**56**(8):884-892

[75] Dawson G, Rogers S, Munson J, Smith M, Winter J, Greenson J, et al. Randomized, controlled trial of an intervention for toddlers with autism: The early start Denver model. Pediatrics. 2009;**125**(1):e17-e23

[76] Howes Oliver D, Rogdaki M, Findon JL, Wichers RH, Charman T, King BH, et al. Autism spectrum

disorder: Consensus guidelines on assessment, treatment and research from the British Association for Psychopharmacology. Journal of Psychopharmacology. 2017;**32**:3-29

[77] Foxx RM. Applied behavior analysis treatment of autism: The state of the art. Child and Adolescent Psychiatric Clinics of North America. 2008;**17**(4):821-834

[78] Boyd BA, McDonough SG, Bodfish JW. Evidence-based behavioral interventions for repetitive behaviors in autism. Journal of Autism and Developmental Disorders. 2012;**42**:1236-1248

[79] Enriquez-Geppert S, Smit D, Pimenta MG, Arns M. Neurofeedback as a treatment intervention in ADHD: Current evidence and practice. Current Psychiatry Reports. 2019;**21**:1-7

[80] Escalona A, Field T, Singer-Strunck R, Cullen C, Hartshorn K. Brief report: Improvements in the behavior of children with autism following massage therapy. Journal of Autism and Developmental Disorders. 2001;**31**:513-516

[81] Mesibov GB, Shea V, Schopler E. The TEACCH Approach to Autism Spectrum Disorders. Springer Science & Business Media; 2005 - Education - 211

[82] Tanaka JW, Wolf JM, Klaiman C, Koenig K, Cockburn J, Herlihy L, et al. Using computerized games to teach face recognition skills to children with autism spectrum disorder: The let's face it! program. Journal of Child Psychology and Psychiatry. 2010;**51**(8):944-952

[83] McCracken JT, McGough J, Shah B, et al. Risperidone in children with autism and serious behavioral problems. The New England Journal of Medicine. 2002;**347**:314-321

[84] Troost PW, Lahuis BE, Steenhuis MP, et al. Long-term effects of risperidone in children with autism spectrum disorders: A placebo discontinuation study. Journal of the American Academy of Child and Adolescent Psychiatry. 2005;**44**:1137-1144

[85] Sharma A, Shaw S. Efficacy of risperidone in managing maladaptive behaviours for children with autistic spectrum disorder: A meta-analysis. Journal of Pediatric Health Care. 2012;**264**:291-299

[86] LeClerc S, Easley D. Pharmacological therapies for autism spectrum disorder: A review. Pharmacy and Therapeutics. 2015;**40**(6):389-397

Chapter 10

Utilizing Transcranial Electrical Stimulation (TES) to Individualize Social Learning Therapy with Autistic Adults and Adults with High Traits of Autism

Joan Esse Wilson and Claudia D. Tesche

Abstract

Autistic adults (individuals diagnosed with autism spectrum disorder or having high traits of autism) without a co-occurring intellectual disability are observed to have reduced social alignment with others and report experiencing reduced quality of life with high levels of loneliness and a desire for improved relationships. While the term heterogeneity is often used to describe the wide variety of symptoms and levels of severity found across autistic individuals, current supports for social learning are rarely individualized to account for heterogeneity. An approach utilizing individualized transcranial electrical stimulation (TES) parameters may have considerable potential to accommodate heterogeneity and improve the effectiveness of current evidence-based social learning therapies by targeting specific brain regions and processes, depending on each person's unique needs. This chapter reviews current literature on this topic and provides direction for the future.

Keywords: transcranial electrical stimulation, social learning, autism spectrum disorder, transcranial direct current stimulation, social communication

1. Introduction

Autism spectrum disorder (ASD) is a highly heterogeneous neurodevelopmental condition with core diagnostic domains of social communication impairments and repetitive behaviors and restricted interests [1]. Successful social communication is a complex process that not only requires the expression and reception of verbal speech, but also the modification and coordination of many behaviors to achieve social alignment [2]. Social alignment is a mostly unconscious phenomenon in which people become more similar to a conversation partner by adjusting communication features such as vocal speech prosody (patterns of voice stress or intonation), facial expressions and gestures [3]. It is also suggested that social alignment reduces the burden placed on the cognitive system, thus making social interactions easier, and possibly less anxiety filled [4]. Research has shown that individuals with ASD have significantly lower social alignment when compared to their neurotypical peers [5, 6]. Social interactions require continual social decision-making based on rapid and ever-changing environmental contexts. With the advent of powerful neuroimaging tools, such as functional magnetic resonance imaging (fMRI) and magnetoencephalography (MEG), we now have a view into the brain's overall metabolism, dynamics, and network-level connectivity during social interactions, further demonstrating the complex and miraculous nature of social interactions [7].

Autistic adults without a co-occurring intellectual disability (hereafter referred to as autistic adults—estimated to be 62% of autistic individuals) report experiencing high levels of loneliness that negatively impact mental health [8], including a longing for improved relationships and social interactions [9]. These relationships and interactions include both personal and work settings, as well as exchanges experienced during psychotherapy, thus limiting the possible benefits of mental health support. Quality of life is also predicted by an autistic adult's employment (reported to be the lowest of any other disability group (cite)), with work settings that are frequently below the intelligence and education of the individual (cite). Quality of life is also predicted by an autistic adult's level of social isolation, as well as by the levels of psychological and/or social supports received [10].

2. Transcranial direct current stimulation (tDCS)

For decades, research utilizing functional and structural neuroimaging, electrophysiology, metabolites and, most recently, gene expression, has informed the neural and physiological bases for ASD and revealed a correlation between differences in brain structure/function with behavioral challenges that reduce the quality of life experienced by autistic individuals [11]. However, current therapies neglect to capitalize on what has been learned about the neural and physiological bases for ASD and have focused instead on behavioral or pharmacological therapies that often provide only modest results for alleviating core social and behavioral symptoms. Approximately 56% of autistic individuals are prescribed at least one psychotropic medication and 30% are prescribed three or more, despite experiencing negative and often serious side effects, suggesting a need for more efficient and effective therapeutic approaches that produce fewer negative side effects [10].

A promising approach to accelerating and/or enhancing traditional behavioral therapies that also provides an alternative to pharmaceuticals is to induce weak electrical currents in the brain. Two methods are now available, transcranial magnetic stimulation (TMS) and transcranial electrical stimulation (TES). In TMS, a transient burst of current flowing through a coil located over the scalp induces "mirror currents" in the brain. In TES, electrodes are placed directly on the scalp, with current flow within the brain determined by the electrode locations and the conductivity profile of the skin, skull and brain of the individual [12]. TMS and TES are known to modulate metabolite concentrations, brain dynamics and behavior [13]. In both TMS and TES, the amplitude of the induced current may be modulated in time to match features of endogenous brain dynamics. TES also provides an opportunity to up- and down-regulate brain activity by applying a constant amplitude current (transcranial direct current stimulation, tDCS) for an epoch on the order of 5–30 minutes. Importantly, tDCS devices are also affordable, lightweight, portable, and safe, making them attractive for clinical use.

DOI: http://dx.doi.org/10.5772/intechopen.1006563

tDCS has been shown to accelerate and/or enhance accuracy of performance involving perception, mood, motor performance, and a multitude of cognitive functions [14, 15]. Research has elucidated many of the underlying mechanisms of tDCS, including the depolarization and hyperpolarization of neuronal membrane potentials during stimulation, a modulation of the threshold for neuronal firing and the strengthening of glutamatergic synapses [16]. Local changes near the electrode site(s) include tDCS-induced decreases in gamma-aminobutyric acid (GABA) that are associated with increases in learning and performance, with long term effects that demonstrate the regulation of neurotransmitters, such as dopamine, acetylcholine, and serotonin [13, 17].

While tDCS devices are currently only utilized in research settings, the U.S. Food and Drug Administration (FDA) has granted an Investigational Device Exception (IDE) for a clinical trial utilizing remotely-supervised tDCS (RS-tDCS) for use in major depressive disorder (*c.f.* Soterix Medical Inc.). This approval suggests the possibility of future clinical implementations of tDCS for use in a range of other disorders. In particular, the use of RS-tDCS may be an attractive option for individuals with social challenges, such as autistic adults, who often prefer predictable settings and routines [18]. RS-tDCS would allow the stimulation to be delivered at a time and place that is comfortable and familiar to the client, such as their home.

3. tDCS parameters for individualized stimulation protocols

While the term heterogeneity is often used when discussing ASD to describe the wide variety of symptoms and levels of severity found across autistic individuals, current social therapies are rarely individualized to accommodate heterogeneity and often use a one-size-fits-all approach [19]. An important feature of TES is that the stimulation parameters may be chosen to target specific brain regions and processes, depending on each person's unique needs. An individualized approach that includes personalized TES parameters may have considerable potential to improve the effectiveness of current evidence-based behavioral therapies. The regions of interest in the brain may be selected by a consideration of previous neuroimaging studies that have shown increased brain activation during a given task or behavior. Modulating brain activity by placing tDCS electrodes over these brain regions has repeatedly shown improved outcomes in those and similar tasks, especially when task performance is conducted also during stimulation [20].

The choice of the tDCS parameters include the number, size and location of the electrodes, the direction and amplitude of the current flow at each electrode site, and the duration of the stimulation session. For example, a traditional electrode montage may include two electrodes, an anodal (tending to depolarize neuronal cell membrane potentials and increase cortical excitability) electrode and a cathodal (tending to hyperpolarize neuronal cell membrane potentials and decrease cortical excitability) electrode, energized by a 9-volt battery. The electrodes are often placed within small, saline-soaked sponges to increase electrical contact with the skin. The current amplitude and duration are controlled by electronics within the stimulation device. The locations of both scalp electrodes matter. In the two-electrode montage, current leading from the anodal electrode must be captured by the second cathodal electrode. There may be significant depolarization/hyperpolarization of neuronal cell membrane potentials induced during stimulation not only in the vicinity of the anodal/cathodal electrode but also in other regions in the brain that lie within the flow of the induced current.

High-definition tDCS (HD-tDCS) may be used to focus the current flow induced in the brain. In HD-tDCS, four small cathodal scalp electrodes may be placed around a central anodal electrode. This limits the induced current to the vicinity of the HD-tDCS electrode array. Care must be taken in the placement of the HD-tDCS array on the scalp and in the choice of the spatial extent of the electrodes to ensure that the induced current does indeed extend down into the cortex. Multiple electrodes may also be located across the scalp to produce complex patterns of current flow.

A personalized map of the current flow in the brain can be calculated in detail for a given electrode montage if an individual's structural MRI is available. Theoretical considerations make it impossible to determine a unique electrode montage from a previously specified pattern of current flow, although an acceptable montage may be determined by trial and error. Finally, the orientation of the current induced in the brain with respect to the orientation of the cortical surface is important. An anodal stimulation that generates an induced current flowing into one wall of a cortical sulcus may become, in effect, a cathodal stimulation on the opposing wall of the sulcus. This can lead to considerable variability in the overall effect of stimulation between individuals for a similar electrode montage depending on the shape of the cortical surface [21].

Functional magnetic imaging (fMRI) may be used to identify brain regions that are either underactive or overactive in a person compared to what may be typically seen, suggesting a potential choice of the locations and polarities (anodal vs. cathodal) of the scalp electrodes. The expectation is often that up-regulation of an underactive region with anodal stimulation will improve function. Evidence that this is the case for a given individual may be obtained through simultaneous tDCS/fMRI. Since the tDCS epoch typically lasts from 5 to 30 minutes, the concurrent fMRI data may be utilized to reveal on-line changes in brain activity occurring under each electrode site, as well as in other brain regions, during task performance. Since changes in brain function observed during stimulation may be dissimilar to that which persists after the termination of stimulation, behavioral and neuroimaging data should also be recorded after tDCS.

Finally, the highly interconnected feature of the human brain suggests that any change in brain function, even one limited by an HD-tDCS montage focused onto a localized neural population, may lead to unintended consequences. There is the potential for the stimulation to affect not only the "target" neuronal population, but also distant nodes of any network that includes this population. In addition, brain networks containing nodes that overlap with those of the "primary network" may also be affected. As a result, cognitive functions and behaviors seemingly unrelated to those of interest in a given study may be affected by the stimulation. This is particularly true if the stimulation modulates activity within a major brain hub in posterior parietal or dorsolateral prefrontal cortex, or subcortical regions such as the cerebellar cortex that are interconnected with multiple regions within the cerebral cortex. Unintended consequences may be difficult to predict and easily overlooked, becoming evident only on examination of results from a battery of neuropsychological tests.

4. tDCS in ASD

Evidence is beginning to accumulate that suggests that tDCS provides therapeutic benefits for autistic adults across a variety of outcomes after employing targeted and individualized stimulation (for a recent systematic review and meta-analysis, see

Liu et al. [22]) One of the earliest applications of tDCS in ASD was based on fMRI evidence that demonstrated the right temporal parietal junction (rTPJ) plays a crucial role in social cognition and may be modulated with transcranial stimulation [23, 24]. Targeting anodal tDCS to rTPJ improved social functioning in healthy individuals in tasks involving perspective-taking and evaluation of self against others, suggesting that anodal tDCS over this region may also improve aspects of social functioning in individuals with ASD. Wilson et al. found that even a single session of 2.0 mA tDCS for 30 minutes with the anodal electrode located over the rTPJ of autistic adults improved performance for empathy, social cognition, and recognizing facial emotions that convey threat when compared to placebo tDCS [25–27]. In this study, the cathodal electrode was located over the ipsilateral deltoid. As a result, the induced current flowed not only within rTPJ but also throughout the right temporal cortex and right cerebellum. Modulation of brain function in all of these regions may have contributed to the improvement seen in social function. Cerebellum is of particular interest, since cerebellar differences are known to occur in ASD. Cortico-cerebellar networks, especially those involving the lateral cerebellar cortex, are known to participate in a wide variety of cognitive functions [28]. Replacing this electrode montage with an HD-tDCS electrode located over the rTPJ would strongly reduce any current flow through the cerebellum. This may reduce the potential for unintended consequences of the stimulation, but also may produce a different therapeutic outcome.

A different electrode montage was employed in a study of attentional bias in adults with autistic traits by English et al. [29] Anodal stimulation (2.0 mA for a mean duration of 9.76 minutes) was targeted to the right posterior parietal cortex (P4, International 10–20 electroencephalography (EEG) electrode location), a region known to participate in attentional task performance. Attentional bias, similar to what is utilized during face gaze to process others' facial emotions, was significantly increased following verum compared with sham stimulation. In this study, the cathodal electrode was located over the vertex (Cz), eliciting a pattern of current flow that was localized to cortical regions proximal to these electrodes. In this case, an HD-tDCS montage located over P4 is likely to produce similar therapeutic benefits.

Recent studies have explored the effects of multiple sessions of tDCS. In a double-blind, randomized clinical trial (RCT) by Han et al. [30], 105 adolescents and young adults with ASD completed 10 sessions of tDCS applied over prefrontal cortex (stimulation duration 20 minutes at 1.5 mA) while completing computerized cognitive training. Electrode placement was motivated by the notion that atypical cortical excitability in the prefrontal cortex contributes to core symptoms in ASD. The anodal electrode was placed over Fp2 (right prefrontal cortex) and the cathodal electrode over F3 (left prefrontal cortex), motivated by the observation of overactivation in left, but not right, frontal cortex in ASD. The results showed significantly reduced scores for social impairment and restricted, repetitive behaviors when compared with sham tDCS.

The dorsolateral prefrontal cortex (DLPFC) is a common target for transcranial stimulation in many studies involving both neurotypical participants and various patient populations. In a study by Zemestani et al. [31], thirty-two children with ASD (7–12 years of age) were randomly assigned to either 10 sessions of verum or of sham tDCS. The anodal electrode was placed over left DLPFC (F3) and the cathodal electrode over right DLPFC (F4), with verum stimulation at 1.5 mA for 15 minutes. Improvement was seen in autism symptom severity with respect to communication, theory of mind and emotional regulation following the last session and at a 1-month follow-up. Interestingly, the choice of electrode polarity in the study by Zemestani et al. was opposite to that utilized in the study of Han et al. [30] Both protocols produced significant improvement in some aspects of social function, but only the Han et al. study reported reduction of restrictive, repetitive behaviors, suggesting that tDCS stimulation parameters may be chosen to address different core diagnostic domains of autism.

5. The future

These studies illustrate some of the challenges of designing potential tDCS protocols for ASD. The parameter space for tDCS is large, with multiple potential electrode montages, each producing a different pattern of current flow in the brain. ASD is a highly heterogeneous neurodevelopmental condition, with the potential for an individual-specific pattern of social communication impairments, repetitive behaviors and restricted interests, as well as other challenges. Individualization of the tDCS protocol, including not only the electrode montage but also the selection of tasks and/or therapeutic environment presented to the individual during stimulation, could be facilitated by a creating profile of each individual that extends beyond a grouping defined by clinical symptoms to include neuroimaging data on brain chemistry, metabolism, dynamics, and network-level connectivity. An important first step has been taken by Buch et al. [32]. In this study, 12 subgroups of participants were identified from resting-state fMRI data from individuals with ASD. Subgroups included 4 verbal IQ dimensions, 4 social affect dimensions and 4 restrictive and repetitive behavior dimensions, each with unique patterns of connectivity between specific brain regions. These results are useful in the present context because the subgroups were extracted by a network-level analysis of the functional connectivity between brain regions, including both cerebral cortex and cerebellum. As a result, the nodes of these networks could serve as potential targets for the design of the electrode montage in tDCS. If resting-state fMRI data for an autistic individual were available, it could be used in combination with clinical symptoms to select a set of these network nodes as potential targets for tDCS. Probing the effect of one or more HD-tDCS arrays onto these targets, or for more complex networks perhaps a more distributed current flow pattern from an electrode montage, based on symptom severity and also on any unintended consequences of the stimulation might usefully precede implementation of a multi-session protocol designed to effect a long-term change of brain function.

Functional connectivity data extracted from resting-state fMRI scans are only one of many measures that may be useful for the personalization of TES in ASD. This approach could also be implemented with data from other brain imaging methodologies such as structural magnetic resonance imaging (sMRI), positron emission tomography (PET) or MEG/EEG. The latter is of particular interest. MEG/EEG arrays have sufficient temporal resolution to image brain dynamics in multiple frequency bands, from slow theta-band activity (3–8 Hz) to high-frequency oscillatory activity in the gamma-band (>40 Hz). For example, measures of local theta-gamma-band coupling and a spectral Granger analysis of causal relationships across frontal and posterior nodes of an extended network could be combined with network relationships derived from fMRI scans to suggest target locations for the stimulation electrodes. In addition, a parsing of an autistic cohort into groups based on the frequency-dependent MEG/EEG measures motivates utilization of transcranial alternating current stimulation (tACS), a form of TES in which the amplitude of the induced current oscillates at a frequency that may either match/enhance local endogenous activity, recruit oscillatory activity across nodes of an interconnected network at a more functional frequency, or selectively increase synchronization across the network.

An indication of the potential power of this approach is shown in a study by Grover et al. [26]. Auditory working memory (WM) and long-term memory store (LTM) are known to be reduced in healthy older compared to younger adults. In this study, modulating brain activity with tACS was motivated by studies suggesting a role for both theta (3–8 Hz) and gamma-band oscillatory activity in DLPFC and inferior parietal lobe (IPL) in WM and LTM. Previous to this study, electrode montages have included HD-tACS localized over either DLPFC or IPL, with inconsistent results. Grover et al. found that WM was improved in older adults following theta-band, but not gamma-band tACS applied over IPL on day 3 and 4 of a 4 consecutive day study, and at a 1-month follow-up in 65–88 year old adults. In contrast, gamma-band, but not theta-band tACS, applied over prefrontal cortex improved LTM on days 2–4 and at the 1-month follow-up. Learning from this study, tACS may provide additional stimulation protocols for the induction of long-lasting plasticity in networks that are atypical in ASD with the potential to induce plasticity in specific networks with characteristic oscillatory activity at the tACS drive frequency without inducing unintended changes in other networks that are functional in the individual. What is needed before implementation of this approach is a characterization of endogenous activity in the multiplicity of networks associated with subgroups identified in the fMRI data (i.e., verbal IQ, social affect and restrictive and repetitive behavior) or perhaps, more appropriately, with subgroups that emerge from a frequency-dependent analysis of MEG/EEG data.

In summary, the search for an individualized, targeted intervention with TES for autistic individuals has just begun. There is already evidence for a significant clinical benefit of this therapy, but also a considerable challenge in developing an optimized protocol.

Author details

Joan Esse Wilson[1,2]* and Claudia D. Tesche[2]

1 Department of Communication Disorders, New Mexico State University, Las Cruces, NM, USA

2 Department of Psychology, University of New Mexico, Albuquerque, NM, USA

*Address all correspondence to: wilsonj@nmsu.edu

References

[1] American Psychiatric Association. Diagnostic and Statistical Manual of Mental Disorders. 5th ed. Washington, D.C: American Psychiatric Publishing; 2013

[2] Wynn CJ, Borrie SA, Sellers TP. Speech rate entrainment in children and adults with and without autism spectrum disorder. American Journal of Speech-Language Pathology. 2018;**27**:965-974

[3] Czoska A, Klessa K, Karpiński M, Jarmołowicz-Nowikow E. Prosody and gesture in dialogue: Cross-modal interactions. In: Proceedings of 4th Gesture and Speech in Interaction (GESPIN) Conference, Nantes, France. Published online. Nantes, France: University of Nantes; 2015. pp. 83-88

[4] Garrod S, Pickering MJ. Joint action, interactive alignment, and dialog. Topics in Cognitive Science. 2009;**1**(2):292-304. DOI: 10.1111/j.1756-8765.2009.01020.x

[5] Lehnert-Lehouillier H, Terrazas S, Sandoval S. Prosodic entrainment in conversations of verbal children and teens on the autism spectrum. Frontiers in Psychology. 2020;**11**(October):1-13. DOI: 10.3389/fpsyg.2020.582221

[6] Hong Y, Chen S, Zhou F, Chan A, Tang T. Phonetic entrainment in L2 human-robot interaction: An investigation of children with and without autism spectrum disorder. Frontiers in Psychology. 2023;**14**:1-12. DOI: 10.3389/fpsyg.2023.1128976

[7] Noonan MP, Mars RB, Sallet J, Dunbar RIM, Fellows LK. The structural and functional brain networks that support human social networks. Behavioural Brain Research. 2018;**355**:12-23. DOI: 10.1016/j.bbr.2018.02.019

[8] Schiltz H, McVey AJ, Dolan Wozniak B, et al. The role of loneliness as a mediator between autism features and mental health among autistic young adults. Autism. 2021;**25**(2):545-555. Available from: https://epublications.marquette.edu/psych_fac

[9] Camm-Crosbie L, Bradley L, Shaw R, Baron-Cohen S, Cassidy S. People like me don't get support: Autistic adults' experiences of support and treatment for mental health difficulties, self-injury and suicidality. Autism. 2019;**23**(6):1431-1441. DOI: 10.1177/1362361318816053

[10] Mason D, Mcconachie H, Garland D, Petrou A, Rodgers J, Parr JR. Predictors of quality of life for autistic adults. Autism Research. 2018;**11**:1138-1147. DOI: 10.1002/aur.1965

[11] Enticott PG. Targeting discrete symptom domains using non-invasive brain stimulation in autism spectrum disorder. Brain Stimulattion. 2017;**10**(2):349

[12] Yavari F, Jamil A, Mosayebi Samani M, Vidor LP, Nitsche MA. Basic and functional effects of transcranial electrical stimulation (tES)—An introduction. Neuroscience and Biobehavioral Reviews. 2018;**85**:81-92. DOI: 10.1016/j.neubiorev.2017.06.015

[13] Antonenko D, Schubert F, Bohm F, et al. tDCS-induced modulation of GABA levels and resting-state functional connectivity in older adults. Journal of Neuroscience. 2017;**37**(15):4065-4073. DOI: 10.1523/JNEUROSCI.0079-17.2017

[14] Mattioli F, Maglianella V, D'Antonio S, Trimarco E, Caligiore D.

Non-invasive brain stimulation for patients and healthy subjects: Current challenges and future perspectives. Journal of the Neurological Sciences. 2024;**456**:1-25

[15] Antal A, Luber B, Brem AK, et al. Non-invasive brain stimulation and neuroenhancement. Clinical Neurophysiology Practice. 2022;**7**:146-165. DOI: 10.1016/j.cnp.2022.05.002

[16] Sousa B, Martins J, Castelo-Branco M, Gonçalves J. Transcranial direct current stimulation as an approach to mitigate neurodevelopmental disorders affecting excitation/inhibition balance: Focus on autism spectrum disorder, schizophrenia, and attention deficit/hyperactivity disorder. Journal of Clinical Medicine. 2022;**11**:1-12. DOI: 10.3390/jcm11102839

[17] Sellaro R, Nitsche MA, Colzato LS. The stimulated social brain: Effects of transcranial direct current stimulation on social cognition. Annals of the New York Academy of Sciences. 2016;**1369**(1):218-239. DOI: 10.1111/nyas.13098

[18] Stark E, Ali D, Ayre A, et al. Psychological Therapy for Autistic Adults. London, U.K: Authentistic Research Collective; 2021

[19] Weisberg HR, Jones EA. Individualizing intervention to teach joint attention, requesting, and social referencing to children with autism. Behavior Analysis in Practice. 2019;**12**:105-123. DOI: 10.1007/s40617-018-0265-5

[20] Jog MV, Wang DJJ, Narr KL. A review of transcranial direct current stimulation (tDCS) for the individualized treatment of depressive symptoms. Personalized Medicine in Psychiatry. 2019;**17-18**:17-22. DOI: 10.1016/j.pmip.2019.03.001

[21] de Berker AO, Bikson M, Bestmann S. Predicting the behavioral impact of transcranial direct current stimulation: Issues and limitations. Frontiers in Human Neuroscience. 2013;**7**:613. DOI: 10.3389/fnhum.2013.00613

[22] Liu A, Gong C, Wang B, Sun J, Jiang Z. Non-invasive brain stimulation for patient with autism: A systematic review and meta-analysis. Frontiers in Psychiatry. 2023;**14**:1-18. DOI: 10.3389/fpsyt.2023.1147327

[23] Krall SC, Volz LJ, Oberwelland E, Grefkes C, Fink GR, Konrad K. The right temporoparietal junction in attention and social interaction: A transcranial magnetic stimulation study. Human Brain Mapping. 2016;**37**(2):796-807. DOI: 10.1002/hbm.23068

[24] Santiesteban I, Banissy MJ, Catmur C, Bird G. Enhancing social ability by stimulating right temporoparietal junction. Current Biology. 2012;**22**(23):2274-2277. DOI: 10.1016/j.cub.2012.10.018

[25] Esse Wilson J, Wilson JK, Trumbo MC, Tesche CD. Improved performance on the empathy quotient in adult autism spectrum disorder after tDCS. Clinical Neurophysiology. 2020;**131**(4):e81-e82

[26] Grover S, Wen W, Viswanathan V, Gill CT, Reinhart RMG. Long-lasting, dissociable improvements in working memory and long-term memory in older adults with repetitive neuromodulation. Nature Neuroscience. 2022;**25**:1237-1246. DOI: 10.1038/s41593-022-01132-3

[27] Esse Wilson J, Trumbo MC, Tesche CD. Transcranial direct current stimulation (tDCS) improves empathy and recognition of facial emotions conveying threat in adults with autism spectrum disorder (ASD): A randomized

controlled pilot study. NeuroRegulation. 2021;**8**(2):87-95. DOI: 10.15540/NR.8.2.87

[28] Pezzetta R, Gambarota F, Tarantino V, et al. A meta-analysis of non-invasive brain stimulation (NIBS) effects on cerebellar-associated cognitive processes. Neuroscience and Biobehavioral Reviews. 2024;**157**:1-17. DOI: 10.1016/j.neubiorev.2023.105509

[29] English MCW, Kitching ES, Maybery MT, Visser TAW. Modulating attentional biases of adults with autistic traits using transcranial direct current stimulation: A pilot study. Autism Research. 2018;**11**(2):385-390. DOI: 10.1002/aur.1895

[30] Han YMY, Chan MMY, Shea CKS, et al. Effects of prefrontal transcranial direct current stimulation on social functioning in autism spectrum disorder: A randomized clinical trial. Autism; 2023;**27**(8):2465-2482. DOI: 10.1177/13623613231169547

[31] Zemestani M et al. The impact of prefrontal transcranial direct current stimulation (tDCS) on theory of mind, emotion regulation and emotional-behavioral functions in children with autism disorder: A randomized, sham-controlled, and parallel-group study. Autism Research. 2022;**15**(10):1985-2003

[32] Buch AM, Vértes PE, Seidlitz J, Kim SH, Grosenick L, Liston C. Molecular and network-level mechanisms explaining individual differences in autism spectrum disorder. Nature Neuroscience. 2023;**26**(4):650-663. DOI: 10.1038/s41593-023-01259-